D1326923

MENOPAUSE

MENOPAUSE
A
POSITIVE
APPROACH

Rosetta Reitz

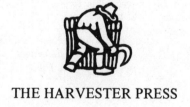

THE HARVESTER PRESS

First published in Great Britain in 1979 by
THE HARVESTER PRESS LIMITED
Publisher: John Spiers
2 Stanford Terrace, Hassocks, Sussex

Copyright © 1977 & 1979 by Rosetta Reitz

British Library Cataloguing in Publication Data
Reitz, Rosetta
    Menopause.
    1. Menopause
    I. Title
    612.6'65   RG186
    ISBN 0-85527-964-8

Harvester Press thank Sheri Safran for all her assistance with the British edition

Grateful acknowledgement is made for the following extracts: p.v From 'Ash Wednesday' in *Collected Poems 1909–1962* by T. S. Eliot, copyright, 1936, by Harcourt Brace Jovanovich Inc.; copyright, 1963, 1964, by T. S. Eliot. Copyright 1963 by Faber and Faber, Ltd.
.p. 11 Reprinted from 'From an Old House in America' from *Poems, Selected and New, 1950–1974*, by Adrienne Rich. Copyright © 1975, 1973, 1971, 1969, 1966, by W. W. Norton & Company, Inc.
p. 25 From *Woman's Mysteries* by M. Esther Harding. (G. P. Putnam's Sons, 1972)
p. 42 From *The Poems of Emily Dickinson*, edited by Thomas H. Johnson, Cambridge, Mass. (The Belknap Press of Harvard University Press) Copyright © 1951, 1955 by the President and Fellows of Harvard College. And from *The Complete Poems of Emily Dickinson*, edited by Thomas H. Johnson, (Little, Brown and Co.) Copyright 1929 by Martha Dickinson Bianchi. Copyright © 1957 by Mary L. Hampson.
p. 79 From 'Diary of a Middle-Aged Divorce' by Ethel Seldin-Schwartz. (*Ms.* Magazine, April 1976)
p. 96 From *The Sacred Fount* by Henry James. (Charles Scribner's Sons, 1953)
p. 103 From *Science and Sanity* by Alfred Korzybski. (International Non-Aristotelian Library Publishing Co., 4th edn. 1958 (1st edn. 1933))
p. 115 Reprinted from 'The Stranger' from *Diving into the Wreck, Poems 1971–1972* by Adrienne Rich. Copyright © 1973 by W. W. Norton & Company, Inc.
p. 138–9 From 'The Laugh of the Medusa' by Helene Cixous, translated by Keith Cohen and Paula Cohen. In *Signs* vol. 1, no. 4 (Summer 1976). Copyright © 1976 by The University of Chicago Press. All Rights Reserved.
p. 236–7 From 'New Discovery: Public Relations Cures Cancer' in *Majority Report* vol. 6, no. 20 (February 5–18, 1977).

Printed and bound in Great Britain by
REDWOOD BURN LIMITED
Trowbridge & Esher

Blesséd sister, holy mother, spirit of the fountain,
    spirit of the garden,
Suffer us not to mock ourselves with falsehood. . . .

T.S. Eliot,
"Ash Wednesday"

Contents

Acknowledgments

In the winter of 1969 I attended my first consciousness-raising group and heard women who were strangers to me speak about their feelings in a way which I had never heard before. I was startled and impressed with their courage, but it wasn't until many weeks later, after I joined a group of older women (35 and over) who became known as the OWL (older women's liberation) group, that I, too, could do the same thing. Without my being aware of it, the seed for this book was sown then. It was the comfortableness I felt with these women that enabled me to speak up, and I thank every one of them for being active participants during that year and a half, for they all helped me develop a new kind of self-esteem. I am grateful for that, for without it, this book could not have been written. Nor could it have been written without the hundreds of women who generously shared their feelings about menopause with me. I am in their debt, for this book is really a collaboration: without their contribution, I could not have known so wide a range of experience.

I am grateful to the women who participated in the individual menopause workshops which I facilitated at various feminist conferences and to the groups which invited me to share the subject with them, especially the NOW chapters of New York, New Jersey, and Connecticut. From the questions that were raised at these workshops and groups I was better able to determine the material to focus on in this book. The women not only added to my knowledge but shaped my determination to try to find answers to the questions we were exploring.

I am especially glad to have had the opportunity to speak at East Meadow Public Library, East Meadow, Long Island, and at the New City Free

Library, New City, New York, because the men in those audiences forced me to broaden the focus of the subject of menopause.

My thanks to Marjory Collins, editor of *Prime Time,* the feminist journal for older women, for asking me to organize the older women's Sunday afternoon workshops in the winter of 1974. They gave me a new kind of confidence, as did the Older Women's Speak-Out of February 2, 1975. The latter confirmed for me my need to be involved in regular meetings about menopause, because there never is enough time to talk out all of the ramifications. I am especially indebted to those women who participated in the menopause workshops at my house during the winter and summer of 1975, for it is their testimony which has enriched this book. Also of prime importance are the long one-to-one interviews I had with many women over a two-year period. These interviews provided me with information that has given this book dimensions and reverberations it could not otherwise have had.

I am most grateful for the trust these women had in me to permit me to share their most secret and sacred confidences, including their greatest fears and anxieties and their greatest fantasies, some of which, out of respect to them, I did not discuss, because to do justice to their complexity would require more time and space. I am referring to subjects such as face lifts, dying hair, money as power, to name a few. It is difficult for me to describe the feeling of sisterhood these meetings imparted to me. I can only say that I felt privileged to witness and share the search for unadulterated truth as well as the tears that were shed and the anger that was expressed, for they deepened my understanding.

I am especially indebted to the thirteen women whose premenopause and menopause I was able to watch closely over a three-year period (you know who you are), but I must single out in particular my valued friend Lynn Laredo. She pointed me to the road of loving your body and faithfully continued to keep me informed of her menopausal changes by telephone even after she moved to California.

I wish to thank Susan Brownmiller for setting a new standard for feminist writing, one which has never ceased to be an inspiration to me. She stimulated me to sharpen my ideas and forced me to reach further in my quest. I am also deeply grateful to Florence Rush, who constantly and consistently encouraged that reach, applying her own high standard to me, and to Margaret Tureck, who, besides having total confidence in me, did not allow me to miss a single New York Times article related to my subject over a three-year period. My thanks, too, to the numerous women who sent me clippings on menopause from journals, magazines, and newspapers which I might otherwise have missed. I sometimes received three of the same article in the mail from three different women—that kind of concern encouraged me during many months of retreat when I did little else than concentrate on this book.

I thank my daughters Rainbow and Robin for their positive feelings and feedback whenever the subject of the book came up and my daughter Rebecca for her uncritical and perpetual "Right on, Ma" for every fragment of an idea I mentioned. My deep appreciation to my niece Marjory Aronson, my sisters Shelly Aronson and Barbara Callen, and my chosen sisters Florence Major, Trudi Vogel, Vivien Leone, and Melinda Schroeder, whose complete faith in my ideas acted like solid bricks of support for me. A special thanks to Alan Benjamin who kept on rooting for me and always knew the right word when energy flagged and to Saul Gusberg for the serious and dignified way he treated me and my questions.

The potential reality of this book became more concrete when my agent, Jim Seligmann, upon seeing the proposal, confirmed the need for the book. I thank Jack Kelly and Benton Arnovitz for wanting it for Chilton, and Glen Ruh, the editorial director whose respect for my ideas made it easier for me to stretch them further. I cannot express enough thanks to Hazel Richmond, my editor. Her understanding of what I was trying to do and her regard for the material made the writing of this book the most pleasurable work experience I have ever had.

There are so many people who have, in one way or another, contributed that to thank them all would take too long, but I must name some: Helen Payne, Lolly Hirsch, Jan Crawford, Colette Lageoles, Jean Bach, Charles Graham, Ruth Greenspan, Laura Hanks, Iris Herman, Louise Silverstein, Sheila Brantley, Molly Wilson, Anna Mutnick, Irving Wexler, Miriam Silverstein, Barbara Mehrhof, Dick Chell, Belita Cowan, Clement Meadmore, Irene Duvall, and Pat Westphal.

A final note of gratitude to my goddesses, Demeter and Dinah, who somehow put the right words in my mouth when I need them to speak about menopause.

R.R.

1
Why This Book?

This is a revolutionary book. It looks on menopause as a positive experience. It is revolutionary because its emphasis is exactly opposite to what we have been taught, consciously and unconsciously, about our bodies. We have been taught to hate our bodies, hide our menstrual blood, fear our menopause, and reject our aging. This book is about loving yourself, enjoying your body, even relishing your hot flashes, and embracing aging. It is a conscious attempt to undo the damage the American culture has done to us as women, especially as middle-aged women, the 35 million of us aged 45 years or over in 1976, who are made to feel invisible because menopause has been so long shoved under the rug. I'm trying to pull menopause out into the open, remove the cobwebs, clean it off, and look at it.

What is menopause exactly? I didn't know at first; the word *menopause* had little meaning for me. All I knew was that menstrual periods would be over. I'd heard of hot flashes and the vague phrase "woman trouble," which seemed to be something that happened to women around that time. But I didn't really know what it was all about. In my early forties, I began to wonder about menopause because for a couple of years I'd been having what seemed to be excessive premenstrual irritability. I wondered if these premenstrual feelings could be premenopausal, and if they were, I should know.

It didn't occur to me that there would be any problem in finding out about menopause. When I had needed childbirth information, for instance, I had only to walk into any bookstore and take my choice from a large selection. I had wanted to know what to expect from pregnancy, what would be happening to my body. I had not been much interested in childbirth, of course, until I was going to have the experience.

Luckily, "natural childbirth" had come back into style when I was pregnant. Having a baby became an adventure, and I went shopping, early in 1953, for a doctor who was associated with French Hospital—at that time the only hospital to permit "lying in." The doctor had to be a sympathetic human being, not one who would promise to take care of everything for me—namely, drugging me and the baby to "save me" from birth pains. I was greedy for every part of the experience, for it would be happening to me and my body, and I wanted to participate fully. I felt that if I could prepare myself, I would be investing in an easier delivery and an altogether better experience. I wanted to avoid the horrors I had heard about from other women. The doctors I rejected were surprised when I told them I'd have to think it over.

I attended my childbirth classes and did my prenatal exercises religiously. Dr. Grantley Dick-Reed's *Childbirth Without Fear* was always close at hand, as well as a number of other books that I constantly reread to follow the development of the embryo and help me look forward to the growth in the coming months. I was meticulous about my diet and vitamins. Seeing my daughter Robin in the mirror above the delivery table as she left my body was the biggest thrill of my life. It was the quintessential orgasm. The release, after so many months of buildup, left me euphoric for a couple of days. I had known what was happening to my body, and I had not been afraid.

I had assumed that when I was ready to find out about menopause, I'd go about it in a similar way. Read books—that's the way I learn when I want information. When I had wanted to understand cheese soufflés, I read about twenty cookbooks. When I'd wanted to become a stockbroker, I read investment books and went to the New York Institute of Finance. When, however, I had wanted to learn about what would be happening to my body in my menopause, I found I couldn't just walk into a bookstore and ask, "Where is the menopause section?" There wasn't any. I felt like I had when, as a teenager more than thirty years before, I wouldn't dream of going into a drugstore and asking for a box of Kotex the way I could a tube of toothpaste—it just wasn't done. You remember, you whispered it to the clerk, and the box was brought to you already wrapped in brown paper.

The absence of books on menopause made me wonder. Books on fishing or gardening were easy enough to find, and what percentage of the population engages in these activities? Even childbirth is experienced by fewer women than is menopause, for every female, whether or not she gives birth, goes through menopause—and that is over 50 percent of the American population. I was discovering that menopause was very unimportant, not as big a topic as history, fiction, or sports. I was getting a message: the book industry may not have any prejudice against menopause; the industry merely reflects our culture.

My menopause adventure did not start yet—it would take a few years. Each time my premenstrual symptoms disappeared with the onset of my period, I forgot about them. My excessive irritability was not a regular occurrence. It came and went, with no apparent pattern. My interest in menopause remained, but it was not urgent. When I heard women speak about the "change of life," I listened more attentively. I continued to look in bookstores. I learned that the actual word *menopause* was rarely used in conversation, and that book titles euphemistically described the contents. I eventually found these five books, *Changing Years, You'll Live Through It, Ageless Woman, Feminine Forever,* and *Woman's Prime of Life,* written between 1937 and 1967.

Since I began writing this book, two books have come out that do use the word *menopause* in their titles, and I am very happy about this. As of 1975, there were four titles in the New York Public Library system listed in the subjects catalog under "Menopause." The Donnell Library, a large mid-Manhattan branch, had six cards under "Menopause" in the subject file.

I read all these books and was very unhappy. Was I really to expect what they described? I had not thought that menopause would be fun and games. After all, I had lived, I was in my forties and had three children. But the attitude toward menopause expressed by these books echoes the Bible's edict: "I will greatly multiply thy sorrow."

Dr. Robert A. Wilson, author of *Feminine Forever,* is the worst offender, for he builds fear while he writes. His chapter 5 is titled "Menopause—the Loss of Womanhood and the Loss of Good Health." Here are some quotations from his chapter:

. . . the ovaries shrivel up and die as a result of menopause.

. . . the woman becomes the equivalent of a eunuch.

I have known cases where the resulting physical and mental anguish was so unbearable that the patient committed suicide.

. . . no woman can be sure of escaping the horror of this living decay. Every woman faces the threat of extreme suffering and incapacity.

. . . most women are well aware of the extent to which menopause cripples them.

I have seen untreated women who had shriveled into caricatures of their former selves.

Though the physical suffering from menopausal effects can be truly dreadful, what impressed me most tragically is the destruction of personality.

Outright murder may be a relatively rare consequence of menopause—though not as rare as most of us might suppose.

. . . this common aberration.

To be suddenly desexed is to her a staggering catastrophe. . . .

... she is incapable of rationally perceiving her own situation.

The transformation, within a few years, of a formerly pleasant, energetic woman into a dull-minded but sharp-tongued caricature of her former self is one of the saddest of human spectacles.

In a maze of longing and delusion they sometimes lose touch with reality, and thus a menopausal neurosis develops.

Enlightened physicians who see menopause for what it is—a preventable and curable deficiency disease—are still in the minority. [Thank the Goddess!]

Instinctively, I felt that such negative programming *must* bring negative results. Menopause, like childbirth, was happening to *my* body, and I wanted to understand it. Giving birth was a joyous experience, despite the weight and pain. Could I not have a similar experience with menopause, despite the hot flashes? It was, after all, the same body.

I can hear some readers ask, "How in the world can you compare menopause and childbirth, when one is a creative act and the other is the end of possible creation?" Well, I am not comparing them, I am merely questioning. Why are the prevailing attitudes about childbirth positive and the ones about menopause negative? What is involved here? Why am I looked on with value when my body is going through one natural function, then, twenty years later, looked on as valueless when my body is going through another natural function? My life changed much more when I became a mother for the first time than when I started to skip periods. It seems to me that "change of life" more accurately describes motherhood than menopause.

As I read those few available books, I began to ask more and more questions. A medical description of menopause is "deficiency disease." I had always thought that a disease was an illness doctors tried to cure. I found that many doctors prescribed drugs for menopause. This began to upset me; I had not taken any medication when I began my menstrual periods or for childbirth. Why should I need drugs when menstruation was ceasing?

My adventure started; I began to search for answers to my questions. My intuitive femaleness told me that the more I could learn about my body and its natural working, the less there would be to fear. Not knowing, not understanding, being taken by surprise, that was the scary part. And the books? Yes, I admit that I learned from them, but I was also disappointed. I didn't like their tone or the way I was talked down to. I didn't like the menopausal language, either. As I continued my search, I began to piece things together for myself, but you can be sure that the first time I came across "atrophic vaginitis," a medical term that appears in almost every article, book, or paper on menopause, I got as frightened as hell. Did that phrase mean my vagina would atrophy?

Two close friends—one was 64 and the other 69—were having active sex lives. I wondered about their "atrophy." Was it different for them than for women who were not sexually involved? Always, of course, underneath my interest in these women was my interest in myself and how their experiences would relate to mine. Sometimes I had a lover, and sometimes I didn't. Was that going to affect my vaginal walls and the dryness talked about in all the books? I not only wanted to know, I wanted to see for myself and later did (see chapter 9, "Me and My Speculum").

The trouble with the books was that most of them were written by male doctors who would never experience menopause. I knew there was more to this business than just the physiological or the descriptions of women's "neurotic" complaining during menopause. I did not trust the authors' patronizing attitudes. Eager to read women doctors, in the hope of getting a little closer to the *feelings* of menopause, I found little difference. If anything, the women writers carried on about the poor husband who was to live through his wife's menopause.

Dr. Miriam Lincoln wrote one of the more popular books titled *You'll Live Through It* (written in 1950, it's still selling in paperback), which many in the medical profession proclaimed as a fine contribution. She wrote:

A considerate woman usually makes a valiant effort to disguise the fact that she is "going through the Change of Life." Sheer pride: pride in keeping young, pride in not talking about bodily ailments, pride in adjusting well to Nature's demands—these keep her lips glued and help her hold her head high through the months when she experiences new, unusual feelings.

On the next page, Dr. Lincoln reinforces the notion of glued lips: "Talk sometimes makes mountains out of molehills."

The psychoanalytic literature leaned heavily on Freudian psychologist Helene Deutsch, whose "presumptive mistakes compounded the errors of her master," for they characterized menopause as a universal emotional trauma marking the end of the "servant of the species" years. Therese Benedek modernized the Freudian view twenty-five years later by emphasizing the menopausal woman's adaptive potential to release energy for new sublimations. However, Benedek still hung onto Deutsch's concept that a woman's hormonal change automatically leads to stress and tension and results in emotional imbalance.

The social psychologists were more interesting to me because they rejected the hormone-emotion equation, which I have always resented as an oversimplication of our menopausal symptoms. These psychologists emphasized the situational stresses of middle age as the cause of our symptoms. That, too, was an oversimplification. Stresses in life occur before middle age, with or without symptoms. Why should symptoms be labeled menopausal when they happen around age 50?

SEARCH FOR TALK

I realized that the real lowdown I was looking for was available only from women who had experienced or were experiencing menopause. Nothing else would satisfy me. I wanted details, subtleties, innuendos, reverberations, not merely that phrase "estrogen diminishes." I didn't even know what the phrase really meant. What were the *real* effects of diminishing estrogen in terms of sex and comfort?

You may wonder why I didn't ask my doctor. Oh, I did. When I went for my regular yearly Pap test, I asked if I wasn't menopausal or premenopausal. My doctor asked if I was getting regular periods. I was. She looked again at my vagina and said, "No, everything is fine." "What about those feelings I get before my period, like wanting to cry?" "Premenstrual" she answered. "Lots of women get it." "How about my bloat and my engorged breasts?" "It's all premenstrual," she repeated. "Look, you're not in your menopause." There is not much room for dialogue with doctors—they are always very busy. You feel foolish taking their time when there are sick people waiting for their attention.

But talk was what I wanted. I wanted to talk at length and listen, too, to what other women were feeling. I began to search out all the women I knew who were in their menopause or had been through it and asked them very clear-cut questions—if they let me. It wasn't easy, for many women didn't care to go into the kind of detail I sought. Unless I knew them well, I couldn't even ask certain questions about their sexuality. A number of the questions I was asking were more than could be dealt with over a quick cup of coffee.

But first, however, I had to learn how to talk about menopause. It is one thing to be told that a woman is having flashes and another thing entirely to have her feelings about having them described to you. One cannot describe a hot flash and what it is all about without knowing that one kind is different from another, how they differ, when the differences occur, how one feels about them when they are happening, and what one is doing for them. Describing them takes time and leads to other things because your reaction to hot flashes is related to the current state of your life. They are critically connected to more than one's momentary level of estrogen.

How a woman feels about her aging always comes up during discussions on menopause. It never fails. And to discuss aging, one must feel safe. When I began talking, at first to my friends, we firmly established that we were talking about menopause. That is the way I learned how to talk about it, by simply stating it clearly. That small amount of structure makes all the difference. It seems to free people.

Talking about menopause is the best thing a woman can do. By talking to a sympathetic listener, you can begin to look at how you feel about it. Our

American culture has not openly acknowledged menopause. It is embarrassed by it, and the general view of it is dim. This has filtered through to us in many subtle, even subliminal, and sometimes not so subtle ways. We have internalized those negative attitudes; openly discussing menopause is the best way to get rid of them.

When I became convinced that talking about menopause would make the experience more positive for me, I found that my life began to change. I went out of my way to invite women to my house expressly for that purpose. I preferred the comfort and privacy of my home, and I was happy to have them over for dinner, or if they couldn't make it, then for any other three-hour period (the time is best open-ended). I was happy to supply whatever refreshments made them most comfortable—wine, coffee, tea. In that environment, woman to woman, with plenty of time and clarity about our subject, with nothing threatening and no one listening who might judge, I was able to learn what other women were experiencing and feeling about menopause, as well as about aging, love, sex, health, and even work and children, for those areas were also involved.

I became fascinated and discovered other women were fascinated too, and I thought perhaps one day I might share the information. I took notes on our conversations. Some of my questions were structured in a very loose kind of way so I could be certain to remember particular points. I spent a few years conducting these interviews, and during that time I became known among middle-aged women as being vitally interested in this subject. I was connected with a group that produced a publication for middle-aged women called *Prime Time* and organized a series of workshops for older women. The meetings took place on Sunday afternoons in the winter of 1974-75.

During this period I was also asked to speak to various kinds of groups. I especially enjoyed the question-and-answer periods because problems came up that I had not thought about. Ideas that I was taking for granted turned out to be "not necessarily so." It was a broadening experience, for with groups a different dimension developed. While it was not intimate, a very positive, open energy was stimulated. Whether the group was 250 women and men in a public library or 20 women in someone's living room, I always began in the same way: "My name is Rosetta Reitz, I'm 50 years old and in my menopause."

I would then explain why I had said that: we have learned to hide our age, for to be aging is a disadvantage, especially in terms of jobs and lovers, and we have certainly been taught to hide our menopause, but we can't even begin to look at menopause and aging unless we are prepared to tell the truth. This explanation always set the tone. It was as if people could relax; there seemed almost to be a collective sigh of relief.

After I decided to write this book, I organized a series of menopause workshops in order to create a climate in which some of my ideas could be tested and explored. Through these groups I was trying to be comfortable with menopause, trying to find harmony with my own nature. We are not used to talking about our bodies in an open way. We have to learn how to do so by speaking with others and listening to them. This helps us remember ideas that have troubled us. In the company of other women who are also trying to deal with their worries, we gain courage. That is one of the chief advantages of these groups.

Each workshop met at my house one evening a week for five consecutive weeks, and had a maximum of ten women. The only requirement was an interest in menopause and a commitment to five sessions. Things came out that were very valuable because by the third meeting enough biographical material had been presented and enough familiarity had become established so that shyness and reluctance flew out the window. We talked about the things we are afraid of, such as the changes that are taking place in our bodies, the wrinkles that are showing, the difficulties of our having sexual relations on our terms, our fears of illness and the reluctance to discuss them with doctors, and our embarrassment about our "women's complaints."

The things that I have learned are in this book; only names have been changed. I was able to tape some of the workshops and some of the one-to-one conversations but not all of them, for some women were sensitive about it. If I judged that women would not mind, I took notes. But in some cases that was not practicable. If note-taking would have changed the ambiance, I waited until we were finished and then typed up the material from memory.

The style we used was consciousness-raising, and I was the facilitator. For each of the five five-week workshops, the technique was the same. The few guidelines were clear. We went around the room in a circle, and each woman would speak on the chosen topic—"How I feel about menopause," or aging, and so on—for about five minutes. No interruptions were allowed. We listened to each other. Pads and pencils were available for note-taking, and questions were put during the conversation after every woman had had her turn. One point was firm: no one was permitted to give anyone advice. That was absolutely forbidden because each woman determines her own rhythm for her own actions, for we are all in our own unique places. Each one of us knows more about herself than anyone else can. What may seem good for Mary may not be good for Helen.

There was one taboo word: *should*. It is a destructive word. Many middle-aged women berate themselves for not doing what they "should" do, and we were having none of that. We respected each woman's particular persona. This was the place where there was space to explore and articulate tentative feelings, perhaps for the first time, and no one would judge these efforts. We were giving each other not only our ears but our sympathetic understanding as well. No one could tell another what she "should" think or do. It's a simple system, for one gave what one hoped to receive, and since there was no one present in a leader or authority role, there was no one to whom one tried to be ingratiating. Such talk becomes creative, although it is sometimes frightening since it involves maximum self-exposure with minimum internal defenses, and most of us have been led to believe we must not express feelings that are asocial.

This opening of one's consciousness has many positive effects for it also amplifies one's mental processes. There is a danger, however, that outside the group this new kind of thinking, and the resulting changes in us, will provoke anxious opposition from the people we are close to.

The results of the workshops were very gratifying. Many of the women in these groups became friends. Moreover, each participant felt very differently about herself and her menopause after the discussions. These women psychologically separated themselves from stereotypes. They were individuals who had spoken the unspeakable and, instead of punishment, received validation for it.

Women have traditionally enjoyed coming together. Historically, we have used all kinds of excuses to do so, like sewing circles or quilting bees. One of the best parts of my children's growing up for me was taking them to Washington Square Park because that was where my friends and I always met. By the time we have lived to be menopausal women, there is a deep sadness in all of us from the pain of life, and meeting together to talk and to dare look beyond the conventional gives us a wonderful feeling of support. We need each other. Few of us have big families with aunts and grandmothers and cousins around us, and we lack the kind of human companionship those people may have provided.

My hope for this book is that it will help us get rid of the negative programming so that we may enjoy our menopause, instead of fearing it. And I mean really enjoy it, for I believe that instead of disliking our bodies—and our minds—we can come to love them and respect them and do good for them, and not harm them in any way, not with sugar or drugs or hateful thoughts.

I would like to define what this book is not: it is not a medical book. I am not a doctor, and I do not claim to have answers. I am a woman in her menopause who had a lot of questions and searched for the answers. Nor is this book a scientific study. At one time, I had thought about mimeographing a questionnaire for women in their menopause, but I was not prepared to make a psychological study of the percentage of women in this or that category who do or do not have hot flashes. I think such work is valuable, and I would like to see more of it done, but it's not my thing. The ideas I developed were largely stimulated by the questions women asked.

When I was reading books about menopause, I chafed at being referred to as "they" or "them." I longed for a book that spoke of "us" or "we." This book is about us, trying to reflect us honestly speaking our feelings on menopause for the first time, openly and with no shame or hesitation.

If, as Gertrude Stein phrased it, you are in your "middle living" and groping and struggling to find a way to survive with dignity and self-esteem and, it is hoped, with joy some of the time, then come along with me. That is what I am doing, and having good company is the best way to share an exciting adventure.

2
Menopause—
What Is It?

Menopause and aging are not myths; they are our realities. How we *feel* about ourselves largely determines the nature of our experiences and the degree to which we suffer. A woman's body cannot prepare itself for the possibility of pregnancy for some 35 years (releasing about 400 eggs in that many cycles) and then stop doing so without her feeling the change. To pretend that nothing is happening to her is not only absurd but does her an enormous injustice. If she is not aware of the change in her body, she would have to be anesthetized or be, at least, an unfeeling person, out of touch with herself. A lot is going on in her body and her head; to deny it is to deny her existence, and that is inhuman. Isaac Asimov, one of the good guys, when discussing menopause in *Human Body*, says, "It is a condition that is all the more frustrating to women in that its existence is either un-sympathetically dismissed by men or completely ignored." Menopause has been shrouded in a mystery of silence; it is time to demystify it.

To start, let's take a look at what menopause is. *The Merck Manual*, a book of diagnosis and therapy used by physicians, is a typical example of our culture's attitude. Immediately, this book communicates something negative. Instead of listing menopause under "Gynecology," where I automatically looked first because menopause is a natural physiological process, it is listed under "Ovarian Dysfunction." The word *dysfunction* means malfunction, impairment, abnormal functioning, or deterioration of the natural action. Since thousands of doctors use this authoritative text, is it any wonder they look on menopause as an illness? Say a 32-year-old doctor, who knows nothing about menopause firsthand, is to treat his first woman patient who mentions it. He looks it up in *Merck,* and what he finds is detrimental to his viewing the woman objectively. The minute it registers in his mind that menopause is a dysfunction rather than part of the normal aging process, he is going to respond to her in an entirely different way, presupposing illness rather than health.

My objection is that a woman's life is not "normal" for the 30 years she ovulates and "abnormal" before and after. That attitude reduces her to a baby-making machine. My ovaries are only one part of me. Why should I not be judged by the alertness of my brain instead of by my ovaries' ability to release eggs? *The Merck Manual* defines menopause as *"the transitional phase in woman's life when menstrual function ceases.* It may be natural, premature or artificial."* (The italics are in the original.) They give "Change of Life, Climacteric" in parentheses, and the older editions continue with "and often is attended by a complex imbalance of the glandular and autonomic nervous system." Phenobarbital and estrogen are recommended under the section labeled "Treatment." The current edition adds, "Uninterrupted estrogen therapy is not good practice," which is a different tone from that employed in the 1961 edition, which recommended "large doses of estradiol benzoate." It is interesting, by the way, that *The Merck Manual* has two numerical references after the word *menopause* and eight listings after the word *prostate.* Only 40 percent of men over 60 develop prostrate problems but menopause happens to *all* women. Can you guess the sex of their editorial board?

Dorland's Illustrated Medical Dictionary (1974) brings men into the picture, too. In it, menopause is defined as a "critical point in human life, the syndrome of endocrine, somatic and psychic changes occurring at the termination of the reproductive period in the female; it may also accompany the normal diminution of sexual activity in the male. Called also climacterium." Notice no mention of diminution of sexual activity in the female. Dr. Sheldon H. Cherry, whose book on this subject was published in 1976, says, "The term menopause means the end or cessation of menstrual periods. However, the end of menstruation is only one of a train of symptoms that marks the gradual transition from the years of reproduction to those of older age."

In a 1976 television interview with four doctors about menopause, Dr. Marcia Storch, clinical professor of obstetrics at Columbia University, noted: "The problem is really a social problem; it may, in fact, be a social disease and not a medical disease at all. It is unfair to women to say that they have psychological problems. This is something that is ingrained in our society so deeply that we have to take another look at women as people rather than as property."

The word *menopause* comes from two Greek words meaning "month" and "cessation," linguistically making the word "menocease," which would seem more accurate. Most of the time, the word *menopause* is used medically to mean "menocease" because, according to the definitions, menopause is the ceasing of the menstrual periods, not a pause in them. The exact meaning of menopause is not clear, however, because there are symptoms of menopause that appear before the periods actually stop. For example, Cynthia, 47, gets hot flashes but also has regular menstrual periods. According to the redefinition presented in this book, Cynthia *is* in her menopause. I believe menopause is the time around the end of the periods and is not distinguished by the last period, as many claim. Many of the symptoms of menopause present themselves both with and without periods. A number of authorities claim hot flashes begin when the periods end, but they are wrong, for I have spoken with too many women whose experience has been different.

One cannot generalize about middle-aged women, one cannot over-simplify menopause, for there are so many variations. For example, Henrietta, 58, discontinued flowing at 51, but when she is upset, she occasionally gets a flash. Is she or isn't she in her menopause? I say she is not in her menopause. Another example: Sylvia, 49, has had no apparent symptoms and menstruates regularly with a flow that is only slightly less than her flow of ten years ago. Is she or isn't she in her menopause? My guess is that she is in her menopause. She may or may not have symptoms for a year or two or three. It seems likely that she is in it, and whether it will continue to be uneventful cannot definitely be predicted. But again, we can theorize. If we were to look at the way Sylvia has handled other changes in her life—marriage, birth, jobs, illnesses, and stress situations—we may reasonably assume that, if she "fell apart" before, she will again. However, if Sylvia met those challenges with equanimity, she will probably not have severe symptoms. If Sylvia has mild symptoms, she will probably handle them comfortably.

Many authorities say menopause takes about five years to complete itself. It is the end of a cycle that began at puberty with menarche, or the onset of menstrual periods. The most common age in Western culture for menarche is 12, while menstruation stops from 45 to 53. A relatively small number of women begin menopause in their early forties and some after 53.

In 1937, the age for menopause was given as 47; in 1965 the national average was 49.2, and in 1975 it was 50.2. However, the range of normalcy is very large, and as 28 days is only an average number for the time between periods, so too, 12 and 50 are only numbers and should not be taken as rigid. Because 28 days is referred to so often, it is accepted in women's minds. If their periods are 25 days or 32 days, they fear something is wrong when nothing may be. Their cycle is normal for *them*. We are all individual, and we all have different rhythms. Numbers are merely convenient reference points.

The general rule that a pattern exists of early menarche–late menopause is questionable. Yet one of our eminent authorities, English gynecologist Dr. Katharina Dalton, says in *The Menstrual Cycle:*

Strangely enough, it is usually just those women who started their first menstruations late, at sixteen or seventeen years, who are likely to finish first, while those who started early are also likely to continue menstruating well into their fifties. There is often a strong family pattern in the timing of the menopause; those whose mothers and elder sisters finished early are likely to finish early themselves, and vice versa.

Women today are much more nutrition-conscious than their mothers were, and I feel that affects every aspect of menopause. I think a healthier diet makes for a later menopause. The shortest menstrual life I ever heard of was that of Christine, now 71, who came to America from Denmark, where she was born. She began menstruating at 19 and ended at 28 and has been and still is a healthy woman.

Dr. Dalton tells us that there "is no ovulation for the first couple of years after the onset of menstruation so, during the last couple of years of a woman's menstruating life, ovulation is absent." These years are rarely reproductive or fertile—even though there is a menstrual flow during most of the time—because there is no ovulation; that is, the ovaries are not releasing *ova,* or eggs. At puberty the ova are not yet mature enough, and at menopause the ova have either been used (that is, released during the over 400 periods in a menstruating lifetime) or have naturally disintegrated, as they do.

We are born with about a half million egg cells in our ovaries. At puberty, the number has dropped to about 75,000. A female has her complete equipment for motherhood existing in her body at birth; it has only to unfold as she matures. Men, however, manufacture their sperm as they go, which is one of the outstanding differences between us.

At menopause, the amount of hormonal stimulation from the pituitary gland—the master gland of the whole endocrine system—to the ovaries and the womb diminishes in the same way that it increased at the onset of menstruation.

The menstrual flow is only tangentially related to the eggs and occurs not because of the presence of eggs in the body but because the lining of the uterus, the *endometrium,* which is a spongy mass, is broken down. This mass develops as a lining during the second half of the cycle, in preparation for the egg to implant itself. However, if the egg is not fertilized or if there is no egg because there was no ovulation, the lining is flushed out as menstrual flow.

SEX HORMONES

In addition to estrogen, the female's most important sex hormone, her body also produces progesterone, the No. 2 female sex hormone. It is responsible for and necessary to the shedding of the walls of the womb, which creates the flow. The female sex hormones are produced in a complex way by the body. The main hormone-producing organ is the ovaries. Notice I said "main," not "only." One can produce estrogen without producing progesterone. Although these two female hormones are related and interact with each other, they are each distinctly different.

Remember what I'm going to say next; it is very important. Estrogen, the No. 1 female hormone in our bodies DOES NOT STOP being produced at menopause. Because of the inadequate language and its sloppy usage, there are people, particularly those who are convinced we *should* take estrogen replacement at menopause, who use terms that imply that we are no longer producing estrogen. *Ovaries fail, estrogen is shut off, without estrogen, castration, senile ovaries, steroid starved, missing hormones, hormone deficiency* are doctors' terms picked up by newspaper and magazine writers and thus brought into popular use. They are 100 percent wrong. Your ovaries do not fail at menopause; they merely go through their natural biological process.

Your body is a superb composition. It is not built like the "One-Hoss Shay," where if one part snaps it all collapses. Our estrogen supply does not stop at 50, and we do not fall apart. Our estrogen manufacture has been slowly decreasing since our middle twenties when our bodies were making the largest amount we ever had; that is also when our bodies are the most fertile.

At menopause it is common for our hormonal output, instead of being produced gradually, to alternately stop and start. There is a general readjusting of the endocrine balance in the body. The endocrine glands are organs that secrete various hormones which, when in balance, cooperate with each other in aiding the regular functioning of the body. When one hormone changes, it affects the other endocrine glands. This readjustment of the endocrine system at menopause is largely due to the change of function of the ovaries, which causes hormonal changes not only in the ovaries but also in the womb, breasts, vagina, pituitary, thyroid, adrenals, and hypothalamus. The unevenness of production is what is meant by *hormonal imbalance;* it is also what is meant by that crude term "raging hormones."

Our estrogen supply eventually regulates itself and reaches a plateau where it remains, some say until we are around 70.

Progesterone is not as important as estrogen because it functionally exists only during the second half of the menstrual cycle. Its supply does diminish to the point where it does not perform its functions, which are to create a comfortable habitat in the womb for a fertilized egg or break down the uterine walls which causes the menstrual bleeding. This means that if you skip a menstrual period it is because your body is not producing enough progesterone to shed the lining of the womb. You may have the same premenstrual symptoms from the estrogen your body is making but pass over the period because there isn't enough progesterone present. The estrogen level remains, albeit in lesser amounts, but that lessening is a gradual process that has long been going on in your body.

Veronica, 52, had not had a period for 18 months but did have her premenstrual symptoms of crankiness and swollen breasts every month, on schedule. Her estrogen level most probably remained the same but the progesterone did not. Selma, 49, had not had a menstrual period for six months but did not have premenstrual signs at all during that time. She only became aware of the amount of time because she checked back on her calendar for the day of her last period. Both of these women's menopausal experiences were different undoubtedly because their estrogen production was different.

The miraculous thing about our bodies is that when one organ slows down, others help out. This is what happens to our estrogen supply, too. As our ovaries, which have been the chief organ related to our estrogen production, lose cells (in a similar way that the rest of our body loses cells as we age) and gradually produce less estrogen, the adrenal glands pick up some of the production; as you will read in chapter 13, extraglandular sources also exist.

MENOPAUSE AND AGING

Language is living and keeps changing. I would like to see the word *menopause* become a common household word, with no negative connotations, eventually with positive ones. Because it now includes men, the meaning of the word *menopause* has broadened to refer to "middle-aged with problems."

There has been a lot of talk about male menopause, as well as a number of articles. Men's bodies go through hormonal changes, too, around middle age. Indeed, it is impossible to disentangle aging from menopause, and sometimes the words are used synonymously.

Climacteric, a medical word for menopause, means a critical period in life due to many changes, including endocrine, somatic, and psychic ones, and is also related to the word *climax.* The word *climacteric* is poorly chosen. By labeling this time as critical, it can become so. Should not adolescence be called a climacteric then? And if menopause is a climax, then is everything else to go downhill? That is not a kind way to view the rest of your life. I feel that I am expanding in my life more than I ever have before. My wisdom, my experience make my judging of situations much richer than when I was younger. The thought of living without perpetual possibilities for continued growth is a negative view of aging. Most menopausal language implies that the best is over, and that affects us and our view of menopause. The best is yet to come, especially sexually, but the men who chose these words didn't know that about us.

The psychological as well as the physiological changes that occur in middle age are covered in the term *menopause syndrome.* The term means many symptoms are occurring concurrently usually because of the original physical symptoms.

The concerns of middle age are neither feminine nor masculine because we all take stock and wonder about the life we didn't live, the time that was wasted, the additional affection and loving we might perhaps have enjoyed and sigh with sadness.

The reality of aging for women stands out in bolder relief at menopause because our long-time ritualistic practice of dealing with our monthly blood with the tampons and napkins and additional bathing is over. The curtailing of any ritual (even if found disagreeable) in which we engaged for over two-thirds of our lives represents a loss. We know it can only happen to us at a particular age. And the American culture does not like age; its attitude toward aging is abominable. Does that make us abominable?

Samuel Beckett's play *Endgame* was advertised on billboards all over New York City some years ago showing the heads of an old woman and an old man, each in their own garbage can. I found that sight frightening. But that is society's view of how we play the end of the game of life: of no more value than garbage. But menopause is only halfway to the end, according to the new gerontological findings. By the year 2000, life expectancy will be between 90 and 100. "Forecasting studies by the Rand Corporation (Santa Monica, Calif.) predict that an increase of 50% in human life span will be achieved by the year 2020."

The idea of problems existing because of age rather than sex strikes me as a move toward androgyny, or, as author Carolyn G. Heilbrun said, "a move away from sexual polarization and the prison of gender." It is a positive move and I celebrate it. It is also why I do not mind the phrase *male menopause.* Some women do; they feel men are co-opting a particularly female function and "won't let us even have that." I think it broadens the perception of menopause and may perhaps help us view more realistically the destructive cultural attitudes toward us. Androgyny is not a new idea, and many great writers have recognized its importance. Shakespeare frequently referred to this concept, and in *Love's Labour's Lost* has Berowne comment, "And gives to every power a double power, Above their functions and their offices." Long before that, the sex of the God Dionysius of Euripides' *Bacchae* could not be clearly defined. "Dionysius appears to be neither woman or man; or better, he presents himself as woman-in-man, or man-in-woman, the unlimited personality." Over a hundred years ago, Coleridge said, "The truth is, a great mind must be androgynous." One always hopes for more great minds on the horizon.

SYMPTOMS

Although the most common age for menopause for women in our culture is around 50, it is not uncommon for women to start noticing symptoms at around 35. These are the premenopausal feelings described by some women who feel and experience accelerated premenstrual symptoms for 10 to 15 years before the actual menstrual flow stops. This does not seem to jibe with the idea that menopause takes around five years to complete itself, but it is the case with enough women so that it is not unusual.

When I was 39, my premenstrual outbursts made me wonder if my body was inhabited by the Greek Goddess Hysteria or at least was the temporary dwelling place of a dybbuk. (The Greeks made a connection between woman's emotions and her womb. Their word for uterus is *hystera*. Did you know hysterectomies were performed as late as the turn of the twentieth century to "cure" women of emotional and sexual ills?) I went to a doctor, because my outbursts frightened me, and he automatically gave me tranquilizers and Premarin. No questions about my life or diet. At the time, I was drinking many cups of coffee with Sucaryl, eating a lot of red meat, and drinking red wine every night with dinner. My three daughters were 8, 9, and 10 at the time; I was separated from my husband and had to face finding a job. Was it any wonder I was scared and nervous? I didn't need too much hormonal imbalance to make me feel shaky. I believe the degree of our stability, security, and self-confidence affects the way we respond to the amount of estrogen our bodies produce.

I didn't know then that Premarin was estrogen and the doctor didn't tell me, but I did know after a month of taking those little oval yellow pills that I didn't like the zombie-like feeling of my body. I stopped taking them. The tranquilizers took longer to get rid of. At the time, I didn't even know what estrogen was. I made no connection between what I was experiencing and menopause. It was not until two years later that I thought perhaps there might be an association. And I do believe there was for me.

A premenstrual symptom I have always had was enlargement and swelling of my breasts, and it has become my major menopausal symptom. My three daughters also get that symptom when they are premenstrual. Some authorities say premenstrual symptoms run in families. One of my daughters has severe cramps, whereas I never did. They also suggest menopausal symptoms run in families, too, but I question that even more than the premenstrual ones for I believe a person's individual nature is more the determining factor in what kind of menopausal symptoms are experienced.

I have become very attuned to the hormonal changes in my body, for my breasts are my barometer; they go from normal to engorged with many stages in between. Midway to engorged, I wear a bra when I sleep because they become heavier and sensitive, and I need the support for comfort. When they are engorged, they become sore too, and then it is painful if I turn too fast. This would happen one night in every two months, and the symptom lasted for almost two years. I accepted it and was more careful about how I turned. I try to walk more when the heaviness is building up, and that helps. I also concentrate on such foods as celery juice and cucumbers, which are natural diuretics and help combat edema.

If I digress, bear with me, for I mean this book to be more of a dialogue than a lecture. Men have written almost all the books on menopause until recent times; and they are the ones who have defined it. Those who supposedly know all about it are the doctors and only 7 percent of doctors in the United States are women and only 3 percent of those are gynecologists. Most of the books tell us that menopause occurs in one of three ways: abruptly, gradually, and irregularly. What they are talking about is cessation of the menstrual flow, not menopause, for many women have menopausal symptoms while they are still having regular menstrual periods and long after the periods stop. We do not know when the periods will stop or in what manner unless it is "artificial menopause," which is the result of surgical removal of the uterus. That is abrupt and predictable. There is also a term "premature menopause," which means the menstrual periods stop before 40. Although it is not common, it does happen and may mean nothing more than merely being out of the usual range.

Abruptly means the period stops and there are no more menstrual periods. Some women claim they were not even aware of it until many months later when they realized they had not used their napkins or tampons. These women usually find menopause uneventful and have few, if any, symptoms. However, upon further questioning I have found that symptoms were present, but these women seem to have a high threshold of tolerance for discomfort. And as we individually and uniquely experience our menstrual periods, so, too, do we experience our menopause.

There is another kind of abrupt ending of menstruation. It is a result of a particular stress situation in the woman's life such as a death in the family, a separation from someone close, new job, new dwelling, and so on. This type of ending of menstruation may not be final, for when the stress situation is relieved or an adjustment has been made, the cycle may return.

Gradually means the period changes by slowly diminishing in amount and length of flow. This is the result of the gradual shift in hormonal balance in the pituitary, a gland at the base of the brain which controls the ovaries and many other glands. A woman may hardly notice the gradual change, for it may occur over a period of time lasting anywhere from six months to three years. For more than 35 years, her menstrual period may have lasted for five days. When it is reduced to two days with a lighter flow, she can be sure she is in her menopause. The periods may become scant, and she may skip a period; or the periods may gradually become irregular but with cyclic regularity. That is, one, two, three, four, or more periods may be skipped, but when the flow appears again, it is in the structure of the cycle. If one woman's normal cycle had been 25 days and another's was 30 days, they will find the time skipped will be multiples of their individual cycles.

Irregularly is by far the most common way for menstruation to cease. The menstrual pattern becomes increasingly irregular. The flow may vary from heavy to scant without any apparent pattern. The number of days of flow may also become irregular. The length of time between periods may become irregular, too. A single month or many months may be skipped, or periods can occur within a shorter range of time than the usual cycle. It is not unusual to go for a whole year without any periods and then get one or more. Some women who have thought they were through with their periods because they had not menstruated for a year or more have had their menstrual cycle return during a stress situation, and periods may return for many months. However, if there have been no periods for a year, it is common to consider the periods to be over. Some doctors feel women cannot be sure until two years have passed.

There is a difference between irregular normalcy and an irregularity in bleeding, also called abnormal bleeding. There are three kinds of bleeding that are not normal menopause: hemorrhaging or flooding, which is an excessive flow of blood that is faster and heavier than a heavy period; lengthy staining outside the menstrual periods; and very frequent periods. These irregularities may not be serious at all and may discontinue by themselves, but they should be closely and carefully watched and checked by a physician. Staining for long periods such as a month, no matter how slight, or periods every other week or every two weeks, even if they are light periods, should be investigated by a doctor. Polyps, fibroids, birth-control pills, or estrogen replacement therapy may be common causes of irregularity in bleeding.

Polyps are small fleshy growths in the cervix and can be easily removed in the doctor's office. Fibroids, common for all ages, are overgrowths of uterine muscle and fibrous tissue in the uterus, also called fibroid tumors. Dr. Sherwin A. Kaufman, a prominent New York City gynecologist on the faculty of New York University School of Medicine, says, "They are so common that one out of three women past the age of 40 has them." More often than not, they cause no symptoms, but if they project into the inner cavity of the womb, they do cause heavy bleeding. Fibroids usually shrink and often disappear after menopause.

Some women have a very heavy period or two during their menopause, but that is different from hemorrhaging or flooding. The abundant flow is containable with a tampon and napkin or two napkins. Hemorrhaging is not. Sometimes there are clots. Tanya, 48, described them "like pieces of liver." Dr. Kaufman says, "Clots are simply the result of more rapid flow, with insufficient time for the blood to liquefy." Any kind of uterine bleeding when menopause is definitely over should receive medical attention.

Although the clearest indicator of menopause is the end of menstrual flow, a woman may stop menstruating after 40 for reasons unrelated to menopause—because she is pregnant or because of a big stress situation in her life, such as the death of someone close, a move to a new residence, or a new job. In such cases the woman is not menopausal. If there are no unusual circumstances and the periods stop, that is menopause. All other so-called symptoms of menopause are questionable. In other words, is menopause the reason for a headache or fatigue or does the pain come from something else in your life? One can have a headache or fatigue at 15 or 25 or any age. How do you know that it's menopause? You don't for sure, you can only guess.

If you are over 40, a good way to guess is by consulting your calendar, assuming you have kept a record of your periods (see the following section, "Menopause Menstrual Record"). If your headache or fatigue has been coming around the time your period is due, and that has not been your usual menstrual symptom, then guessing they are menopausal is reasonable but not certain. If your premenstrual symptoms are exaggerated, they are probably menopausal symptoms, except for stomach cramps—which we don't get at menopause.

I have seen figures specifying that 10 percent and 20 percent of American women have no symptoms at all, but where those figures come from is anybody's guess. Some women do not get detectable symptoms; some women have many symptoms. Some of the symptoms are so mild as to hardly be worthy of notice. However, to know what they are, once you've gotten over the initial alarm that there can be so many, is a comfort when one does occur. You can recognize it as, "Oh, a menopausal symptom" and not the beginning of a dreaded fatal disease.

The symptoms I mention below are culled from my reading and from talking to women. There is not one symptom, except the menses stopping, that I believe can be attributed only to menopause. Not even the symptom most notoriously menopausal of all, hot flashes, is convincingly due to our hormone changes alone, for women long finished with their menopause get them occasionally, even twenty years later. I have mentioned all of the symptoms that I have become aware of so that you will know what the current thought is. I mention even those that I believe are due to aging rather than to menopause. (I have tried unsuccessfully to separate the fear of aging and menopause. It can't be done.)

The most talked about symptom of menopause is hot flashes. Chills are also a symptom, and when they appear, they usually follow flashes. Sweating and night sweats are common too. In technical language, these are referred to as vasomotor instability; a hot flash is a vasomotor symptom. There is talk, too, that men get them in middle age.

Nervousness, irritability, excitability, and anxiety are high on the list of menopausal symptoms, but, like headaches, who knows when it's menopausal or something else? Again, we can make guesses. If swelling breasts are one of your symptoms that lets you know your estrogen level is out of balance, and if you are irritable, it's very likely menopausal.

Weight gain ranks as the second symptom most discussed by women but it is not much discussed in the printed material. Bloat, too, is a symptom that is not much written about.

Depression, blues, lassitude, lethargy, emotional outbursts, temper tantrums, feeling fragile, crankiness, and crying appear a little lower on the list, and one can only guess, depending upon their intensity and frequency, whether they, too, are or are not menopausal.

Menstrual irregularity or disturbance, and breast changes are symptoms of menopause. Osteoporosis (bone changes) can also be a symptom, as can backache, leg pains, vertigo, dizziness, palpitations, faintness, numbness, tingling, feelings of suffocation, mouth sores and swollen gums, dry mouth, momentary swallowing problem, hair loss or gain, insomnia, urinary frequency and incontinence, nausea, indigestion, lack of appetite or excessive appetite, flatulence, constipation, arthritis, freckles, skin spots and skin changes, and vaginal changes. *Pruritis* is the medical term for itching skin in the vulva or genital region. *Senile vaginitis* is pruritis plus an irritating discharge which may or may not be blood-tinged (although this is sometimes called menopausal, it rarely occurs until long after menopause).

The Merck Manual lists some that sound bizarre because of their names, but they are only additional symptoms: *arthralgias* is a pain in a joint; *myalgias* is pain in a muscle or muscles; *formication* is the sensation of small insects crawling over the skin; and *desquamative gingivitis* is an inflammation of the gums with some gum tissue loss.

MENOPAUSE MENSTRUAL RECORD

The following table is a record of my menstrual periods for 32 months during my menopause. Mine is an example of the irregular type, the most common way menopause is experienced. The record begins when I was 50.33 years old. My cycle was around 30 days, and my flow lasted for 5 days. As you will see, there is neither a 30-day listing nor a 5-day listing here. I was 50.5 years old when I missed my first period. My menstrual flow had been lessening gradually for the previous five years, and I feel that I had had premenopausal symptoms for some ten years already.

I very strongly recommend keeping a record of your periods. It is part of the whole system of taking care of yourself and caring for your body. I don't mean only the date, but the kind of flow and length and the symptoms that show themselves, as well as changes in mood, appetite, and energy. You will be surprised when you look back a year later. You may find you had a headache with a couple of periods that you forgot about or any one of a number of symptoms. The realization that you have had the same symptoms before becomes comforting.

The chief value of marking the date is that it removes the guessing. You don't have to wonder, you *know*. You will know, too, if those *Weltanschaung* feelings you're experiencing are due to the human condition. If you

MENOPAUSE MENSTRUAL RECORD
32 months

Date of Period	Amount of Flow	Days from Last Period
1975		
February 12— 50⅓ years old	4 days	29
March 8	4 days	25
April	no period	
May	no period	
June 21	3 days	105
July 21	3½ days, heavy	31
August	no period	
September 28— 51 years old	no period	
October	no period	
November 15	4 days	118
December	no period	
1976		
January 5	3 days	52
January 30	2½ days	26
February 26	3 days, light	27
March 16	2 days, light + 1 day stain	20
April	no period	
May	no period	
June	no period	
July	no period	
August	no period	
September 28— 52 years old	no period	
October 13	1½ days, light stain	212
November	no period	
December 9	3 days, regular + 2½ days stain	58
1977		
January	no period	
February	no period	
March	no period	
April 1— 52½ years old	3 days, regular + 2 days stain	113
May	no period	
June	no period	
July	no period	
August 9	2 days stain	131

know you become fragile when you are premenstrual, and you have your own record keeping to confirm the time, then you can guide your behavior and take it easy. Rest more. Be good to yourself. Respect the fact that your body is doing its special female thing. Don't fight your body. This is all part of loving yourself and loving your body. Allowing for the changes that take place in it is accepting the rhythm that is you, your special, separate, individual, unique self.

You will be surprised how others around you will regard you when you regard yourself. Pat, 47, told us at her fourth workshop session: "I was going to get my period and when I came home from work I was so tired and cranky, I told my husband and two kids I didn't feel like making supper and they said, 'OK, we'll make it.' I almost dropped dead from shock. I had never done that before."

A very good way to come to know yourself and accept yourself as you are is to keep a journal. It doesn't have to be a rigid thing, but if you write in it when you are feeling new or different feelings or confused emotions, it will help sometimes to sort them out for yourself. It gives yourself to yourself in a wonderful private way. You become less afraid of the negative feelings inside yourself. We all have them and, somehow, putting them on paper makes them less terrible.

*By facing her own emotion, love, fear, hate,
whatever it may be, in stark reality, no
longer camouflaged by the assumption of
indulgence and maternal concern, she becomes
once more one-in-herself, dependent only on
the goddess, truly a Daughter of the Moon.*
                                    M. Esther Harding

3
Hot Flashes

The first thing to know about hot flashes is that they are harmless. They pass quickly and are nothing to be afraid of. I have them and I have talked to over 500 women who have had them. Usually they last from 15 seconds to a minute, sometimes up to two minutes. They vary as much in size, shape, and intensity as women do. Just as no one can describe a "typical" menopausal woman, so, too, there is no such thing as a "typical" hot flash.

I searched to find out exactly what a hot flash is. I looked in the two medical dictionaries in my library, and neither one had a listing for hot flash. As I scanned the names of editors, contributors, and consultants I could understand why—there were practically no women among those long lists of doctors.

I couldn't believe that the most talked about symptom of menopause didn't have its own entry. But I don't give up easily. I hunted around under *endocrine* and *flashes,* and finally, way down under numerous other definitions in the entry *flush* in *Stedman's Medical Dictionary,* I found: "hot f. a vasomotor symptom of the climacterium; sudden vasodilation with a sensation of heat, usually involving the face and neck, and upper part of the chest; sweats, often profuse, frequently following the f."

The medical books defined hot flashes as vasomotor "disturbances," "instability," or "irritability." But what is "vasomotor"? Vasomotor is any element or agent that affects the caliber of a blood vessel. The chemical and hormonal changes that are taking place cause the tissues, particularly the blood vessels and the nerves, to be irritable, which is sometimes the reason they "overreact." The nerves respond to this, causing the blood vessels to overdilate. This creates a hot flash.

The medical profession does not claim to understand hot flashes or their exact nature, since the range of variation is so great. But Dr. Katharina Dalton says a hot flash "is caused by a temporary error of the thermostatic control due to diminishing and uneven hormonal output." The hypothalamus largely regulates our heat-producing mechanism. However, what triggers it is a good subject for research candidates. My theory is that a hot flash is the result of blood vessels dilating abruptly. The vessels dilate and the flash appears; then it leaves in a flash and you feel flushed. A flush is like a blush only more so; the redness is deeper and the heat is hotter. It is common to feel hot in the head too. About 10 percent of the women I spoke with reported chills after a flash. The words *flash* and *flush* are used interchangeably.

Hot flashes usually begin at about the time menstrual flow begins to wane and usually continue until after the periods have stopped. Most women who experience them—once they have come to accept them—are not very troubled with them, for flashes most commonly are relatively mild. A small percentage of women do experience heavy and frequent flashes, often accompanied by a tingling sensation. The tingling may appear in the fingers, toes, or head, or it may appear in the toes and move up through the body to the top of the head. Sometimes flashes come singly and sometimes in series. Their frequency is completely unpredictable; one woman may have a flash once in a while, another might have them in series of threes for a few hours, another might have single ones every 15 minutes for a couple of hours. The variety is endless.

Our glands send messages to each other through our bloodstream, but because our bodies are readjusting and re-regulating themselves, sometimes the complex network of receiving and sending slips up for a moment. If a message to the vasomotor system is the one that's interrupted, we get that uneven spurt of blood which we experience as a flash.

All women do not get flashes or flushes. Some women merely sweat more than they did before, and they do not have the redness of flushing. Hot flashes may be mild and totally unnoticeable to others. It may simply feel as if the room has begun to get too warm suddenly, or it may be extreme, causing deep redness accompanied by an enormous amount of sweat literally pouring from your body. I repeat: flashes are harmless and pass immediately. The worst thing about them is that they may be uncomfortable, but they are never accompanied by pain.

If you have sweated a lot during your life as your normal condition, due to an active thyroid, for example, you may hardly be able to distinguish a flash from what you are accustomed to normally. I have been a "sweater" since childhood. Summer or winter, if I have been rushing to leave my house, my face gets flushed and I sweat as I go out of the door, into the elevator and onto the street. Some of my menopausal flashes are of the same intensity, but I know they are flashes because they happen when I am sitting quietly in a room.

I also get a clamminess or a cold sweat, especially when the weather is humid. I haven't read much about this but other women have also experienced it. It is a cold wetness around the forehead and on the head. My hair gets damp, sometimes wet. It is not in the flash or flush category, for its buildup is slower and it remains longer, but it is definitely related, for although I do not feel flushed, removal of clothes changes the condition. Since I've been in my menopause, a cold sweat can be provoked by a stuffy room. I have noticed it especially when I am attending a concert or lecture, and it also seems to be related to feeling closed in. When I can change my seat to one on the aisle, that helps. It is not uncomfortable and it's amazing how well we adjust. Knowing what it is, of course, makes all the difference.

Flashes can come at any age from normal behavior that causes our heat-regulating system to step up its activity—from eating too fast or eating heavy, spicy food, from exercise, from rushing around, from vigorous love-making, from heavy blankets or excessive clothing. Linda, 51, wears clothes in layers. In the middle of a conversation she may take an outer shirt off and I know she is having a flash. We speak of it. When her body cools down she puts her shirt back on. Betty, 54, has not had a period for five years but she still wears sleeveless dresses with jackets or sleeveless blouses with sweaters so that she can take the long sleeves off when she gets an occasional flash.

Diane, 50, called to tell me how her flashes changed. Her daughter had undergone a serious operation, and Diane had been sitting at her bedside for long periods. She said she knew when the flashes were coming because she would get a warning. They would begin with a tingling in her toes. The heat gradually worked up through her body to her head, and zing—a huge one. Because she had attended the workshops a few months before, it didn't frighten her. We had talked about the tingling, but the "warning" part was a new experience and it gave her a chance to prepare herself.

Minnie, 62, remembered her flashes as a feeling of heat "washing up over me." Margaret, 48, says, "I feel I have to catch my breath." Julia, 50, claims, "I get energy from my flashes and use it."

My friend Lucretia, 49, who knew of my interest in menopause, called me up one day with great excitement to announce she had gotten her first hot flash and what a "biggy" it was. "You wouldn't believe it," she said. "I can't wait to tell you all about it." "I'll believe it," I said and invited her for dinner. She told me every detail. "I was reading a book and suddenly this wave of heat came over me. I couldn't believe it was happening to me. I rushed to the mirror, and my face and neck were as red as a beet. It was *my* face, but I was so shocked and while I was looking and touching my face, it started to disappear and in a minute it was all gone. It wasn't really scary—but it was."

TALKING HELPS

One of the best ways to handle hot flashes is to talk about them. *They are nothing to be ashamed of.* The more we talk about them the easier they are to cope with. I joke about them and ask friends, "Is it too warm in here or am I having a hot flash?"

I cannot overemphasize the importance of discussing your hot flashes. Tell the people around you: your family, your friends, your co-workers. It is a wonderful thing to share for many reasons. By sharing the fact of your flashes you no longer feel ashamed or try to hide them. Most often, we are the only ones who know we are having a flash, but the fact that others know we do have them makes our feelings about them different.

To speak about your hot flashes helps you accept them more easily. It is amazing how marvelously people respond when you are open. There are exceptions, of course. Gertrude, 43, a friend of mine, is an extraordinarily handsome and mischievous woman. She was having dinner out and said to her escort, "I'm having a hot flash now." She later told me, "He flushed so hard, it looked like *he* was having a flash." "What were you doing?" I asked. "Are you in your menopause?" She laughed and answered, "I don't think so but I'm practicing. I wanted to shake the guy up a little."

Shirley, 47, a demure woman, surprised us when she revealed that she had told the women she works with—there are 17 of them of all ages—that she gets hot flashes at the office. They were not only interested, but a quick grapevine developed and the word passed fast when it happened. They all wanted to see what it looked like when Shirley was having a flash. "Who would have thought I'd be so popular because of my hot flashes?" she laughed.

The point I wish to stress is to accept yourself. Accept your menopause and your hot flashes. They are a part of you.

WHAT TO DO WHEN A FLASH COMES

There are simple ways you can help yourself if you are having a hot flash. First, *don't panic.* A hot flash is a normal phenomenon for a woman in middle age. Sit quietly and make yourself comfortable. Take off outer layers of clothing if you can, loosen your belt and unbutton your blouse at the neck. Take a few deep breaths—be certain to exhale deeply, too. If you can take your shoes off, do so; if not, loosen the ties. Loosen all clothing that is restricting. If you have hairpins, clips, or a rubber band in your hair, remove them; they may be pulling your scalp. Remember, the best thing about a flash is it passes quickly.

"What about estrogen?" some women ask. "Haven't we been reading for years in *The Ladies' Home Journal* and *McCalls* and all those magazines that if we take estrogen we can avoid hot flashes and aging?" Yes, we have been reading that. Women have found help from hot flashes by taking estrogen but the risk of cancer has been so closely linked to estrogen replacement that it is almost foolhardy to take it unless your condition is so completely uncomfortable that you can't stand it. Then, perhaps, and only then, does taking it make any sense, and for only a short period—hopefully, a mild dose for no longer than six months. But I wouldn't recommend taking estrogen until the alternative other women have found successful has been tried. That is vitamin E.

Many women have found relief in two days from taking 800 International Units of vitamin E complex, also known as mixed tocopherols. I have seen flashes disappear completely when the vitamin E is also accompanied by 2,000 to 3,000 milligrams of vitamin C (taken at intervals throughout the day) and with 1,000 milligrams (also at intervals) of calcium from dolomite or bone meal. When the flashes have subsided, usually after a week, the women reduce the vitamin E intake to 400 International Units.

Most physicians are not sure exactly in what way our estrogen level is related to hot flashes, or if it is at all. The medical thought in this area is changing because our hypothalamus, our heat regulator, is also critically involved.

The women in the workshops decided since flashes are involved with the flow of blood, it follows that the blood vessels should be kept as clear and open as possible. That is the reason they were interested in vitamin E, for it not only helps the blood to carry more oxygen, but it also helps break down cholesterol buildup on the walls of the arteries, allowing the blood to flow more easily.

Whether a woman does or does not take estrogen, the flashes eventually disappear. The flashes are like everything else about us. They are a part of us, and the more we fight them the longer they seem to remain. As for aging, I have seen women "hooked" on estrogen who have more wrinkles than women who do not take it. Estrogen does improve the vaginal dryness that happens to some of us, but other alternatives exist. They are discussed in chapter 15, "Estrogen Replacement Therapy"; chapter 11, "Masturbation" and the section "Yogurt Therapy" in chapter 17.

Some doctors are convinced that a woman's estrogen level drops suddenly, and the only way to save her from the "ravages of old age" is to pump her full of estrogen by needle or mouth. I do not agree with them. The only time the estrogen level drops sharply is when the ovaries are surgically removed. When this operation takes place during the menopausal years, it may cause immediate and severe hot flashes, but the same operation does not seem to cause flashes in younger women.

Women whose estrogen level decreases very gradually do not experience flashes at all. As Dr. Sheldon H. Cherry notes, "About 60% of women get distinct hot flashes or other vasomotor symptoms." I think that's a pretty good guess but I would make it a little lower. I think about half of the women who go through menopause get hot flashes, so there's a 50-50 chance you will. Many women have only a few mild flashes during this transition period, and most women learn to live with them and continue their daily lives without interruption. Although many women miss work because of menstruation, I have not heard of women missing work because of hot flashes. At least two reasons exist for this: There are no cramps or abdominal pains, and the menopausal symptoms are so unpredictable one doesn't know when they will show themselves. A hot flash comes and goes, usually within a minute. If you get one before going to work, you might not have another all day or for a week or a month or ever again.

Alida, 46, a dress designer, was in a conference showing her sketches. "Suddenly I became a mass sensation of hot pricklies. No one said a word, I'm not even sure they noticed, because I was so excited about the designs and you all know what an excitable type I am anyhow." Eleanor, 48, told us, "When my husband and son go off in the morning I get a hot flash." "Do you go to work?" I asked. "Oh yes," she hastily replied, "it doesn't last." Some women's flashes are still more accommodating. They come in the evenings and on weekends.

There seems to be a connection between one's estrogen level and stress. As the estrogen in our bodies is re-regulating itself, the additional element of stress seems to trigger the symptoms.

Michele was 54 when I interviewed her, and she had gone through menopause eight years before. At that time she was a social worker and lived in the suburbs; she was having serious marital difficulties, as well as coping with four teenaged children and taking care of a sick mother. One winter, when she was between jobs, she had severe hot flashes. Her experience was difficult: "I was like a lunatic," she said. "On one cold night, when everyone was freezing, I was burning up. I went outside in a summer dress (I had been wearing them that winter because of the flashes) without a coat and patted snow on my face and arms. It was the only way I could cool off." She was living on donuts, coffee, and cigarettes and was not taking vitamins. Finally her children grew up, her mother moved out, and Michele separated from her husband. She thought she would not have had such a rough time with her menopause if her life had not been so full of problems.

The workshop women were concerned about stress and agreed the B complex vitamins were necessary for menopausal women to keep the nervous system functioning normally. We know that women who have long been through with their menopause may get hot flashes in stress situations. I wonder if for these women it is the heat-regulating system of the body rather than the estrogen level that causes this effect. Heather, 67, returned for a visit to Scotland, where she was born. She hadn't been there since she left as a child. She had finished menstruating at 50, and had had occasional flashes for seven years. Since then, she had not had any at all for ten years. However, she got flashes at Prestwick Airport—coming and going.

NIGHT SWEATS

Although flashes and sweating go together for most women, some have hot flashes without sweat while others have sweat without flashes. Sweating during the night is called night sweats and may or may not be accompanied by hot flashes. Virginia, 49, had mild ones. "During the night I'd find myself taking my covers off for a few minutes, then pulling them back up. I got so that I hardly woke up." Priscilla, 54, had a different experience. Her story is interesting, for she had been bothered by night sweats and hot flashes for two years. They were so severe that she not only was awakened, but "was drenched. My pajamas were soaked and so were the sheets. I had to change everything." This was before she took vitamin E. After two days of taking it she was astounded at the relief. After a week of taking it she was sleeping through the night. A month later, after three weeks without a flash, Priscilla went to see her doctor and told him about this miraculous change. He said it was nonsense. On the spot, that instant, Priscilla had a huge hot flash. She tells me her present condition is not as good as it was during the three weeks before she went to see that doctor, but that it is a lot better than it used to be.

This kind of story sounds unbelievable, but I have heard so many of them from people I have come to know and trust, as well as from my friends, that I believe them all. For example, Maryann, 49, came to a workshop series and after the first session her flashes stopped, and she had no flashes during the next four weeks. However, the day after the fifth and last session she got one. Maryann called on the phone to tell me, "I just can't believe it." I can.

It is treading on delicate ground to make generalizations about hot flashes, but I am going to risk it. It seems that women who feel they have their lives under their own control have fewer and milder hot flashes than women who feel confused and frustrated in their lives. I have also noticed that women who are nutrition-conscious and take exercise have an easier experience. I strongly believe there is a clear relationship between a healthy body and an easier menopause.

*You not only are what you eat—
you age by what you eat.*

AMA

4
Weight Gain Is Not a Crime, Only Dangerous

"She's fat because she's frustrated" is true. This statement of derision about us makes as much sense as accusing a mother of small children of always being tired. Of course we're frustrated. Most of us haven't had the opportunity to choose work we would like; we aren't paid as much money as we think we deserve for the work that we are doing. Do we get as much love as we think we deserve, or as much attention as we would like? We receive too little respect for our experience. In fact, instead of being regarded and recognized, we are ignored. We are not addressed by the culture. On the contrary, we are made to feel invisible.

Eating makes us more visible. It validates us for ourselves and we occupy more space when we are bigger. Psychologically, it also acts to insulate us from more hurts.

When nurturers grow tired of nurturing and do not themselves feel nurtured, they feed themselves. Taking care of oneself by feeding is a way of trying to take control of one's life and not being dependent on others to be fed. Also, there is the fear we may not be fed; we are not certain we can trust others to feed us. Perhaps we do too good a job—and that is why we put weight on.

In the United States, weight gain is the chief problem of middle age for both women and men. Our bodies now need less food; also our metabolism (body chemistry) works more slowly. The trick is to do the nurturing job differently so that we don't put weight on, but when one is lonely and hurting and blue it is difficult not to reach for the fast comfort (cheap thrills) of sugar and carbohydrates.

Many of us, too, lose weight, only to regain it. What is operating in our brains when this happens? Why is a pastry resistible one day and not the next? This is the mystery we must explore and confront. What is taking place? What secret lies in our brains? How can we learn to expand the capacity to say *No* to destructive or excess food? I believe these questions to be much more relevant than a discussion about the fewer calories in celery. We are plenty aware of the calories when we are eating bread and butter, yet we do it.

We want to understand the need in us that is being served when we eat cookies. For someone to tell us we eat ice cream when we are troubled—just as an alcoholic drinks—is no help to us. We know that. We will show concern and respect for ourselves when we look at the fact that some craving is definitely being satisfied. There is no question that among the complexities operating, something in us becomes momentarily fulfilled. That something has a value. That something is worth looking at.

A hundred theories exist about weight loss and they all hold some truths. But what good are they if we cannot use them to serve us, to help us from putting food in our mouths? We all know plenty of good weight-loss ideas, and most of us have tried them many times. The behaviorists tell us to change our behavior, and they have a point, but not enough of one. We all know that when one is busy getting ready to go to a concert one doesn't eat so much. Life, however, is not mostly getting ready for concert going. Clever directions are thrown at us: "Reach for your mate instead of your plate." Not everybody has a mate. If you do, the chances are your mate may not feel like loving you at that moment.

Slick answers have not worked. We must, each one of us, personally find our own, not to please the people around us, but for ourselves because we all know it is healthier to be thinner than fatter and statistically our chances for living longer are better when we are not overweight.

The health reasons against being fat are numerous. We all know it puts a strain on our heart and an extra burden on the digestive system, overburdens the bones and joints, and taxes our total metabolism more, altogether forcing us to use ourselves harder. For every pound of fat above your normal weight, there must be an expanded system of blood vessels, which in turn requires one's heart to pump extra gallons of blood over longer distances. Extra fat is also associated with diabetes and high blood pressure. In the article, "Live Longer and Like It," prepared by the American Medical Association, we are told, "If you can control your diet, you can significantly control your aging."

Excess weight after menopause increases one's risk factors for coronary heart disease and arteriosclerosis. Doctors warn fat people who have the high risk factors of high blood pressure, high blood sugar, and high cholesterol to be under the care of their physicians. Fat people are more susceptible to maturity-onset diabetes; it is the most prevalent complication of obesity and can cause serious consequences. One of the most frequent complications of diabetes is hardening of the arteries, which doubles the possibility of a coronary heart attack. Endometrial cancer, which is cancer of the lining of the uterus, is linked with obesity because during and after menopause extraglandular estrogen has been found to be at higher levels in fat women. When this high level is sustained for a substantial period it has been discovered to be closely related to uterine cancer.

When are you fat or obese or overweight? The concensus is that overweight describes a person who weighs more than an average person of the same sex, height, and body build. It also can be translated as consuming more calories than the body uses. Obese, however, is defined by some as a person weighing more than 20 pounds over the figure listed as "average" on height and weight tables.

Body weight is closely linked with self-image. In the culture of twentieth-century America, it is a social liability for a woman to be fat. It is also a concrete liability in the job market. In the hiring for many kinds of jobs—and I don't mean jobs as fashion models—discrimination against fat women is practiced but rarely spoken about. We know that job applications are marked "too old" and "too heavy." This means a double-decker prejudice is working against *us*. This was apparent in the case of 47-year-old Betty Rose Hall. In the spring of 1969, she was denied a job as a $75-a-week teller by a Fort Lauderdale, Florida, savings and loan association. The U.S. Labor Department scored one of its first victories in enacting Title VII of the antidiscrimination act which became law in 1964. The case's issue was actually age discrimination, for there is no law against weight discrimination. However, the transcript of the case noted that Betty Hall "was on the plump side, five feet five and something over 145 pounds."

In America, the idea of fat has taken on such gross proportions in people's psyches that no matter how fat or thin some people are, in terms of health and averages, what fat means to them personally is much more significant. I have listened to women who weighed 110 pounds carry on about their weight gain, or their need to watch their figures as much as women who weighed much, much more. Weight is relative, like age. I've heard women in their early thirties worry about getting old.

Some people seem to have natural tendencies to be more plump than others, but the quest for the ultraslim figure has grown way out of proportion because too many women can never find satisfaction in being themselves. They are constantly trying to be a thinner person, thereby never finding pleasure in themselves, never accepting themselves as they are.

Eminent authorities—among them Dr. Jean Mayer of Harvard, Dr. Albert Stunkard of Pennsylvania, and Dr. Jeremiah Stamler of Northwestern University—agree that a moderate degree of overweight is neither dangerous nor a liability for most people and is far better than a continuing weight loss and gain pattern. Diets, in fact, may be dangerous unless you're under a doctor's care, and then some of those are dangerous, too. Diets can cause headaches, dizziness, diarrhea, fatigue, indigestion, skin disorders, and constipation, as well as irritability and depression. At a recent nutrition symposium, Dr. Judith S. Stern of the University of California at Davis said the relapse rate after dieting is very high: 95 percent of the subjects regain lost weight. Exercise, however, was found to be very useful, because through exercise it is possible to manipulate caloric utilization over and above the amount taken in. She does not recommend diet regimens that depend on a low carbohydrate, high fat and protein intake because they work primarily through the loss of water, which is readily regained. Also, they can result in undesirable side effects such as tiredness or raised blood cholesterol levels.

Adelle Davis tells us that "the craving for sweets disappears when the blood sugar is kept high." Translated into practical terms this means eat protein, a handful of sunflower seeds or unsalted peanuts. Yes, they are high in calories if you compare them to carrot sticks. However, we all know that the substitute for ice cream, cake, or candy is not carrot sticks. Those sweets are desired for reasons other than hunger and we are not going to pretend we can ignore those *other* reasons. They are there. However, as a transition technique, the eating of healthy food instead of harmful food is taking a big leap in self-love. If you must buy snacks and nibblies in the grocery store, buy items that you know are good for you, so that you have the better alternative available.

The book, *Fat Can Be Beautiful,* by Dr. Abraham I. Friedman, tries essentially to take the torment out of being fat. We are told women are by nature more inclined to be fat. The body of a normal male has only 14 percent of fat compared with 25 percent in the average female. Moreover, an editorial in the San Francisco *Medical Society Bulletin* stressed that "We can allow ourselves to be plump and contented, rather than neurotic over a few pounds. The time has come to stop the war against fat, and admit that people can be fat and healthy. Stay fat and live happy."

I am not suggesting we don't continue to work on change and growing as healthy human beings. What I am talking about is the self-contempt and constant finding fault with oneself that is so destructive. It is as if we sometimes lose perspective about ourselves as whole human beings with many assets and focus in on the "fault" of being too fat. Loving yourself as you are is the chief message of this book. I strongly believe that, if you can accept yourself, you can more easily change yourself.

IS IT OUR HORMONES?

Is there an actual connection between menopause and weight gain? It is common for women during menopause to put on weight for so-called menopausal reasons, related to the changes that are taking place in the endocrine system. The hypothalamus, our heat-regulating mechanism, which we have learned is related to hot flashes, also has a relationship to our eating patterns. Dr. Solomon H. Snyder, professor of psychiatry and pharmacology at Johns Hopkins University, says in *Madness and the Brain,* "In the hypothalamus there are also specialized 'hunger' and 'satiety' centers." Something undoubtedly is happening to our satiety center as a result of the hypothalamus, which controls the pituitary gland. Both the hypothalamus and pituitary are involved with releasing hormones, but their stimulation of the ovaries to release estrogen is no longer getting the same results. We know that in this transition period, the pituitary must learn *not* to stimulate the ovaries as it previously had, because the ovaries are not responding as they had been; they are much slower and are putting out much less estrogen. Until the pituitary learns to stop making this demand, things are not synchronized in the brain. One wonders whether, until the pituitary learns its new role, and the hypothalamus changes its directions to the pituitary, the hunger-satiety centers are also askew?

When women are premenstrual, many feel like eating more. It seems the same factors are operating during menopause: the hormonal level changes seem to trigger these hunger-related centers. We have also learned that premenstrual symptoms often become exaggerated at menopause. From my own experience and from observing closely and talking to other women I think there might be a relationship between the amount of estrogen and progesterone the body manufactures and our "hunger." After my periods became irregular and my buildup of estrogen was high—which I felt clearly from enlarged breasts and the general puffiness of my body that comes from water-logged tissues, or edema—my appetite increased. This was very much like my premenstrual behavior. Then, until my estrogen level dropped, that *fat-hungry* feeling remained. When we skip periods, we do not get the relief that comes from the menstrual flow, and I believe all of this is connected with our bodies' producing less progesterone, for it is the progesterone that is one of the chief elements involved in causing the sloughing off of the lining of the uterus which creates the period. Therefore, do we feel like eating more because we are not producing enough progesterone? Until our bodies adjust to this change, some of us feel like eating more. Don't fight it, just be conscious of it. It will settle down.

We are more concerned with a healthy way of eating for the rest of our lives, a way that will naturally be self-regulating, rather than going on and off diets. We know how important it is not to be too overweight for our health but it is not an easy thing to deal with. The way we live in this world is so alienated from our food supply. I am certain that if we could have gardens and be more connected to the earth where the food we consume comes from, we would be able to regulate ourselves more easily. Less of our food would be harvested prematurely; we would also have the benefit of its being ripened by the sun. So much of our food looks like manufactured plastic objects with shiny coats of wax.

I can hear some mumble, "She's looking for excuses for menopausal plumpness." My answer to that is *No,* but I am looking for more avenues to explore. We're too old for smart-aleck answers or ones that don't work. We have to figure out our own systems for ourselves. If a sense of alienation from nature is felt because most of our food is packaged, then that alienation exists. And if our relation to the whole cosmos has to be realigned because we no longer mark our months with blood, who dare laugh at that? Those are legitimate areas of search about our weight gain. Our minds and bodies are sensitive and we respond to many different kinds of stimuli. Looking in as many places as possible makes more sense to us than someone telling us to pull ourselves together so we'll fit into their idea of how we should look.

There is agreement among authorities that adults require at least 1,200 calories a day for good health; any less may be risky. However, like all generalities, a person's individual metabolic rate and activity level, as well as one's current weight, are also factors. The calories that we don't use to maintain our body processes and our movements are converted into fat. As a general formula, it has been figured out that for every 3,500 excess calories we take in and don't use, we store one pount of fat.

After the age of 20, our calorie requirements diminish at the rate of 1 percent a year, which means we must cut down on the quantity of food we consume as we grow older.

Our fat problem grows as we age, according to Dr. Marci Greenwood of Columbia University. In women between 55 and 64, over 30 percent are obese. Dr. Sami Hashim, director of the Nutrition and Metabolic Research Center at St. Luke's Hospital in New York, found from experiments that normal-weight people have a fixed satiety level, which is controlled by a mechanism geared to maintain body weight. Obese people do not have the same satiety level. It appears that fat people eat because of environmentally generated signals, not because of hunger. "Factors such as smell, taste, social setting, conviviality, relief of boredom, relief of tension, etc., are important in governing food consumption in the obese," said Dr. Hashim.

Some people have found success in controlling their weight by keeping calorie consumption and activity or energy output in harmony, a little like balancing scales. Others have found that eating three meals is harder on the total digestive system, whereas eating the same amount of food spread over a longer period of time made a difference. Studies of both animals and humans have shown that frequent small meals make weight control and weight loss easier, tend to reduce levels of blood cholesterol, and improve glucose (sugar) tolerance. One of the practices some women follow is to eat from smaller plates. Other practices include such obvious things as eating one egg instead of two, and one slice of toast.

Carol Munter, a feminist therapist in New York, specializes in working with the overweight. Her therapy helps women to get in touch with their stomach hunger, which is different from what she calls chewing hunger or mouth hunger. Ms. Munter claims we are not enough in touch with our true hunger and can learn to be. She also emphasizes self-acceptance as one is, not to wait until you become thinner. She recommends looking at your naked body in a mirror and accepting it; in that way you "energize" the heavy parts.

HOW WE TRY TO LOSE

In the menopause workshops, we discussed our weight in relation to how we felt about ourselves. So much has been written about self-image connected with self-loathing and fat and although there was some of that, there was also the reverse attitude: "I'm tired of trying to be something I'm not," and "I can't be bothered to try to please others," and "If someone won't like me because I'm ten pounds heavier but will if I'm not, then I don't need that person."

We didn't come up with any pat solutions but we did hear a lot of ideas. Gloria, 50, said she has observed her weight gain in direct proportion to her sexual activity. When she becomes celibate, she puts weight on. Cynthia, 49, related her weight gain to the pressures of her job; when the pressure lets up, she loses.

Linda, 47, noted that when she felt really good about herself she lost weight, because she wouldn't eat things that weren't doing her good. But she could not define for us what the circumstances in her life were when she felt good. Rachel, 52, however, could tell us. She said that when she was feeling like a successful person, she automatically ate less. Her standard of success for herself was being effective on her job and feeling intimate and close in her love relationship. All of us agreed that those elements together could work for all of us. This prompted Helen, 51, to remember when she was at her best weight. She, too, told us of feeling successful with her work, socially, and as a mother; her marriage, however, was not giving her satisfaction. "That was before the Women's Movement," Helen said, "and I really didn't know that one could dare expect more from a marriage. I was almost unconscious of that because superficially everything looked like it was going well. But I felt unconnected to my husband." This led to further discussion about what middle-aged women want from intimate relationships but that is another book.

The following weight-loss ideas were presented in the spirit of sharing. There seemed to be general agreement that getting one's digestive tract cleaned out was primary to losing weight. The obvious diets and the obvious commercial weight-loss programs are known to all of us; there is no need to go into them. We are as much interested in eating healthy food as in losing weight. The idea of using synthetic sweeteners heavily loaded with inorganic chemicals does not make any sense—not when we're trying to love our bodies and keep junk out of them. These suggestions worked for the women who were using them. They are listed as idea material and practical examples of what other women do to stimulate their weight consciousness. No one ever, under any circumstances, suggested that another woman use her system. I want to emphasize that these ideas were used by healthy women and are not to be taken as suggestions by people who may be ill or are under a doctor's care.

Your own plan, your own method of proceding, is much more likely to work for you, for you can tailor-make it for your comfort and taste. The more personal the approach, the more likely are the chances for success with it. You know better than anyone else what is making you fat. You know that cutting a specific portion of cake for yourself and putting it on a plate is safer than leaving the cake, pie, bread, or cheese in front of you— then "just evening it out." You know what I mean—to cut a little sliver so that the food can be put away neatly. Those slivers have a way of building up into another big portion. How do I know? I'm a sliver slicer.

It was common among the women to cut down on carbohydrates and sugar, even honey. They all agreed that the summer is an easier time to lose weight because of the abundance of local fresh fruit and vegetables. We can learn from the cultures where people live to be around a hundred years old as a usual phenomenon. Those people are not involved with the concept of "well-balanced" meals; that is an American idea that goes with packaging. The mountain people of the Andes, the Hunzas of the Himalayas, and the Azerbiajans of the Georgian USSR eat the seasonal foods when they are available, and the populations are not fat. They are also more active than are we of the "advanced" culture and walk much more because they don't have cars and public transit systems. Eating a lot of tomatoes, or cucumbers, or watermelon when they have been ripened in the sun seems to have a more positive effect than does concern for balanced meals. I strongly believe in "shocking" the system by using an abundance of the foods that are available and cheap.

Kathy, 48, has what she calls a "citrus purge" every spring. For two days she eats only grapefruit and oranges. She feels this puts her on the road to better health because she watches herself more after it.

Helen, 52, starts eating a couple of tablespoons of yogurt upon arising and continues every two hours throughout the day until retiring. She feels this corrects and cleans her digestive tract and creates a slimmer consciousness.

Dale, 54, fasts for a day when she decides to take some weight off and drinks only water.

Alita, 46, fasts for two days and drinks liquids, mostly juices, whenever she wants them.

Rebecca, 51, prepares a bottle of apple cider vinegar, honey, and water and keeps taking "slugs" from it throughout the day, especially before meals. She does this for a week and watches her food intake very carefully.

Linda, 45, changes the furniture in her house, especially her bed. She feels this always creates a change in her eating habits.

Colette, 42, cleans out her closets and drawers and altogether tries to think slim, neat, and pared down.

Virginia, 55, tries to do something exciting and different in her life when she starts to put on weight. She strongly believes such changes create changes in her metabolism and her body responds differently. She observed this whenever she traveled or was interested in a new lover; her body responded in some way that was different. She is very much for getting shaken-up, out of one's usual pattern.

Mandy, 47, said she loses weight when she walks a lot. She doesn't think it is so much from the walking as from the way her metabolism responds to the walking.

Marge, 62, found that if she ate nothing after 7 P.M. she could lose those extra pounds.

Jessie, 44, found that when she uses her juicer, she loses weight, and when she's "too lazy" to use it, she puts weight on.

Peggy, 56, stops eating bread.

Willa, 50, loses weight, she says, when she puts yogurt on everything for a few days at every meal. She eats the yogurt with fruit and honey but also eats rice and potatoes with yogurt on them. She uses yogurt for her salads, yogurt on everything, and that works for her.

Gertrude, 49, loses weight when she eats grapefruit before every meal and as her snacks instead of anything else. The Mayo Clinic diet uses grapefruit or its juice at every meal because it acts as a catalyst that starts the fat-burning process.

Margot, 54, claims when she stops eating a large salad every day, she puts weight on. When she goes back to the salad she gets herself back in shape.

Barbara, 44, says her eating becomes a problem at night and if she masturbates instead of snacking, she can control her weight.

Julie, 57, takes an enema every morning while she is trying to lose weight.

Frances, 51, says she tries to program herself and keeps repeating: if I don't eat it, I don't have to feel guilty.

Dawn, 49, told us that her system is to cut everything into very small pieces. This gives her the illusion of eating more. She keeps her knives very sharp so that she can cut things very thin. We have seen her eat an apple and the whole ritual lasted for about an hour.

Belinda, 53, told us the only way that worked for her was to keep a notebook. She wrote down everything she put in her mouth and when she wanted to eat and felt she shouldn't she wrote her feelings in her notebook. She said this took a lot of time, but the act of writing helped lessen her food intake. She could not, however, tell us the reasons why at times she could keep her notebook and other times she couldn't. She didn't understand it herself, except she said, "I could never do it for more than a month at a time."

Whatever way you find that works for yourself—and you may have to try various methods or a combination of them—it can work for you for the rest of your life. We're slimming down for ourselves because it makes us feel better and healthier. Doing everything out of choice is the way we want to go. The best place to start is with our own bodies.

5
Other "Symptoms"

SKIN AND HAIR

Will I lose hair on my head? Will I grow hair on my face? How can I prevent wrinkles? How can I keep my complexion? Women think about and ask these questions around menopause. As with all the other questions about menopause, the first answer is: a healthy body is directly related to such factors. And a body is more likely to be healthy if the kind of nutrition it gets is body-building rather than body-destroying. A hamburger on a white roll with French fries and coke for lunch will give you greasy hair and a puffy, pasty complexion. A salad and a yogurt will make you beautiful. You hair and skin reflect the food you eat.

Because it is an external part of the body, skin shows age before any other part. Around the age of 35 our skin gradually becomes thinner and loses some of its flexibility and elasticity. Women's skin is thinner, less resilient, and less stretchable than a man's skin. Although one doesn't think of skin as active, it is in fact a very busy collection of interrelated body organs that protects our bodies against invading bacteria, against harm to sensitive interior tissues, against the sun's rays and, very importantly, against our losing moisture.

Skin consists of three layers. The deepest, subcutaneous layer, contains nerves, fat, and blood vessels. It rests between the next layer of skin, the dermis, and the tissues which cover bone and muscle. This deepest layer also acts as an undercover for the two outer layers—the dermis and the epidermis—and is also related to wrinkles. The fat lobes of this underskin decrease as we mature and the underskin doesn't support the other two layers as well as it did originally. The loss of this fat affects our insulation; therefore, our body temperature is not as constant.

The dermis, or middle layer, is thicker and thinner in different parts of the body. It contains the oil and sweat glands, which for many women function less vigorously after menopause. This action, or lack of it, by the oil glands can create dry, uncomfortable, itching skin, for oil gland loss is critical to the health of the skin. We must, therefore, add oil or moisture to prevent wrinkles and cracks.

The epidermis or top layer is made up predominantly of dead skin cells which fall off all the time; these are more noticeable when they soak off in the bathtub. Underneath these dead cells are living cells which are nourished by general circulation. The sloughing off process is functional, for it is a self-cleansing mechanism which casts off bacteria, dirt, air pollutants, and other potentially harmful substances. The texture of this outer layer, these dead cells, is largely determined by the amount of moisture it holds; so that the skin surface may be dry, rough, and covered with lines or soft and smooth.

A person's skin represents about one sixth of the body's weight, contains one quarter of the blood supply, and covers approximately 20 square feet. It is hard to imagine that one square inch of skin contains some 15 feet of blood vessels; by dilating and contracting these are our most important temperature regulators.

As we raise our skin-consciousness, we come to realize how much shows through it. For example, a feeling of well-being is evidenced by color, whereas sadness is usually manifested by paleness, sickness by pallor, shyness by blushing, anxiety by sweating. One can say our skin speaks for us. And in the vernacular we use skin as metaphor, as in the tune made famous by Dinah Washington, "I've Got You Under My Skin," or the strong expression of feeling like "jumping out of my skin," or as a description of cowardice when a person acts "to save his skin." The concept of "laying on hands" emphasizes the skin as receptor for sensitivity and healing. Goose pimples is a loud statement of skin response. A furrowed brow is wrinkled skin showing grave concern but a big smile is wrinkles with an upbeat message.

Like everything else about us, our skin, too, must receive our attention and care. Living in steam-heated apartments dries out our furniture, the binding of our books, and our skin. Air-conditioning also dries the air and is detrimental to skin. It is helpful to keep plenty of moisture in the rooms you occupy. I own a large fish tank because I like fish and because it is an excuse to have a large body of water in my living room. Leaves and evergreens in large vases of water, particularly near radiators, help enormously. So does keeping your bathtub full for many hours at a time. You will be surprised how much water evaporates. One of the women keeps her tea kettle simmering a few hours a day because she wants the moisture from the steam.

Soaps and detergents dry skin out and many dermatologists suggest bathing less after age 45 to preserve natural body oils. Water, however, is a healer so bathing is fine, but cut down on the use of soap; use it more sparingly. Try to use glycerine soaps rather than perfumed soaps. Dermatologists agree that lubricating the skin is important: because "the glands of the skin begin to decrease their activity and there is insufficient sebum to keep the skin as soft as in the teen years, external emollients provide part of the oil the skin needs."

In practical terms, oil your body. Use your kitchen oil because whatever soaks into your skin eventually finds its way into your bloodstream. I don't like commercial cosmetic oils or baby oils because they contain petroleum and other nonorganic chemicals. We like natural, cold-pressed unsaturated oil with no preservatives. This oil can be bought in health-food stores. My favorite is safflower oil, and when I'm extravagant I use apricot kernel oil. Sesame and almond oil are superb too. Anoint yourself lavishly, rub it in, it's a fine way to massage yourself while you're at it. Close your eyes and get those wrinkles in the corners and don't forget any parts like between your toes and between your legs and all around your fingernails. Let it soak in for an hour or longer, then soak in a hot bathtub. This is healing yourself. It is loving yourself.

Oil your body before going to bed so it can soak in overnight. When you shower the next morning don't rub too hard because the oil is good for you. If you haven't done this before, it may take some getting used to because overcoming the greasy feeling seems to take a little while for some people. Do try; it's really worth it for the good it will do your skin. Aesthetically it becomes smoother and softer to the touch and looks and feels better. Use a drop or two on your hands after dishwashing. Women have been anointing their bodies since time immemorial. It's a good idea for men, too, especially if they have hard, dry, scratchy feet. That's unpleasant for everyone.

Why do we stay away from corporation cosmetics? For two reasons: first, women are insulted by the advertising that tells us unless we use their products we're smelly and dirty, that the odor under our arms and between our legs is offensive, having a "natural, foul smell." Curiously enough, they have not invented genital sprays for themselves or their brothers. Does that mean male genitals do not "smell funny," or if they do, that it is acceptable? Would you believe that in 1971 the profits from vaginal deodorants were estimated at $53 million?

By masking vaginal odors with perfumed deodorants many women have not been able to detect serious infections that are best treated before they can spread. We cannot support a destructive, hateful attitude toward us. Second, we don't trust them because we know about too much damage that has been done to women because of these products. We have seen the hair texture of our friends ruined from hair dyes and home permanents which have caused chemical burns, conjunctivitis (eye infections), nausea, blisters, scalp sores, and facial swelling. Recent research suggests a link between hair dyes and cancer.

It is against our way of trying to live our lives, for there is a huge difference between *caring* for your hair and skin and violating them with harsh chemicals. We are trying to avoid artificial preservatives and unnatural chemical additives both inside and outside our bodies. In 1970 the National Committee on Product Safety reported that 60,000 people were injured each year "so seriously as to restrict activity for one day or require medical attention." Beauty aids were the No. 2 cause among all classes of products reported to cause injuries. A 1973 report of 1,031 eye cosmetic products showed that 50 percent were contaminated by bacteria, 10 percent by fungi.

A 1975 survey showed 40.5 injuries per 10,000 deodorant and antiperspirant applications; 40.2 injuries per 10,000 uses of depilatory and hair remover; and 14.6 per 10,000 applications of hair spray and lacquer. The Food, Drug and Cosmetic Act of 1938 does not require safety testing, ingredient labeling, registration of manufacturers, or the reporting of consumer injuries.

Wrinkles can be controlled up to a point. We can follow three guides: (1) don't smoke; (2) drink plenty of water for moisture, and consume some salad oil every day to keep the skin from drying out; (3) remove the flakey top skin debris by scrubbing so the pores can breathe more easily, then apply oil regularly to retard the evaporation of the skin's own moisture. As for estrogen cream, it is the oil in the cream, not the estrogen, that helps. Ruth Winter tells in *Ageless Aging* about experiments verifying this fact.

What about the appearance, around and after menopause, of freckles and brown spots, sometimes called liver spots or "beauty marks," or blotches or little red flecks? These are all involved with pigment and no one seems to be sure about their origin. A pigment, melanin, influences skin color and acts to prevent the dangerous rays of the sun from harming the skin. As we age, melanin "builds up in our skin, generally, but more particularly in spots." Some think there is a relationship between these spots and "rancid" body fat. Vitamin E is supposed to prevent or help such rancidity. Others think they come from poor early nutrition or the body's inability to assimilate some vitamins. As the melanin spots increase, we also get wartlike growths, seborrheic keratoses. These are thought to be related to a change in the functioning of the sweat glands, causing seborrhea. The result is oily coating, crusts, or scales on the skin. As the melanin builds up over the years, the skin gets darker; the top layer thickens while the underlying layers of the skin thin. This accents the lines and wrinkles.

Our skin is very individual and sensitive. Therefore, what may work for one person may not for another. These are some of the things the women discussed for skin discolorations: to lighten dark spots, apply diluted lemon juice or cranberry juice (unsweetened) before going to bed or dab on yogurt or buttermilk, let it dry and keep repeating the process for an hour. For marks and warts, apply vitamin E oil or wheat germ oil morning and night.

If you have stretch marks because you have lost weight, try sesame oil. Some women have found the marks eventually disappear after a large number of applications. If you shave your legs, use any unprocessed kitchen oil instead of soap. If you expose your body to direct sun, protect it with PABA (para-aminobenzoic acid) cream against the ultraviolet rays. If you're already tanned, organic kitchen oil with a little natural apple cider vinegar is a mild protective shield against the sun. If you have too much sun and are feeling stingingly sensitive, make a paste of baking soda and water and apply to the sunburned area for relief. Then use aloe vera gel for healing. When you're at the beach, be sure your body is oiled for many hours of each day.

Light, air, sun, and water are healthy for your body if taken in moderation. The sun triggers your body's production of vitamin D. Try to be uncovered, and expose yourself to these elements if possible, for the increased respiration of the skin aids the respiration of the lungs and increases metabolism. If you can, at home, for example, it is best to wear less clothes whenever possible. Stockings, underpants, all clothes keep air from circulating on your skin; the more you can remove, the better. Being naked whenever possible is much better for your skin than being confined. Loose clothes are certainly preferable to tight ones. Be conscious of two tightly closed areas which need air, under your arms and between your legs.

Nurture Baths

You can take marvelous baths to nurture your skin. Cleopatra was wise, because bathing in milk and honey makes sense. Use half a cup of honey and a cup or two of dry powdered milk in your bath. While you're lying in it, use some honey for a facial; it is full of nutrients and very good for wrinkles. Or try the oatmeal bath. Cut the foot off an old stocking. Place a cup of uncut, natural (not instant) oatmeal in the toe; then knot the stocking. Rub the oatmeal mitt all over your body and face. The slippery texture is very sensual and leaves your skin silky. You can do the same thing with miller's bran, which contains oils and other nutritious goodies for your skin. Brew some herbs and let the witch in you out for an herb bath. Find your own combination. My favorite is a half cup combination of dry rosemary, thyme, and lavender flowers. Simmer, covered, in two cups of water for 20 minutes, then let steep for 20 minutes more. Pour the essence through a strainer into your bath. Your house will smell beautiful too.

Cook a pot of pine needles that you have stripped from their branches, and pour the pine "tea" into your bath. Or, if you're longing for the beach, pour a cup of sea salt into the tub. The minerals are a tonic for your skin. If you want the smell of a perfumed bath in any of these, add a few drops of scented oils.

If your muscles are aching or your skin is itching, use a cup of natural apple cider vinegar in your bath water. Get used to pampering your skin in this way, because it is most relaxing. Remember, though, don't wash off the nutrients with soap. Use the minimum amount of soap and get used to rubbing your body with a loofa sponge, complexion brush, or hard washcloth instead of soap. Most soaps are alkaline and rob the skin of its acid mantle which protects it from bacterial infection, thus leaving it vulnerable to surface outbreaks. Friction refreshes and tones your skin, cleanses and refines the pores. The dried dead cells are removed from the skin so that it can breathe more easily and the pores are not clogged. As the vigorous action increases blood circulation, those tiny capillaries near the surface of the skin respond. You'll see because your skin will look flushed from the flowing blood.

Kitchen Facials

Nurturers in their middle-living have to think about nurturing themselves. One of the ways to do this and keep fat off our bodies is to feed our faces—not our mouths, but our skin. Facials are a trip that can easily be taken in your own kitchen. They needn't be a big deal or take a lot of time but can be done in a minute while you're doing other things. One merely has to develop one's facial consciousness. We want to keep this channel open to throw off the daily accumulation of waste which is funneled through the skin ducts. Our faces get dirty from the polluted air, especially from the lead that cars exhaust.

One of the skin's functions is to help rid the body of toxins from food that contains additives and preservatives and other nonorganic chemicals, as well as the poisons from sugar, coffee, and alcohol. It's a good idea to wash your face with a loofa sponge, a complexion brush, or a heavy rough washcloth before you cook. Then, if you are slicing cucumbers for a salad, rub a slice or two on your face and let it dry; it is especially good for tightening the skin to correct large pores. If you're peeling an avocado, mango, or papaya, rub the inside skin on your face. Don't throw out the herb teabag or herbs in your teapot. Let them drain overnight, then empty the herbs from the bag or from the pot into your palm. Spread them on your face and let dry. By lightly touching your face, the dried herbs will come off easily.

If your facial skin is dry, pour a drop—one goes a long way— of salad oil in the palm of your hand and spread it on. Don't forget yogurt. Warm a teaspoon in your palm for a moment, then spread it on your face, and let it stiffen. Those constructive bacteria soak into your skin and fight the destructive ones. Rinse your face with warm, then cool water, and *no soap.*

Honey is superb for wrinkles, especially the tiny ones around the eyes, but we limit that to the bath or just before it because it's so messy. However, even though egg whites are sticky, too, they can be used in the kitchen. When you crack an egg, remove the white that sticks to the shell and apply it to your face; it's a perfect skin toner, feeds your face protein, and is also supposed to be good for wrinkles. If you're eating an apple or a pear, rub a slice over your face. They are good astringents and contain disinfectants. Watermelon juice cleanses deeply and tightens pores. Squeeze a grape and apply the juice for the same reasons.

Oatmeal has a high vitamin and mineral content. If you are cooking oatmeal, reserve a teaspoon of the gluey liquid for your face and apply it. An oatmeal pack or mask takes time but it's worth it once in a while. Add boiling water to three tablespoons of organic oatmeal in a bowl, moisten it, making it pasty, not runny. Let it stand, covered, for a few minutes, and then apply it to your face. (Lie down for this treatment, because the oatmeal is heavy and will fall off.) Leave it on your face for 15 minutes—oatmeal is a superb skin softener that will bring a magnificent luster to your face *if* it has had time to work.

Facial masks do take time, but they deeply revitalize the skin. The stimulation they create brings circulation to every pore. Fruit masks of mashed apricots, papaya, mango, avocado, or banana are also extremely beneficial, but mean lying down for 15 minutes.

Aloe Vera Plant

If you don't know about the aloe vera plant, let me acquaint you with this succulent, a member of the lily family. It is a vital health and beauty aid to have around the house, and it has been used for centuries. Many people call it the Medicine Plant. It is a superb natural healer "cosmetic" for skin and hair. The long skinny leaves are filled with a gelatinous substance which is used for cuts, burns, insect bites, chafing, itching, sunburn, and more. Tear off a leaf and slice a strip. The jelly will run out. If only a speck to heal a cut or bruise is needed, wrap the leaf and store it in your refrigerator. If you can't find this plant locally, you can order through the mail from Vera Products, Inc., P.O. Box 1863, Taos, New Mexico 87571. A two-month old plant costs $1.50, a six-month old one $2.00. This company also sells aloe vera gel (99½ percent pure); a pint is $3.25 if you can't find it in your health food store.

As a general skin and hair conditioner, it is in a class by itself. It's a nongreasy cleansing agent and has astringent and skin freshening properties as well as being a moisturizer for the skin. Put it all over your body, mixed with your good organic kitchen oil as a moisturizer.

Use the jelly as a suntan lotion—the properties of this desert plant have the remarkable ability to protect the skin from the harsh rays of the sun and still enable you to acquire a deep luxurious tan. The lotion screens out the burning (erythemal) rays, 93 percent of them, but allows 78 percent of the tanning rays to penetrate the skin surface. Use it mixed with your shampoo, a teaspoon of each, especially if your hair is dry and brittle; it will not rob you of your natural oils and will help repair split ends. Use it as a hair conditioner, especially if yours needs added body (it brings out the natural sheen and is the best "set" around). For a really good job of conditioning, squeeze a whole leaf on your hair or use a generous tablespoon of the gel from the bottle and rub it into your scalp. Wrap it with a hot towel and let it "cook" for about 15 minutes, then rinse with clear water.

Your Crowning Glory

If the crown on your head starts thinning down, there are things that you can do. I know, because my hair has changed in the last few years from being quite fine to being full bodied. My change in diet is largely responsible, and positive nutrition is the first requirement. Thinning hair as a result of aging or baldness, more common with men, is largely hereditary, but the bloodstream determines the condition and strength of the hair. I have seen dramatic changes among women my age who stopped wearing their wigs. Their hair became thick enough so that they did not need wigs anymore. Hair reflects one's internal condition of health. So do skin and nails. I have seen women's hair which might be described as dry, dull, mousey, thin, greasy, or scraggly change to healthy hair when they took vitamins with emphasis on the Bs, calcium and zinc.

If you are interested in reconditioning your hair, the first absolute rule is *no junk* on your head: no dye, no permanent, no lotion, no spray. Do not tease it either. Keep your hair and scalp clean and breathing. Do not wash more than twice a week, because the natural oils and conditioners must be given a chance to work, and sebum must be secreted by the scalp. Be very careful with the shampoo you use; use no harsh chemicals like preservatives and additives. You want a healthy pH balance. After you wash your hair, continue massaging it for five more minutes (preferably with a plastic thing called a shampoo massage brush) to give it and your scalp exercise. Massage your head every day because it loosens the dead layers of the skin that block the natural processes of the scalp and you want those tiny capillaries on the top of your skull to work for you to supply the hair with a nourishing supply of blood. If you don't or cannot stand on your head, touch your toes so that you change the gravity flow which encourages the blood to circulate.

If you are interested in a reconditioning process for your hair, a good natural haircut will dry fast *without* a hair-dryer. Dry hair and scalp are problems in themselves, and we're trying to eliminate them. You can avoid curlers, rollers, pins, rubber bands, barrettes, combs, and anything that might break ends, pull your hair for long periods (pulling for a couple of minutes is good exercise for your hair) or scratch your scalp. Hair is very alive and that kind of activity traumatizes it and makes it porous.

Remember, in this book we're loving ourselves, and part of that process is not to do violence to any part of us, our hair included. To nurture your hair is to love yourself and in the same way we don't put junk in our bodies, we don't put it on our heads either.

A hot oil once a month is an excellent idea for healthy hair maintenance, especially if your hair is dry or damaged. Warm a couple of tablespoons of your unsaturated kitchen oil (like safflower or sesame oil) by putting it in a pyrex cup and place that in very hot water. When it is comfortable to the touch, massage it into your scalp. Wrap a hot, wrung out towel around your head, turban style. When it cools down, repeat the hot towel wrap a few times, allowing about half an hour for the oil to penetrate. Wash the hair thoroughly and use an apple cider vinegar (two tablespoons to a quart of water) rinse. Pour through your hair and catch in a bowl about five times. Work it in and do not rinse out.

Another health treatment is two tablespoons each of oil and honey, mixed together and massaged into the hair and scalp. Wear a plastic bag and let it "cook" for half an hour. Then wash thoroughly and use the vinegar rinse. These treatments nourish the scalp, put bounce into the hair, strengthen it, give it sheen and gloss, make the hair more manageable, and will rid the scalp of dandruff.

An egg yolk shampoo is an old-fashioned and direct way of feeding protein to the hair and scalp. Beat the yolk in a half cup of water and massage it in well. Place a plastic bag on your head for five minutes or so, then rinse with clear water. Do not use soap or vinegar for this one.

Herbs are a fine tonic and will restore brilliance. Brew a cup of herbs for half an hour over low heat to make your rinse. Then use as your last rinse, catching the water and repeating at least three times. For light hair, use camomile flowers; dark hair, sage. Rosemary stimulates hair growth. Make some strong brew of rosemary and add it to your vinegar rinse. Use a few drops of pure rosemary oil—careful, only a few drops—on your hair for a smooth sheen. It will also prevent splitting ends, and, amazing as it may sound, it does not feel or look greasy on your hair. You can use it every other day. The smell is strong but it evaporates. If you don't care for it, add a drop of lavender oil to the rosemary.

If you hair gets greasy easily, you're eating too much animal fat. Cut out red meat (eat fish and chicken instead), butter (change to margarine), and rich cheeses (change to part skim cheese) and you'll see a difference. The primary nourishment for hair comes from within the body. Healthy hair depends on a delicate balance of protein within the hair shaft and oils on the outside of it. Dry hair may be the result of not eating enough vegetable oil. Be certain to take two tablespoons a day, on your salad or in your cooking if your hair is dry. And of course, don't dry this type of hair further with heat from a dryer.

Hair is constantly being renewed below the skin surface. We keep the hair on our head from two to six years, and it falls out at about the rate of 60 hairs a day, which are replaced by new hair sprouts from the same bulb. Hair generally grows at about the rate of half an inch a month, slowing down as we age. Many women lose hair on their bodies as they age, particularly in the pubic area and under the arms, as well as on their legs. Some women have an increase in hair on other parts of their bodies as they age. Medical jargon calls this hirsutism. It may appear in one or more places, such as around the chin and upper lip or around the nipples and from the navel down. Hair increase, like hair loss, is hereditary, and the increase is more likely to occur in women who have darker or olive skin, particularly those who have Latin or Mediterranean backgrounds, even if many generations past. This, and hair thinning on the top of the head, is considered to be due to a hormonal shift. Some authorities believe it to be caused by an increase in the amount of androgenic (male) hormones. If individual hairs grow around the nipples or on the chin will cutting cause them to grow faster? Authorities agree that the rate of growth will undoubtedly not be affected—and you will probably feel more comfortable. If there is a growth on the upper lip, you may want to bleach it with lemon juice. However, if it is upsetting you, you might visit a dermatologist and check out other techniques such as electrolysis.

Graying hair is the absence of pigment in the inner layer of the hair shaft. When hair is gray or white, air replaces pigment in the cells. Old hair does not lose pigment; thus one does not "turn" gray but new hair grows in without it. Adelle Davis thought the lack of pigment in hair is related to the B vitamins. "Deficiencies of at least four B vitamins, PABA, biotin, folic acid and pantothenic acid, appear to affect hair color." If this idea stirs you to taking these B vitamins, I would like to encourage you, for the Bs are especially important for stress, too.

However, I do want to warn you about folic acid if you're in a menopause year when you're skipping periods. First, folic acid is produced by intestinal bacteria, which presumably supplies all we need, while the other B vitamins come largely from the food we eat. Thus, avoiding extra folic acid is not serious. If you take brewers' yeast, the richest food source of the Bs (and the cheapest), a B complex, or a multiple vitamin tablet, you're getting some folic acid that way. My concern and reason for caution with folic acid is that I believe it to be a precursor to the formation of estrogen in the body. I have read that in a number of places and my own experience with it bears it out. I was taking folic acid with numerous other vitamins, and I strongly believe my estrogen level did increase. It can be very uncomfortable to be producing too much estrogen but not enough progesterone to cause a menstrual period. This creates those premenstrual bloated feelings with sore breasts, if you are prone to that. Therefore, use great caution with folic acid.

PABA, short for para-aminobenzoic acid, is known as the gray hair vitamin, and I have read of cases where large doses have caused a change in hair color. Linda Clark in *Get Well Naturally* tells about some interesting cases of hair color changes from the use of blackstrap molasses. A particularly interesting case was that of a 51-year-old man whose hair had become gray and was falling out in patches. After he changed his complete diet, his hair grew back, black, in a few years. He thought, though, that his hair improvement was due to the blackstrap molasses. Every morning he mixed a batch of two tablespoons each of blackstrap, natural honey, and apple cider vinegar, and gradually consumed it during the day by adding it to his drinking water. Ms. Clark found seven people who also believed that their hair color change was due to blackstrap, which is rich in B vitamins and also contains many minerals, particularly iron and copper (all used to recolor animal fur). Acid helps iron to become assimilated, which may have been the function of the vinegar. Two warnings about blackstrap molasses: it must be taken diluted, because it can harm your teeth, and it is a powerful laxative. If you want to try it, do so gradually.

Nails, although not skin, are an outgrowth of the epidermis and an important body cover. They are made chiefly of keratin, fibrous proteins that form the basis of the horny tissues. Nails contain calcium, and defective ones can be a sign of calcium shortage or defective calcium metabolism. Look at your fingernails. They, like your hair, reflect your nutrition. I hope they are pink with white nails above the fingers, not a gray color. I also hope they are not cracked, striated, ridged with lines, or have white specks on them, and that the skin around the nails is not ragged or torn. If they are any of these, you probably need more zinc.

Finally, a word about the skin on your feet. Give your feet more attention—they are what you need to stand firm on. Therefore, make them strong through touching. You may not believe this, but it is true for me. The more I love my feet and the more attention I give them, the healthier they become. They are precious because the 72,000 nerves in the body have their endings on the bottoms of the feet. Foot massage with oil can relax your entire nervous system. Give that to yourself—a strong base to stand on will keep you firm and strong.

CONSTIPATION

Constipation, if a sometime problem for you before or during menstrual periods, is likely to appear around menopause. If constipation has been a problem unrelated to your cycle, it will probably recur as your body readjusts to the physiological changes. If it has never been a problem, it may become one temporarily. Our whole metabolic process slows down a little as we age, and, in addition, your body is searching for its new estrogen plateau. Together, these may cause temporary constipation.

Some women find that when they add more calcium to their diets, it causes constipation. If we have upped our intake for the benefit of our bones (see chapter 17, "Nutrition and Middle Age"), we have to compensate in another way for the benefit of our colon. Constipation may result from—beside many other reasons—a lack of coordination in the nerve and muscle functions of the colon and other bowels. This sluggishness of bowel action means the muscles of the intestinal walls are not able to push the waste material from the body to eliminate it.

The bowel is the most obvious eliminative channel of the body, but we also eliminate wastes from the kidneys, lungs, and the pores of the skin. The kidneys excrete the end products of food and body metabolism from the liver and other organs. The bowels eliminate not only the food waste but also waste matter known as body waste, in the form of used-up cells and tissues. This residue is the result of our physical and mental activities and if not eliminated would cause protein putrefaction resulting in toxemia (poisonous substances in the blood).

Strangely enough, constipation can result from positive changes in the diet such as eliminating sugar, coffee, or alcohol. It is only temporary, however. Since we are all so individual, what one person may call constipation another may consider healthy evacuation. Some women move their bowels three times a day and some women move theirs every three days—daily is the most common. Your comfort and your knowledge of your own body will help you determine your "normalcy."

Laxatives, we all agreed in the workshops, were a dead-end method. They wash away the friendly bacteria in the colon and can cause constipation to become chronic. The women were interested in trying to get natural stimulation. Some of the ideas may or may not strike you as workable, but trying natural methods and natural foods which the body can handle more easily than cathartics is worth considering. Many of the women found success with the following methods, and I list them all. You may find one or a combination that works for you.

If when you try a new food, you find it is helping but you are also experiencing flatulence and distention, don't be discouraged, for it is only temporary, and it will not last. It is part of the transition until your system becomes accustomed to its new reflex. Give yourself a few weeks to get used to it, until the new reflex becomes natural. This is important, for some of the women gave up after only a few tries.

Nature's Way

Acidophilus, a natural culture, is alive with millions of live organisms which assist in the maintenance of a favorable acidic intestinal flora. Take it as liquid, in capsules, or drink a glass of acidophilus milk daily.

Blackstrap molasses has the reputation of being the most laxative food there is. The taste is terrible, but if you can disguise the strong taste, you'll have an extra benefit from the iron in it. Take a teaspoon or more daily (rinse your mouth immediately—it's bad for your teeth).

Bran is in commercial cereals, but those are processed and contain malt and sugar which can offset the beneficial effect of the bran. Look around in a few health stores for bran, known as miller's bran. It is inexpensive when bought in bulk, without the commercial packaging. Take a tablespoon one to three times a day.

Bran is a natural food fiber. Fiber, the structural part of plants, is composed of complex carbohydrates: cellulose, heim-cellulose, pectin, and a woody substance called lignin. Bran builds soft bulk which absorbs many times its own weight in moisture. It stimulates the colon and passes quickly, thus helping your digestive system to regulate itself. Plenty of liquid must be taken when bran is used. Most processed foods have had the fiber removed in their manufacture. People on a high-fiber diet are less prone to digestive problems than those on a diet of low fiber.

Some of the women take bran in water or juice before meals; others put it in yogurt and add honey, and some sprinkle it on cereal or salad. Others have it with milk as cereal, both warm and cold. Be certain you buy only the unprocessed bran.

Brewers' yeast was suggested by Clara, 51, who found it worked for her. However, I have also known it to help diarrhea. Since it is very rich in B vitamins, I can only guess that there is some general regulating strengthening benefit.

Buttermilk is another cultured food that creates a positive flora in the intestines. Drink a glass daily.

Enemas have their champions as well as their foes, and they both feel strongly on the subject. If the use of some mild warm water makes a person feel more comfortable, it seems like a harmless aid during a transition.

Flaxseed is best put in a blender for a moment—to chew those seeds would take forever. Some take it like bran, a tablespoon in liquid, one or more times a day. Ruth, 46, soaks some overnight with oatmeal and then cooks it on a low flame for a short period for breakfast. It does get gluey, but she doesn't mind that.

Fresh fruit and *vegetables* are the best foods we can eat at any time. Sonya, 45, eats nothing else for a day when she wants to "clean myself out."

Herb teas as well as hot water with lemon works for some and not for others.

Kefir is a cultured whole milk drink that contains Lactobacillus Caucasicus and comes plain or in fruit flavors. It causes constructive bacteria to flourish in the intestines. Drink a glass daily. It is especially effective if only liquids are taken, and no solid foods.

Liquid fasts are becoming popular. Rose, 53, says she likes it because it gives her body a rest and "straightens her out." A few of the women were fasting regularly once a month, and one woman was fasting one day a week.

Massage is also becoming popular. Lynne, 48, discovered that if, before getting out of bed in the morning, she massaged her lower intestine, to the left and below her naval, she had what she called "a more finished movement."

Prune juice, prunes, and apple cider vinegar work for some but not others. Some people take quantities that are too small to be effective.

Walks are a method most women found useful. Phyllis, 55, has a desk job and claims her constipation is helped in proportion to the number of blocks she walks a day. She keeps count and tries to walk at least 20 during her lunch hour and walks part of the way home, depending upon her tiredness and hunger.

Wheat germ, raw, untoasted, is recommended by Dr. Joseph D. Walters, former director of the American Academy of Nutrition and a pioneer in the field of metabolic nutrition. Irma, 48, downs a tablespoon neat before her dinner and says, "It's the only thing that consistently does it for me."

Yogurt, like the other cultured milks, benefits the activity in the intestines. Cynthia, 49, added prunes to hers which she soaked first, then pitted and put in the blender. She thinks it's "the best medicine."

Lorraine, 53, told us that since she religiously eats a salad for lunch every day with two tablespoons of oil, as well as an apple during the afternoon, she has become "regular."

Yvonne, 55, says she "doesn't worry about constipation anymore" since she has been using a heaping tablespoon each of bran, flaxseed, and wheat germ warmed in skim milk for her morning cereal.

Grace, 46, shyly said, "You may laugh, but I find if I masturbate, it makes everything move in my body, including my movement."

The last thing we want to do is strain. Vivien, 49, uses a foot stool in her bathroom because she thinks it approximates the more natural squatting position. Ingrid, 56, told us she uses one, too. Instead of leaning forward, she finds that placing her feet on the stool cooperates with the gravity of the body because it makes her sit up.

Corrine, 57, found that a technique "will work very well for me, but after six months or so it becomes less effective and I have to try something else."

I didn't list honey because none of the women brought it up and I only came upon it in one place in my reading, but I think it is worthy of mention because Dr. D. C. Jarvis of *Folk Medicine* fame says honey "has a natural and gentle laxative effect." And don't forget water. Drink plenty of it. Constipation may be caused by dehydration.

All of these techniques derive directly from women's experiences. They've given it serious thought and experimented. Perhaps there's relief for you in some of the methods reported in their testimony.

BACKS AND BONES

Sometimes when you feel very tired and feel as if your bones are aching, it is not in your head, it is in your bones. Our bones can ache as we age, for very good reasons—they, too, are going through changes. In medical literature, it is called *osteoporosis*. This is a condition in which bone tissue becomes porous and increasingly fragile as a result of calcium loss. The affected bones become brittle and can fracture easily. "Osteoporosis is the commonest chronic disorder of the skeleton and is largely a problem of the aged, especially postmenopausal women," says Dr. Robert P. Heaney, a bone authority who is chairman of the Department of Medicine at Creighton University in Omaha, Nebraska.

The significance of osteoporosis to us is its connection with bone fragility. That is why we worry so much about old women falling, for the decrease in bone mass doesn't produce any definable symptoms, but it does lead to fracture. And fracture is very scary because around one quarter of all white women over 60 (the percentage is not so high for black women for they do not lose as many bone cells) have spinal compression fractures. The risk of hip fractures is at least 20 percent by 90 years of age. Almost 20 percent of the women die from hip fractures within three months of injury.

The medical literature discusses the fact that the loss of bone calcium is more rapid in women than in men. Both men and women reach their peak bone mass around age 35, after which a plateau is maintained or a downward slope begins. Spinal osteoporosis is four times more common in women than in men; hip fractures are more than twice as common in women. This loss of calcium from bone tissue starts with us around menopause, and scientists believe osteoporosis may be sex related, and therefore possibly estrogen related. Sex related indeed! And why not? What has given the embryo its bone structure? Mother's calcium. When I was a child, living among immigrant parents, it was said, "a tooth for a child." The implication was that mothers give a hard core part of their bodies to each infant.

In spite of the threatening promise by the estrogen pushers that estrogen replacement therapy (ERT) can "prevent," "relieve," "cure," and "correct" osteoporosis, it has been clearly stated by Dr. Heaney at the biggest conference on menopause and aging to date (May 1971) that "plainly estrogens have not proved successful in treatment of osteoporosis." Moreover, Drs. Chull S. Song and Paul Beck, hormone specialists, agree there "is no definitive evidence that osteoporosis and bone fractures are a direct consequence of estrogen lack." They also note that estrogen treatment may provide symptomatic relief (so will aspirin) and *perhaps* (italics mine) prevent progression.

Other problems, such as backaches, abdominal distentions, and more can also be associated with this bone condition, according to Dr. Louis V. Avioli of the Washington University School of Medicine who considers osteoporosis to be a major orthopedic problem. When discussing the possibility of prevention, the maintenance of healthy bones was stressed. Dr. Avioli believes day-to-day muscle pull (which is exercise) and plenty of calcium in the diet are of prime importance; so is getting enough vitamins, especially vitamin D. A high meat and low calcium intake may result in a calcium-phosphorus imbalance. Protein is required, says Dr. Avioli, but not entirely in animal form, and "maybe we should all be vegetarians." Also, alcohol consumption seems to be causally connected to progressive bone loss.

Dr. Leon Root, author of *Oh, My Aching Back,* says, "Women who have passed through menopause tend to lose the *collagen,* or protein matrix, of the bones in their spines. Thus the bones become thinner. This lessening of density shows up very clearly on X ray."

Many gerontologists emphasize that osteoporosis is not a natural part of aging. It is an abnormal condition. Some even claim that tooth loss in later years is not due to decay or plaque but to insufficient calcium. This idea certainly bears looking into by women who are menopausal now, because it is possible that many of us who have grown up in the Depression of the 1930s had inadequate diets, which would make the case for taking calcium now an extreme priority. One wonders why so much of the medical establishment is insistent on estrogen replacement for osteoporosis instead of calcium. The US Food and Nutrition Board stated that, "in many osteoporotic individuals, calcium supplements have induced calcium retention and improved bone density . . . and inadequate calcium intake over a period of years may contribute to the occurrence of this disease." Dr. Harold Rosenberg, former president of the International Academy of Preventive Medicine, notes that besides being crucial to our bones and teeth, calcium has many "other bodily functions as well. It is necessary for proper blood clotting, muscular activity, and the functioning of the nervous system. Calcium has powers as a nerve tranquilizer to overcome irritability and grouchiness, as a calming and sedative agent to help insomniacs sleep better, and as a painkiller." Bones aside, these other reasons are certainly convincing enough to take calcium every day.

Osteoporosis may be a cause of backache but there are many other causes too. Remember that to avoid a rounded back and backaches when you age, you must stand, walk, and sit straight. Don't hunch or lean forward, because this can put your back out of alignment.

Good carriage develops more elastic muscles in the shoulder area. Instead of carrying packages with one hand, it is better to use both hands and center the package, or else carry two bags instead of one heavy one. When doing anything—dishes, typing, reaching, bending—be conscious of your center and try to keep your spine straight. This is especially important because our muscles and tendons lose elasticity in the normal aging process.

The most common cause of back pain is from strain in the lumbar region or in a ligament. If your back aches, it can be from emotional strain, because tension can create very real cramps in the muscles. Fatigue and irritability also can affect your back. So can sitting for long periods without changing position or sitting in an uncomfortable chair. The best remedy, if the pain is not from a disease such as infection or arthritis, is exercise—especially walking—particularly if one normally sits for a large part of the day. High heels can give you backaches, too.

Another kind of back and shoulder ache that is common comes from what I call *hitting* and *wanting*. So often we want to strike out at people and situations that hurt us and we can't for a variety of reasons, economic, social, and personal. That hitting feeling or the desire to "punch you in the nose" must be released, and if you have no better way, do it at home alone. Punch into the air, or punch a pillow—it exercises those tense muscles. An opposite feeling is reaching for something you want. How often do we want things we don't dare reach for because of fear, being unwilling to take the risk, not wanting to get hurt or rejected again? We've got plenty of reasons *not* to reach out, but the *wanting* to seems to remain.

Extend your arms right now, while you're reading this, palms upward, and let the feelings flow. Close your eyes and reach out. I almost always cry when I do this and even if I don't get what I want, I do get release for it brings forth feelings of deep sadness. These are very simple exercises that move energy and bottled up feelings. They help some backaches.

Dr. Hans Kraus in his book *Backache* tells us back pain occurs most often for two reasons: underexercise and tension. He is adamant about preventing disease through exercise and stresses that organic disease causes only a small percentage of back pain.

When we become tense and do not release the tension, our muscles, heart, blood vessels, glands, and other organs become strained from wanting to act. If we don't act, we get back pain, a stiff neck, or a tension headache. This unreleased strain, if repeated often enough, says Dr. Kraus, develops into high blood pressure, ulcers, or heart disease.

HEADACHES

Should we talk about headaches at menopause? They're not unique to menopause. Two leading headache doctors from Harvard and Columbia universities tell us that headaches "may afflict as many as half the people of the world—thus, possibly some 100,000,000 Americans." Since we do get them, however, perhaps we should take a look.

A headache comes from nerves in the walls of the blood vessels that supply the brain and the head. When these blood vessels expand or shrink, and the nerves stretch or contact, we get a headache. Do women get more of them at menopause? I don't know, but it's been on every list I've ever seen. Like most of the symptoms, however, I don't think headaches are specifically connected with this time, except possibly those related to bloat or premenstrual tension. We have learned that the latter frequently becomes exaggerated at menopause, particularly when we are skipping periods for then we don't get the dramatic relief that comes with the menstrual flow.

Gay Gaer Luce suggests in *Body Time* that "monthly changes in water retention may account for headaches and blurred vision." At menopause, when we skip periods, we have many of the same symptoms experienced when we were completing our menstrual cycle. Many woman produce increased aldosterone prior to the time when they would normally start their flow. This causes salt retention and leads to retention of fluids in the body. Therefore, it seems reasonable that extra fluid may also be retained in the brain and is perhaps a cause for headaches at the time. If your blood vessels are swollen, because your whole body is, "blood coursing through swollen vessels causes a throbbing pain with every pulse beat. At the peak of headaches from swollen vessels, even the slightest movement brings sudden pain." In this case, stay away from monosodium glutamate (MSG) which is used in Chinese food, among other things, and avoid red wine, because it contains tyramine. Both of these make blood vessels expand and can cause headaches if you are particularly sensitive to their effects.

What is certain, however, is that about half of all headaches come from muscle tension. The muscles of the head and neck contract and stay contracted, creating a problem with the blood flow into your brain. The best thing to do for a headache is get to bed, or try to relax. Migraine sufferers may find that attacks at menopause are more frequent, but if they try to get in touch with the headache before it takes hold, and try to relax, it may not last as long.

BLOAT

Bloat, edema, or swelling is definitely a symptom of menopause. We are more used to hearing it called a premenstrual symptom, however, and little is written about bloat as a menopausal symptom. Like hot flashes, it doesn't happen to everyone, but it can be a nuisance and, at times, very uncomfortable. If bloat has been a premenstrual symptom of yours, and if you are dark skinned and large breasted, the chances of getting it around menopause are pretty good. It seems that tall, thin, light-complected women are not as prone to this kind of swelling and breast expansion.

In the new style medical thinking about menopause, which is partly a reaction against the old-fashioned one which labeled "menopausal" everything that happened to a woman from 45 to 55, the symptoms, other than the end of menstrual periods, have been reduced to two: hot flashes and dryness of the vagina. All women don't get either or both. Only about 50 percent get hot flashes, and most are usually mild. An estimated 20 percent have a problem with the thinning walls of the vagina after menopause. I firmly add bloat as a definable symptom. It has been my prime one, and I have interviewed many women who have experienced it, too. I believe it to be hormonal because sore, sensitive, or swollen breasts are the result of fluid retention and we know that when the estrogen level in the body rises, the breasts get fuller. When that level falls, the breasts soften and shrink.

Dr. Hans Selye, the stress specialist, informs us that stress, too, creates hormonal changes. Aldosterone is the corticosteroid hormone produced by the adrenals, whose task is regulating the water and salt content of the body. "This means," notes Dr. Katharina Dalton, a leading authority in the field of female cycles, "that excess aldosterone or deficient aldosterone-antagonist causes water retention." My guess is that when we feel bloated at menopause, aside from producing unopposed estrogen (we don't produce enough progesterone which acts as an antagonist to estrogen), we are also producing excess aldosterone or not enough antagonist to it, thereby causing an unbalance in our body chemistry.

There is a temptation, when we feel bloated, to think about taking diuretics, particularly because they are often prescribed. Dr. Dalton is cautious about them because "when diuretics are used to remove excess water in the body, they tend also to remove potassium and to leave the excess sodium" which is upsetting to our balance. Potassium depletion can be immediately corrected by eating a banana, orange, peach, apricot, dates, figs, prunes, or raisins.

Dr. William D. Snively, a distinguished authority in the field of body fluids, warns us not to use too much salt if we "tend to swell . . . during menopause." By limiting our salt intake, we will then avoid or lessen the waterlogging of our tissues. Another thing that helps is to take a long walk and build up a good stride. Walking stimulates all sorts of action in the body and it does help bloat. If you can't walk—inclement weather, perhaps, or you must work indoors—lie down and breathe deeply for a few minutes, then exercise, something mild like knee bends or touching your toes and stretching.

The women in the menopause workshops had many suggestions for foods which are natural diuretics instead of taking a drug: celery, parsley, watermelon, grapes, fresh pineapple, cantelope, asparagus, and cucumbers. If you have a juicer, you can consume more celery and cucumbers by drinking the juice. Add a carrot or two for taste. Stay away from carbohydrates and sugar, other than what exists naturally in fruit. The women also take large amounts of vitamin C to lose bloat, thousands of milligrams, as many as 5,000 a day. Dr. Linus Pauling takes 10,000 milligrams a day regularly, more if he feels something coming on.

It is possible for a woman whose tissues are waterlogged to gain as much as five pounds in a day and lose it the next. Dr. John M. Ellis, author of *The Doctor Who Looked at Hands,* strongly recommends pyridoxine (vitamin B_6) to remove fluids from the body and control bloat, edema, and swelling.

ACHES AND PAINS

Everybody has aches and pains, but that doesn't mean one has to run to a doctor every time they occur. In this book we have been stressing the benefits of being acquainted with our bodies, so we can know them better and respect them and love them as well. This takes being attuned to yourself and not living as though your body and mind are two separate entities.

Every little ache and pain is worth looking at because it is your body's way of telling you something. Listen. It is communicating a warning and telling you to "look here, where I hurt." The bravado that goes with ignoring these signals and warnings may cost you your life. Any illness is treated more easily before it gets a chance to take hold. I believe many would not take hold if given attention. A difficult idea for women in their menopause to grasp is the idea of giving in to yourself, giving in to your body. One of the best ways I know to do this is to give it plenty of rest. Last year, when I was 51, I found myself taking naps, something I can't remember ever having done. It was hard for me to give in to that idea but I knew it was important. I trust my body to know what it needs rather than my head. That I am entering a new cycle is a most reasonable idea, and a new cycle demands a new way of being. Something new is happening to my body, and I must respect that. The napping lasted for about ten months. Is tiredness menopausal? Maybe.

Dr. E. Vincent Askey, a past president of the American Medical Association, gave his opinion of self-help in *This Week* magazine a long time ago: "Home remedies always will have a place in the treatment of mankind's aches and pains. Physicians do not expect and do not desire that patients shall dash to the doctor with every minor discomfort, every trifling injury, every small ache and pain. It is sensible to care for such things by simple, safe home means."

There is developing, mostly on the West Coast of the United States, a New Medicine, sometimes known as "holistic health," whose diverse practitioners range from established medical professionals to psychic healers and feminist healers. The goal of this New Medicine is *positive wellness,* not just the absence of overt disease but *good health.*

The followers of this burgeoning health movement believe the causes of most illness are to be found in environment, life-style, and emotional-sensory balance. They argue that *all* disease is related to personality, to the way you handle your emotions. This idea has been carried further by a number of researchers who have independently arrived at what might be called a "cancer personality." They have observed that cancer patients tend to be rather rigid, self-sacrificing people who repress their feelings and hold onto resentments. More conventional researchers reject this thesis.

Prevention of illness, according to the New Medicine, lies not in yearly medical check-ups but in the transformation of your life so as not to abuse it. Dr. Phillip R. Lee, one of America's most distinguished health-care experts, suggested, "If all abuse of tobacco, alcohol, and automobiles could be magically erased with the snap of a finger," he said, "at least half of all hospital beds in this country would suddenly be empty." As for chronic diseases, practitioners of the New Medicine believe many are merely ameliorated by the Old Medicine and that long term healing may take place without the use of powerful drugs.

Illness is not necessarily bad, according to New Medicine practitioners, who see it as an imbalance in your life. In noncritical cases they prefer to let the malady run its course, allowing the body, mind, and spirit (the three aren't seen as separate) to achieve balance, perhaps at a level higher than that before the illness.

The ultimate responsibility for your health lies with you, not with your physician. This simple, radical shift of responsibility, and power, underlies every aspect of the New Medicine. The precise role of traditional medicine has not yet been defined. However, Dr. Leonard Duhl of the Health and Medical Sciences Program at Berkeley says, "Doctors haven't been trained for health, but somehow have been held responsible for it. That's not right! Health is the responsibility of the society. Doctors should be connected to holistic health, but shouldn't control it."

How much of your aches and pains can you control? Perhaps the limit is infinite.

WASTED LIFE BLUES

I've lived a life but nothin' I've gained
Each day I'm full of sorrow and pain
No one seems to care enough for poor me
*   to give me a word of sympathy.*
Oh, me! Oh, my! Wonder what will my end be?
Oh, me! Oh, my! Wonder what will become of
*   poor me?**

Bessie Smith

6
Blues Ain't Necessarily So

Bessie Smith, Empress of the Blues, sang about the way all women feel sometimes, young, old, and in-between. She was doing the same thing that I recommend in this book. Talk about what ails you. Give it space and let it show instead of trying to hide it and allowing it to get all stuck and tangled up inside you. Bessie sang instead of talking. That was her way, and a fine way it is indeed. By singing the blues she knew she would get rid of them.

The best way to handle the blues is to acknowledge them. Say to yourself, *I've got the blues.* Or whatever it is you call it: depressed, being down, anxious, irritable, out-of-sorts, sad, or lonely. My best medicine is to put a Bessie Smith or Dinah Washington or Billie Holiday record on and let them sing the blues for me. They moan and wail and whine and cry, and so do I. They give expression to my feelings but more than that, the act of sharing takes place too. I get strength and power from them and the music. Some of the old love lyrics are embarrassing, but I have learned to ignore those that are and concentrate on the sound and feeling. Try it. Maybe it'll work for you too.

Or call a close friend and tell that person you are hurting inside. It could be for any reason. Maybe you're not being acknowledged on your job or maybe a friend who was supposed to call didn't. The reason doesn't matter; your feeling does. A way *not* to feel helpless or impotent or powerless is to do something about it. Talking is doing something.

---

* From "Wasted Life Blues" by Bessie Smith. © 1929 Frank Music Corp., 1350 Avenue of the Americas, New York, NY 10019. © Renewed 1957 Frank Music Corp. All rights reserved. Used by permission.

I know how difficult it is. One does not want to be a "whiner," to call someone up to cry the blues. It's very hard to show oneself as being "needy." Besides, women have always been accused of being "cry babies," so in our maturity we sometimes try to bend over backward to be "strong and mature." That bending can kill you. True maturity is seeing each situation on its own merits and not stereotyping them as we have been stereotyped. No matter that everyone seems to dismiss us impatiently with "it's all in your head," or "you're imagining it." Of course it's in our imaginations and our heads. Where else could the blues be? We know that when we are unhappy it is for valid reasons. We have, after all, lived through enough pain for enough years to know it well. We are *not* making it up. We are trying to deal with it.

As middle-aged women we're low on the cultural totem pole, and we know it. Carol Nowack, an assistant professor of psychology at Wayne State University, presented a report of her study before the Midwestern Psychological Association in May 1976. She showed that all ages regard middle-aged women as the least attractive people, including middle-aged women themselves. Ms. Nowack found that "middle-aged women concerned about wrinkles and gray hairs class themselves as unattractive." And guess who the young college women considered to be the "most attractive" of any age group? You guessed it, middle-aged men.

For many women, one premenstrual symptom is feeling "fragile." At menopause the feeling intensifies and appears with or without a period. It is an uneasy feeling. Nothing is specifically wrong, and you're not incapacitated. But you're not walking on sure, firm ground either. Maybe after you've gone out you wonder if you turned off the stove? Or did you leave the lights on? Or did you really lock the door? You know you did— but you are just not sure. You go back to check, and you did what you were supposed to. Silly? No, it's not silly. It happens to us. Or maybe "fragility" makes you feel teary. This is not as strong as crying but, even when there is nothing provoking you, no one around, you just feel teary. It is the kind of thing we hesitate to mention, but when we do speak to each other about it, it is comforting to know other menopausal women feel this way too. When "fragility" becomes established as a symptom, it seems to have a structure. Not all women get it, but for the ones who do, it usually begins before the periods stop and continues to appear during what would be the premenstrual time even when periods are skipped. It is generally associated with sadness and loneliness, even though a woman may not be alone or normally feel sad.

When one is entering a major new cycle with a different body rhythm, it does not seem unreasonable to feel these variations, these new feelings. We have been living with one cycle for around 35 years. That whole host of messages traveling through our body fluids and nerves to our organs has been dispatched according to a regular time schedule. But now, as our rhythms change, not everything works in the same way. It's no wonder some of those messages and responses are a little confused. Our menstrual periods are related to the phases of the moon, and when we become irregular that long-time relationship between us and the cosmos is disturbed. So why shouldn't *we* be disturbed a little? The word *lunacy,* remember, comes from strange behavior at the full moon. We don't hide from these bigger connections or fear them. So just be patient with yourself as your complex system finds its own new harmony with the universe.

HEAL YOURSELF

If you feel fragile, that's the way you feel. There is nothing wrong with it. You will not fall apart. You are not failing anyone. But your body is telling your something. Your body is telling you to take care of yourself. It is giving you a warning. Listen. Go along with it, give in to it. Try to avoid stress, take it easy, get some extra rest, be good to yourself, be your own nurturer, your own self-healer. Women have always been healers. We have been called witches for brewing our herbs, and we have been burned at the stake for it. But this is a good time to connect with your historical past as a woman. Brew yourself some herbal tea of mint leaves. If you're at work and can't do that, drink a glass of water. It is one of the best neutralizers there is. "Healing occurs whenever energy is directed toward healing." To heal is to have power, and to get in touch with your own power will help you get over feeling fragile.

Dr. Phyllis Chesler, feminist psychotherapist, says in *Women and Madness,* "Women become 'depressed' long before menopausal chemistry becomes the standard explanation for the disease." She points out that U.S. national statistics and research studies show "a much higher female to male ratio of depression or manic-depression at all ages. Perhaps," she continues, "more women *do* get 'depressed' as they grow older—when their already limited opportunities for sexual, emotional, and intellectual growth decrease even further."

Our women's blues has baffled the healing establishment for a long time. When we read about the cruel and irrational attempts to "cure" us of our distemper, one wants to weep. We are still being given shock treatment and dangerous drugs. Our wombs, ovaries, and clitorises have been cut out. We have been banished to isolated huts, sometimes even banished in our own homes in great luxury and turned into invalids because of our blues. We have been starved and we have been force-fed, given vomitives and purgatives. Our heads have been shaved and we have been plunged into cold water and hot water. We have been whipped, beaten, and punished to make us obedient, to make us behave the way we are "supposed" to. Having the blues is not the way we are "supposed" to behave.

The cause of the blues, hormonal or cultural, seems not to matter. Everything that used to be lumped together as "nervous disorders" is now lumped together as "emotional problems." But "treatment" has long been aimed at the symptom. Barbara Ehrenreich and Deirdre English describe in *Complaints and Disorders* the ways women were "treated" in the nineteenth century: "Bleeding, violent purges, heavy doses of mercury-based drugs and even opium were standard therapeutic approaches." The unbelievable but common medical practice of bleeding by means of leeches is hair-raising. "In some cases leeches were even applied to the cervix despite the danger of their occasional loss in the uterus." This makes Lydia Pinkham's Little Pills sound like peaches and cream. (Women are still buying those pills, by the way, for menstrual tension and menopause.)

Feeling fragile, feeling blue, feeling depressed are emotions women experience around menopause, but that does not mean we are crazy or going mad. Some women concerned about menopause remember hearing as little girls about "a woman who went crazy" or "an Aunt Sarah who was a problem" during menopause, and this memory makes them worry for themselves.

Remember, though, that years ago the world of women was vastly different. Those Aunt Sarahs were usually "old maids," then a term synonymous with "failure." No wonder that poor Aunt Sarah went a little mad. Can anyone feel good about being a failure? A woman's "success" 40 years ago—and 30, 20, and even 10 years ago—was based on her being married. A drunkard, a gambler, a philanderer, or a wife-beater was at least a husband and that was socially more acceptable than no husband. Young women today have no idea what the social pressure was like on us to marry. Fortunately, the failed-old-maid idea is disappearing, along with the husband-at-all-costs syndrome and the stigma attached to divorce.

Women do not go mad at menopause from menopause. Women have had nervous breakdowns, but menopause was *never* the cause in any of the cases I know about; it was always harsh life circumstances that were too overwhelming to cope with.

When does depression become serious? Dr. Solomon H. Snyder explains in *Madness and the Brain*, "Everyone is depressed at one time or another. . . . Depression becomes a form of psychosis only when it is severe enough to interrupt a person's activities at work and at home."

Women who were depressed before menopause have a harder time during menopause, but if they make some changes, the nature of the depression changes also. A good example of this is Ingrid, 51: "I have always been a negative, depressed personality. I thought menopause would put me in a panic and a year ago it did, for a short period, until I decided I was damn sick of it. Sick of the things that were depressing me. So after 25 years of marriage I moved out. I'm not happy, but at least I'm not living on the bottom anymore."

The conspiracy to make us feel dissatisfied with ourselves is so totally ingrained in our culture and so thoroughly taken for granted that to begin to list the many ways our inadequacy is constantly thrust on us is over-whelming. But let's have a go at it:

You look at yourself in the morning and you look like you've slept all night, not like Ginger Rogers or Joan Crawford who awake with hair in place, make-up perfect and nightgown unrumpled. Go to the bathroom and there's a ring in your toilet bowl. Go into the kitchen and your floors are not waxed mirror-shiny. Put the coffee on and your pot's not sparkling clean. You thought you bought the right cleanser but maybe you skimped on the elbow grease. Thumb through the ladies' magazine you picked up in the supermarket because of an article that will tell you the secret of getting thin. None of the women pictured look like you. They're all thin, beautiful, and 25. Do only young women use sewing machines or scouring pads? Thumb some more. There's a pretty table setting. Think why doesn't your cake come out as gorgeous as the one in the picture? That cake was baked under the most expert conditions possible by professional bakers. The shiny gloss on the frosting could come from plastic spray or agar-agar in the icing.

I could go on, but you know the story. We don't measure up, all along the line. It is worse for menopausal women because we have had more years of this kind of intimidation. A cumulative effect develops and, one day, you yell out, *"Enough!"* That is called a menopausal outburst. It can be for any reason. Enough times making the dinner, enough times cleaning up after people, enough times going to the supermarket. Enough of the countless, repetitious, unthanked jobs, done without joy, often without acknowledg-ment, let alone reward.

The interesting thing about these outbursts is they do not come out of the blue, they are not "crazy." They come from a clear-cut buildup of feeling put upon. They are honest expressions of our reality, and we must learn to respect them rather than fear them. We are conditioned to behave in a certain manner so that when we blow up we shock ourselves as well as the people around us. But take a close look at the outbursts and you will find they are justified.

Rachel, 48, shared this experience: "I had to go to the bathroom. My 14-year-old daughter, Perry, was brushing her beautiful long blonde hair in front of the mirror. I asked her to step out; she continued brushing. I asked her again and I asked her a third time. She still continued to brush. In the foyer outside the bathroom I squatted and dropped a load of shit. Perry and her two sisters were shocked. They wondered if their mother was going crazy. I cannot tell you in what matter-of-fact way I did that. And of course I cleaned it up immediately. I was in group therapy at the time and couldn't wait to discuss it. Funny, I wasn't worried about it, but I was very interested in it for I had never done anything like that before. Luckily, the therapist was an older woman with children, and she was very reassuring. She said you had to go and you went. She also pointed out the difference between doing a thing once and doing it every time you're frustrated. Later, I talked about it with the kids and explained it."

Molly, 45, tells another: "It was one of those unexpected hot days in May. Work had been difficult—you know, one of those demanding days—and I had spring fever or something like that and could hardly stand the job. All the way home on the bus all I could think of was getting into my house, out of my sweaty clothes and having a nice cold can of beer. As I approached my door I heard loud rock and roll. I walked in and there were what seemed like hundreds, but I think it was about nine or ten, teenagers spread all over the place with empty bottles and cans and nowhere was there a can of beer for me. The refrigerator was empty. I could have cried. If I had only known I would have picked up some beer before I came in. All I could see in that room were long, sprawled legs. I could have killed my son Ralph. All I could say was, 'Out! Get out of here, every single one of you! Out! Out! Out!' I knew I wasn't crazy. I was only hot, exhausted, frustrated by a job where my boss, a younger man, was earning $100,000 a year and I was getting $145.00 a week as his assistant."

Rachel and Molly may be menopausal, but menopause was not the cause of their behavior. Women in their twenties don't have teenagers, so they are not provoked into these kinds of outbursts. I think the repetition of frustrations, the cumulative effect, makes the significant difference. Neither one of these women was crazy but each acted in what might be called a crazy way.

"Mini-menopause" is a phrase that is sometimes used to describe premenstrual tension. One might also say that menopausal tension is premenstrual tension enlarged, because similar things are taking place in our bodies, only more so. The mildest manifestation of this tension is feeling touchy, slightly irritable, nervous. This can move on up to cranky, and, in its extreme, a ready-for-a-fight feeling. Have you noticed, perhaps when you are watching television or a movie, you feel like crying at situations you normally would not respond to in that way? It is as though anything could make you cry and you're not even feeling sad. (By the way, when you feel this way, it's good to cry—it's a marvelous form of release.)

Chemical changes take place in the body and are the cause of these changes in our personality. Not enough is known about it because there has not been enough research done (money to explore our endocrine system is not as readily available as money to explore the moon because possession of our bodies is a *fait accompli* whereas the possession of the moon is still a struggle). Dr. Katharina Dalton tentatively presents an explanation which she calls a working hypothesis:

It is suggested that if, during the premenstruum the ovary produces insufficient progesterone for the requirements of the womb, some progesterone is taken from the other source, the adrenal glands, leaving them short for their production of corticosteroids [other hormones]. The balance of corticosteroids is temporarily upset and may result in water retention, imbalance of sodium and potassium, failure to control allergic reactions, alteration of the blood sugar level and lowered resistance to infection. All these mechanisms could account for the presence of the various premenstrual symptoms.

I believe that the same theory applies to the menopausal feelings. They too can be caused by a hormonal change in our bodies. Until the body adjusts to the change in progesterone production, until it gets used to the different chemical ratio, we experience these intensified blue feelings.

Adelle Davis looks at our blues from another angle: "The amount of calcium in a woman's blood parallels the activity of the ovaries; the blood calcium falls to such an extent during the week prior to menstruation that nervous tension, irritability, and perhaps mental depression result." Again, with us the condition becomes intensified. Ms. Davis continues: "During the menopause, the lack [diminished amount] of ovarian hormones causes severe calcium-deficiency symptoms to occur; at these times unusually large amounts of calcium should be obtained." (See also chapter 17, "Nutrition and Middle Age.")

All of this underlines the fact that where we are in our cycle is related to how we perceive ourselves, for when one is feeling confident and strong, the blues can't get a foothold. Knowing where your cycle is, by keeping a calendar record, puts you on guard, so that you know what is happening in your body, and this physical knowledge of your body will give you a better understanding of yourself.

Aside from the chemical changes, entering your menopause is a concrete sign of aging. This idea throws women into depressions more than any other. We know how the culture looks upon aging, and some women go into a slump, a down-in-the-dumps place, where those vague forties (which somehow imply the option that 47 can pass for 43) are starting to feel too close to 50. And when we think of middle age as being somewhere between 40 and 60, 50 is definitely middle age. And why is 50 so much more terrible (to some) than 40? There are many good reasons. If you've never had a child your possibility of having one is becoming increasingly slim. If you have had children and are vaguely thinking about maybe having another under "better" circumstances (someday when there's more love, or money, or time), that decision cannot be deferred until that someday. If you were waiting for the kids to grow up before doing "your thing," they're grown up now, you don't have that excuse anymore. That's pretty scary. If you want to go to school, or finish school, or get a degree for a better job, you have to do it now. The longer you put it off, the more difficult it will be to get a new job. And that's scary.

Years ago many women were depressed around menopause because there was so little reliable information about sex. Some women—afraid they would not be able to please their husbands, that they might develop a sexual inadequacy—worried themselves into a decline. I have never heard of a woman going into a depression because she was afraid her husband would not be able to please her. Factually, that would make more sense.

Many men between the ages of 45 and 55 are at their highest points in their careers. They are occupied but their wives are excluded. Without the distractions of taking care of the children, many women feel ignored by their husbands. I have heard this complaint frequently. Along with this there may be the anxiety that he, in his success, may want a younger, more attractive woman. Menopausal women with this fear are not being paranoid. It happens.

Some women who have younger lovers are concerned about telling them about menopause. It seems to be very difficult, particularly if the man is much younger, in his early thirties. I was surprised to come across this problem as often as I did. Lucinda, 51, didn't know "what to do if I ever got a hot flash in front of him. What would I say? I'd have to tell him." Violet, 49, whose friend was living with her, was becoming embarrassed about not having menstrual periods. "He must notice it," she said with grave concern. Vinnie, 48, was sure "I'm not ovulating and it's such a drag to keep using the diaphragm, but I'm afraid not to, because then he'll know I'm an old lady."

Melinda, 58, who had long been finished with her menopause, remembered that relationships with your husband and children are changing at that time. "When the youngsters were small there was this body contact with the kids that was very satisfying. You couldn't hold them and comfort them when they were bigger, and that I missed. I wanted to transfer that to my husband, but he was carrying his heaviest load at work then and wasn't interested."

When children grow up and leave home, it is only reasonable that mothers miss them. Especially when those mothers have spent full time caring for them and their husbands and the house. I do not like the terms used to describe this condition: empty-nest blues, or empty-nest syndrome. The concept of a woman as a hen on a nest is offensive to me.

It used to be thought that women became sad when they realized they could no longer bear children. This male-oriented Freudian concept was laid down by Dr. Helene Deutsch, surely before she was in her menopause. Would any woman in her menopause speak this way? "Woman has ended her existence as bearer of a new future, and has reached her natural end—partial death—as a servant of the species." This is outrageous, and the realization that it was taken seriously makes it worse. Dr. Deutsch had no insight at all into this phenomenon. The depression of the menopausal woman was not coming from wanting more babies but from wanting more life for herself; not more diapers to change but regret for the waste, for the life not lived, for the time spent hoping for love and not receiving it.

Women with not enough to do because their children have grown and gone are people without jobs. The family has been their occupation for 20 or 25 years. Unlike a baker or a butcher, these women cannot easily find another job—they can't go find another family to raise and wouldn't want to. Remember, most women in their late forties and early fifties today were "Homemakers" with a capital H. Once World War II ended, women were not encouraged to work outside the home. If anything, it was discouraged. Rosie the Riveter was sent home.

When this Homemaker takes a typing test for a job today, her experience of 25 years as wife, mother, and nurturer is no help to her at all. It is hard to face a snippy personnel interviewer who says "But what can you do?" It is as though there was no value in the life she has lived. A kind of paralysis of will sets in when a woman thinks "How can I compete?" (I remember getting my hand on the doorknob to go out to look for a job but being unable to turn it.) When society looks upon us as useless and is reluctant to hire us, where do women gain strength and confidence to face new challenges? Where does our sense of self-esteem, our sense of worth come from? When, as it too often occurs, a self-image is based on how others treat us, menopausal women become depressed.

Finances can be a cause for depression around this time. Parents of college-age children are anxious about tuition increases. And, if it's paid, will the kid drop out? Single women start worrying about retirement plans. Many working women worry about being fired from those companies known to be miserly with retirement benefits.

Because of the complex changes in our bodies and minds, and in the way our culture treats us at menopause, it's small wonder we get depressed. On top of it all, the existential question comes up: How will I spend the rest of my life? As it has been spent? Nothing more? We know by now, no matter how much we may have been valued (if we have been) as daughters, mothers, wives, or lovers, it has always been the male who has been thought of as more valuable on human and spiritual grounds. When you become introspective this cannot help but create a deep sadness and give you a case of the blues. We have known subliminally for a long time that, as Dr. Phyllis Chesler says, "women are in a continual state of mourning—for what they never had—or had too briefly, and for what they can't have in the present, be it Prince Charming or direct worldly power." She argues that women are called crazy or mad if they do not conform to the male chauvinist ideal of a woman, that is, a woman "must be" passive, doll-like, a good housekeeper. She "must be" without intellectual presumptions but smart enough to acknowledge his. She "must be" no threat whatsoever to the dominant position of men in our culture. To deviate from this stereotype is to be crazy.

Thomas Szasz, an eminent psychiatrist who has written extensively about madness, says, "Society labels as crazy anyone with deviant behavior in so arbitrary a fashion that the categories of mental illness become nothing but semantic artifices for maintaining the social order."

The British psychiatrist R. D. Laing questions the culture too, and he speculates about the possibility that conditions of life in our time may be more "mad" than the people accused of being mad. He claims, from his clinical observations, that people can go mad and be reborn: "Madness need not be all breakdown. It may also be breakthrough. It is potentially liberation and renewal as well as enslavement and existential death."

The question, then, is, are we crazy when we reevaluate our lives around menopause and find, as Lolly Hirsch, publisher of *The Monthly Extract*, claims, "We have been had."

VALUE YOURSELF

What do we do then at menopause? We can consciously create a shift in values, at least for ourselves. This is where the adventure comes in: you begin to value yourself as important, even though the culture doesn't. Many women have done this. *Woman's Prime of Life*, written in the 1930s by a London doctor, Isabel Hutton, has some interesting advice: "The climacteric is the time for women to review their daily lives and consider whether they should alter them in any way. Let them not regret lost opportunities, for alas, too much time is wasted thus, and too many tears are shed for the days that are gone." Her style has an old-fashioned quality but it's "right on." She continues, "Let no woman repine, but go forward and begin her own development."

Another doctor, Madeline Gray, updates the same idea in her chapter, "You Won't Lose Your Mind," from her book *Changing Years*, which she wrote just before the dark 1950s set in: "Above all, we can learn to love ourselves; never underrate ourselves. Be good to ourselves; don't keep forever looking back on the supposed 'sins' we committed far in the distant past." She cautions us against feeling guilty when we look back: "guilt for some reason wells up especially strong around the time of the menopause, and we sometimes magnify it into something twice as big as we should."

These women were trying to confront menopause and middle age and the blues that is built in to them. Clara Thompson, the Interpersonal Relations psychoanalyst of the Washington School, looks from another view: "Anything which tends to limit a person's free development tends to make them rigid and prematurely old." She sees middle-age depression as a state of mind that can take place at any age. "A person tends to remain young if [s]he has a future, that is, if [s]he can continue to grow and develop." After Ms. Thompson acknowledges the physical changes, she considers them minor compared with "the serious emotional upsets of the middle years." These, she says, "are due, not primarily to physical conditions per se, but to the awareness more or less consciously of the unlived life." Ah, there we have it. How many of us have not thought, *If only I had done (whatever), my life would be so different,* and wept.

Eda LeShan, a self-actualized woman writing in the 1970s on an upbeat note, sees the tensions of menopause as "a time for finding *one's own* truths at last, and thereby to become free to discover one's real identity." She sees it as the time of our greatest opportunity: "Because we have such a sensitized awareness of how precious time is, we can appreciate the urgency and importance of our quest, for if we don't take this opportunity—if we don't really search for ourselves, now—we may never do it." She sounds like my sister: "The wonderful opportunity of middle age is that once and for all, we can begin, with the wisdom and maturity and perspective of our experiences in living, the tough job of sorting out whom we want to please—and in this quest, we discover that until we learn to please ourselves, free of the 'shoulds,' we can give little genuine pleasure to anybody else."

These mature women are telling us to grow and develop, but it isn't easy after we have spent so many years putting the house in order, the children in order—we begin to feel guilty about putting ourselves in order. It is hard to make that transition from taking care of others to taking care of oneself. I try, but sometimes I feel self-indulgent and narcissistic. My monthly ritual bath, replacement for my monthly cycle, takes a lot of time. I have to brew the herbs and oil my body before lying in the tub, and then I take more time for release after all that sensualness. I feel less guilty each time, and maybe by next year I won't feel guilty at all. If I went through those preparations to give a lover a bath or as preparation for a meeting with a lover, guilt wouldn't enter the picture. But taking time "just" for myself, that's hard. I'm still learning about my own importance.

When you become important to yourself you can more easily take control of your life. You can go from feeling helpless to taking command. But wanting to be in control is not enough. You must be able to imagine yourself in the role. The act of independence must be credible. An independent person in control is not a good candidate for depression.

A good way to begin is with a fantasy. How will I behave in a situation that I want to be in? Call it a game if you like, but this is no children's game; this is very grown-up and is a part of the struggle of getting up from under. There are two goals to this fantasy. The first is creativity—the conception, to conceive of being in another job, life-style, and so forth, is a creative thought. The second is attainability—it is crucial that the idea becomes for you an imaginable act, one that *could* be accomplished. Get familiar with the idea. Get comfortable with it so that it loses its strangeness. Your fantasy must be not only conceivable but functional as well.

The best way to get on with it is to position yourself with women you can identify with but who appear to be more in control of their lives than you are. By being in their company your ideas for yourself can take on a reality sooner, since they have done it. You will be astonished to find out they are no different from you. And when they take your ideas seriously, you will too.

One thing *not* to do when you have the blues is take tranquilizers. That may be the first thing your doctor will recommend. Clara, 54, felt trapped by them. Her doctor had been prescribing them for ten years, but she felt they were doing her harm and "keeping me dopey. But I'm afraid to stop taking them," she said. "I'm afraid I'll fall apart." Ida, 57, asked, "Have you considered going to another doctor?" Clara looked astonished. "No," she replied. This question was asked with sympathetic concern. Clara did go to another doctor, and she made other changes too. Her being "stuck" with the doctor was symptomatic of her feeling "stuck" in other areas of her life.

In the United States, the medical profession has recommended Valium and Librium, the two most popular tranquilizers, to the tune of more than $2 billion to date. Tranquilizers are the most commercially successful prescription drugs ever made and are largely responsible for making Hoffmann-La Roche Inc. what *Fortune* magazine calls "one of the most profitable enterprises on earth." Don't buy those across-the-counter tension relievers, either. Some $58 million was spent on them in 1975 alone, according to *Newsweek*. However, a panel of experts working for the US Food and Drug Administration analyzed the ingredients of these spurious sedatives and reported in December 1975: "Of the 23 major active ingredients of the pills and capsules, only the stimulant caffeine could be considered both fully safe [sic] and effective." The nighttime "aids" they studied were Nytol, Excedrin P.M., and Sominex; the daytime sedatives, Compoz, Miles Nervine, and Quiet World, as well as the stimulants No Doz and Energets. The experts were concerned about the daytime tension relievers because they could cause drowsiness and impaired coordination. They also were critical of claims that the drugs produce a "relaxed feeling" or "gently soothe away the tension."

Drugs are very important to the U.S. culture. They are especially important in keeping menopausal women quiet and out of sight. One of the medical profession's functions, it seems, is keeping this society going as it is. Do you know what would happen if all the women between 40 and 55 started making demands? My adrenaline begins to burst forth at the excitement of the idea.

Anxiety during menopause is a difficult symptom to figure out. Every age group suffers from it, for it has become an integral complication of living in modern society. The symptoms of anxiety—vague uneasiness, irritability, tension, slight nausea, shortness of breath, and palpitations—get in the way of the sense of well-being for which we are striving. To relieve these symptoms, as well as the general free-floating kind of anxiety without clear-cut symptoms, many menopausal women take tranquilizers or mood-altering drugs. Yes, they are effective in changing one's feelings, and, because they are easy to get, most women think they are harmless. They aren't. It would be bad enough if their only disadvantage were that they merely help one manage rather than master difficulties. However, like alcohol, they also are central nervous system depressants and muscle relaxants, and have "been associated with a battery of unwanted side effects [such as] fatigue, drowsiness, and ataxia (staggering gait). It is also suspected that Valium can produce lower blood pressure, changes in sexual drive, nausea, slurred speech, headache, blurred vision, tremor, vertigo, confusion, apathy, hallucinations, skin rashes, and constipation. Valium can elicit emotional reactions which researchers speculate are normally 'anxiety bound'—among them irritability, overexcitement, irrational antisocial behavior, hostility, even rage." These symptoms are frequently blamed on menopause, but often they can be traced to tranquilizers. Tranquilizers, along with the tension relievers, are really poor pacifiers. They rob you of the ability to look at what is really happening to you and why. Even if you don't take drugs, depression alone produces changes in the body which in turn causes more symptoms. It gets to be a vicious cycle.

DE-FEAR YOURSELF

I know how hard it is to turn down that "pacifier" when you are feeling rotten, but the self-healer in you wants to help. She wants you to function at your best. Give her a chance. Give her some space so she can try. I am not being mystical, I am being realistic. I am suggesting that you can uncover a power you have within you, a power with a deeper knowledge of your body and feeling. It is a power that can *de-fear* you, *de-terrorize* any sense of disaster such as going mad or dying. For example, when the anxiety builds, it may or may not be accompanied by a headache. It feels as if you are going out of your mind into a nether world of unreality. But you don't need to run for help from a pill. Go along with the feelings; do not try to deny them. Even if you check them out and find that you're really scared or angry, let them flow, for to negate them is to suppress them, and those feelings are as much a part of us as are others. By allowing "uncomfortable" feelings their full range, you are experiencing a fuller range of yourself. That is a way to get in touch with yourself. What we are doing is accepting ourselves in our various dimensions instead of trying to erase those deep dark places by keeping ourselves falsely tranquil or sedated in a gray area of nonfeeling. It is a way to learn not to be afraid of yourself and your feelings. And it works to help you accept yourself more, all your bits and pieces, and eventually to like, even love, yourself.

Your body is giving you signals. This means your mind is also, for it affects the complex machine that is your body. Do not dwell on what is making you feel this way—just respect its demand for quiet. Try to empty your mind and feel only your body. It is very difficult to do, and if you can't manage it, then do the next best thing: put pleasant thoughts in your mind. Try to remember good experiences and try to make up fantasies of joy. Project yourself into the most happy situations you can imagine. Go into detail: what are you wearing, what is the weather like, who is with you, rehearse the dialogue. This is not escapism, this is healing yourself. If you continue to think only of the problems that put you in this state you'll be hurting your body. This respite will help you become stronger and you will better be able to deal with your problems. You will not have run from yourself, and that is a step in accepting yourself.

We are revolutionizing our "psycho-chemistry" and actually allowing changes in our bodily secretions as well as in our lives by allowing ourselves to *feel* or to plumb our own depths. We are not courting death or pain, but becoming more familiar with it and thus not fearing it so much. This is all part of the new discipline to *know your body* to the fullest. Tranquilizers, sedatives, alcohol, even aspirin, dull the pain. When I talk about accepting the pain, I am not suggesting you take a masochistic "trip." (We know only too well where that leads.) I am asking you to negate your previous security devices. When you do, you are acting in a revolutionary manner. You are trusting yourself to take care of yourself. You will not lose yourself in the pain, rather the reverse. You can transform yourself so that you will be able to transform the world around you to serve you better.

Once you begin trusting yourself you will find that underlying your pain or fear you have a sense of wholeness. That female survival quality, based on our greater stamina, will see you through. The self-destructive part of you may make your valiant effort seem foolish for a moment. But you really can get acquainted with your own healing force, become intimate with it, and use it. If, when that moment of doubt or pain comes, you have made your promise to your healing self, you will not need to take a drug.

This then becomes a *significant experience.* You have altered your life, and by changing the way you respond to yourself you are changing power as it relates to you. You are functioning out of strength, out of being in control, rather than from weakness. You can feel yourself fully; you won't want a pill to muddle your feelings. What you have done is face death in life and then restructured your life with new awareness. This is in the true tradition of heroism. And where should we begin, if not with ourselves?

When our bodies are under the stress of anxiety or depression, hormones from the adrenal glands become activated to supply energy for this sustained tension. These hormones help mobilize the brain, influence nerve transmission, and release extra blood sugar. All this mobilization also seems to create a body fluid imbalance and may even alter our daily rhythm of excreting water and minerals. Our total nervous system is involved in this activity. Bed rest helps slow down some of these processes, because the physical activity of your body is greatly reduced and there is a general deconditioning. By not taxing your body's metabolism it can begin to straighten itself out.

NURTURE YOURSELF

During these sensitive blues periods, food is important. Our bodies are experiencing new stresses, and if we ever needed to be strong and healthy it's now. Man-refined sugar robs you of vitamins from the other foods you eat, and constant intake of caffeine can turn you into a nervous wreck and ruin your whole metabolic process. The B vitamins are important for our nervous system's proper functioning. Adelle Davis tells us that "cumulative menstrual losses, pregnancies, and the long use of deficient diets cause anemia to be prevalent in women at and after the menopause. Besides causing needless fatigue, mental confusion, and depression, anemia can bring about such forgetfulness that these women often become convinced they are losing their minds." Ms. Davis has also called calcium a "natural tranquilizer." Unquestionably, natural supplements such as calcium will not pollute your body like Valium. Are you getting enough calcium? Gay Gaer Luce, in her book *Body Time,* suggests calcium may play an indirect role in our blues:

> Like sodium and potassium, calcium has a profound influence upon the functioning of the nervous system, since it appears to be essential in the transmission of nerve messages. Calcium deficiencies are known to affect the parathyroid and thyroid glands, and thus indirectly influence the entire endocrine system. When people have had too little free calcium they have shown symptoms like those known as "anxiety neurosis."

It would seem sensible if some of those doctors who patronize us with "it's all in the head" were to check our potassium levels. Many alert physicians believe irritability and depression can be the result of an imbalance of sodium and potassium in the body fluids. It is also one of the reasons we must watch our salt intake, because salt (sodium) causes water retention. Potassium is essential to keep our nerves functioning normally. However, "emotional, mental, or physical stress can cause excessive potassium loss," says Dr. William D. Snively, a distinguished authority on body fluids. (Potassium can be very quickly replaced in the body by eating an orange or a banana.) Depression can also be caused by too much fluid around the brain, another reason to watch salt. (If you want to know how your body is doing, remember to ask your doctor the results of any and all laboratory tests performed on you.)

Reducing diets without supplements can also cause irritability. Our brain, like the rest of our body, needs nourishment, too. Without the proper kind there are subtle behavioral changes. Carlton Fredericks, in discussing victims of dietary deficiencies, says, "It is as though the emotional brain grows hysterical when its fuel supply is inadequate or cannot, for lack of vitamins, be properly utilized." He further describes the condition as ranging "from a vague feeling of uneasiness and apprehension to severe and clear-cut attacks of unjustified anxiety, with marked heart and breathing symptoms that lead, understandably, to fear of impending death. . . . They are melancholy without knowing why and cry without cause.''

I have a feeling that the nonnutritive sweeteners may be related to depression, too. I don't know of any scientific evidence to support this idea, but I was a heavy user, over a long period of years, of chemical sweeteners in coffee, tea, and soft drinks, as well as in cooking. My reasoning was that man-refined sugar is bad—besides, the sweeteners had no calories. It was a false economy of calories, because since I stopped using chemical sweeteners I feel much better. They do not exist in nature and are produced in a laboratory, which makes me wonder if anyone really knows how the body handles them. Since honey is sweeter than sugar, you use less, and it has only around 20 calories a teaspoonful. I also have an idea about honey and the blues which I can't substantiate either but it feels "right" and works for me. When I feel sour, I take a teaspoon of honey in something to feel sweet. I know it can't hurt.

Maybe our symptoms are not menopausal at all, but dietary.

I am hoarding anger
and stuffing it into pockets of discontent.
I once thought that this kind of anger
would flare up and burn the innocent—
my children. I know now the innocent
is me. I have slid back on this whole
difficult business of expressing anger.
Youth has not cornered the market
on crises of identity.
Ethel Seldin-Schwartz

7
Let Loose Anger—
Learn to Love Yourself

The quotation above comes from a woman's diary. She is 45 years old and has become her own true friend through writing in her journal. It appeared in a story in diary form by Ethel Seldin-Schwartz in *Ms. Magazine*. The story is based on the experiences and feelings of several women and expresses poetically what many of us have done.

We cannot be women aged 40 years old or over in the culture of twentieth-century America without experiencing anger on a constant basis. How do we deal with it? What do we do with it? Where do we put it? We must come to some resolution of these questions in order to survive, for we accept the medical and psychoanalytical idea that suppressed anger becomes something else—physical or mental illness.

We have not been taught to express anger. It embarrasses everyone around us. Clear-cut constructs exist so that we do not express it, so that we remain in the realm of being "civilized"—rather than making known our feelings and becoming socially unacceptable—which leaves everyone comfortable. Everyone but us, that is.

A relationship exists between normality and the various modes of madness. Expressing anger is frequently looked upon as on the way to going mad, behaving like a madwoman. No one wants us to go mad, because if we do, too many people around us will feel like failures.

Growing up in a family and being related to one as daughter and/or sister, we have conformed to what is expected from us; thus our "primary socialization" is deep-rooted. Our "secondary socialization" to establish the extrafamilial society was easily accomplished through school and job.

By giving the appearance of conforming, i.e., by not showing our anger, we have in a sense given up the chance not to conform. By that I mean, the price was so high, we did in fact conform to avoid confrontation.

Our profile is a layering of oppression, repression, and suppression. Oppression is the most obvious and has been spelled out clearly by others. With repression, however, a secondary awareness comes into action so that we become particularly aware of our oppression and, as a consequence, we repress actions, even thoughts, that may endanger our relationships. We have learned from everyone around us, by their examples and their judgments, clearly when to repress even the most primal fears. For example, if, when we were younger, our menstrual period did not conform to 28 days, there must be something wrong with us, we thought. That there is something wrong with the world's telling us 28 days is a woman's cycle would not have occurred to us. With suppression, a different kind of awareness comes into effect so that we do not even allow the first awareness of oppression to emerge. Don't you remember the 1950s as a young woman, or young mother? We were dulled into our roles, so we didn't make waves. We submitted.

"Being a woman" meant never to allow the child in oneself to show. Thus one pretended she didn't exist, which wiped out neatly those feelings of helplessness, fear, or exuberance. Instead we acted strong, giving emotional support to the husband or boss or children or aging parent. As Susan Brownmiller has articulately spelled out in *Against Our Will*, "being a woman" has meant being a man's property, for his use, regardless of job or career. Women have had to fit in jobs or careers, but our main place was the home.

Now that we are in our menopause, many of us are trying to rid ourselves of these complex constructs like repression, for we are learning that life must be more than surviving, more than existing. Life becomes for us, we hope, a matter of being. Being ourselves in relation to our potential as individual human beings means we cannot be the same conforming women. We do not want lives of seeking ways to fill in time. There is not enough time for all the wonderful things to learn and do. We must, therefore, unequivocally speak to the points that create anger in us. Our structured roles have acted too long as self-policing devices that rob us of our differences, our originality, our vision.

We each took a turn, during the workshops, to talk about "what makes us angry and what do we do about it." The hardest areas, those that evoked the most consternation in the women, were at work on the job, and speaking to husbands or lovers who "cut-off," who didn't want to hear the bitching. The fear is of losing the job or the mate; yet many women expressed outright hate, along with the anger, and freely used name-calling in describing the people who were making them angry. They expressed the wish to leave those situations. Many felt they had been "stuck" for years.

The feeling was one of being humiliated on a day-to-day basis, of not being regarded fully, of being taken for granted. These emotions came out over and over.

It is not unusual to feel one way and act another. In fact, it has been most common in this culture for women to act contrary to their feelings. That the women were in situations that were making them angry, yet remained in them, is not surprising. There is a big difference between speaking and acting, but speaking is a step. They are way ahead of the women who claim everything is fine but who in the privacy of their own bedrooms suffer migraines and insomnia.

ANGER AIRED

The following are statements chosen to illustrate the different places women find themselves in, in relation to their anger. Some women have been "working on it," while others are only beginning to get acquainted with their anger.

Linda, 48: I'm very careful about anger because it frightens me. When I allow myself, I fantasize doing terrible things. I fantasize blowing up buildings, tearing men apart, castrating the ones who have hurt me. I fantasize my anger because I'm afraid to let it escape, so I turn a lot of it against myself.

Tillie, 50: When I became 50, it was a looking back: why didn't I do this, why didn't I do that? What did I do for the last 10 years? The anger builds up. I try to deal with it. I'm in therapy.

Sally, 46: Usually I get angry when I can't see my way out of a situation.

Liz, 57: For a long time I never knew how I felt about everything because I didn't allow myself to know. I didn't allow myself to feel. I was angry, I was so angry and didn't have anything to do about it, so I became depressed. I'm feeling better because I can say some things now that I wasn't able to say before. I can allow myself to feel.

Ruby, 53: I can't stand it when men call me dear, especially in business, and I am asking them not to. It's hard though. You know I can't be as free at my job as I'd like to be, and when I can't come out with it plainly I have noticed I articulate more carefully and use that as a kind of one-upmanship.

Dorothy, 45: Rather than hold back my anger and feel guilty about it, I'm trying to express it. I'm trying to work out ways and means. What's wrong with going up to someone and saying, "You're making me angry," instead of smiling and seething inside.

Clare, 50: I would like to find ways of directing my anger at the circumstances that brought me here—age 50, powerless, moneyless—rather than at me, saying to myself, you're a fool, it's your fault. The things that have happened to me have happened to millions of women.

Olive, 47: I was living alone with my daughter and I couldn't take it out on the kid. This unexpressed anger has been compounded. I'm not dealing with it, but I'm aware of it.

Emily, 50: My mother never got angry. I never saw anger, so I don't know how to direct it. I was ashamed of it. It's panicky and makes for terrible anxiety. This age thing—when the number 50 hit me I was really surprised. This damned number. I was furious.

Irma, 43: My life situation gave me no place to put the anger. There was no legitimate way to release it.

Ida, 55: When somebody makes me angry now, I just tell them plain and straight.

Grace, 54: One of the ways I try to deal with my anger, and I work very hard at it, is never to let a situation escape. I don't care how small it is. In New York delicatessen counters we are addressed: "Yes, young lady?" It drives me up the wall. I say to the clerk, "I'm not a young lady, I'm a grandmother. Please don't say that to me." It takes a lot of energy, I'll admit.

Constance, 44: I wish I'd have lost my temper more.

Lorraine, 59: I was angry and didn't have anything I could do about it so I developed an ulcer.

Sarah, 50: My boss used to call me on the intercom. I'd go up in that damned elevator and be trembling. What did I do wrong? What do I have to answer for? I don't tremble anymore. Once I became 50 and realized two-thirds of my life is over, I just decided nobody's gonna make me tremble anymore. I don't care who it is.

Emma, 62: I used to get so mad, but I don't pay attention any more. It goes off me like water off a duck's back. Let them get sick, not me.

Sadie, 51: I just feel that I don't care about being nice anymore. I've been that for too long and it hasn't paid off. Anyone who can trigger anger in me, where I feel I'm not getting the respect for a mature, intelligent, authoritative woman that I feel that I am, will hear from me. I come from the authority of my experience and that is valuable. I'm not going to be a little helpless mumbler. I've made that decision. There's nobody I'm going to kowtow to, it doesn't matter what the circumstances. I am learning that I have an authority. Nobody is going to give me authority, I have to take it. I have to seize it.

Mildred, 63: I used to wait when I was angry. Wait for the right time, when the other person was in a good mood, you know, not to create tension. It's turned me into an invalid. I'm always sick with one thing or another.

Babette, 52: When I married my husband I thought we were equals. But when I got mad and began yelling he said I sounded like a fish wife.

That shut me up and gave me a spastic colon. It took me 13 years but when I got rid of him I got rid of the spasms, too.

Eleanor, 42: The thing that made me the most angry in my life was when my husband would talk about an idea of mine as though it was his own, right in front of me. I didn't know what to do about it, I became silent in company, like a dummy. He did the talking for both of us. I'm not a dummy anymore. No one will ever do that to me again.

Our anger also comes from the way the culture misperceives us. The communications industry presents a misinformed image of the menopausal woman. They tell us we are no longer desirable. That message is unmistakable—it comes at us a hundred times a day. Yet, in our feelings, we don't feel undesirable; in fact, quite the contrary. We feel we are better suited, more equipped to handle situations, including love affairs, but our opportunities are more limited than they ever were before. We are feeling sexually vigorous while the men of our age are more often not. This presents problems. There is a biological difference in the sexual rhythms and energy between men at 45 and 50 and women at that age. The culture frowns on women having younger lovers but does not frown on men doing that. Angry-making? Yes, indeed!

According to the rules, we are not "supposed" to be having the feelings of anger we are experiencing. When this was kept hidden and unspoken, women suffered more. Today, however, the women are talking to each other about these feelings and trying to figure out ways to behave so that they will not have to suppress them when they emerge. We haven't had enough studies. Why haven't women been asked what they are feeling? All kinds of theories, ungrounded in fact, have become part of an academic structure which has worked to the detriment of middle-aged women. A misconception, which is more a superstition, has been to connect women's child-bearing ability with her sexuality.

It makes us angry when mature women of accomplishment are not treated with the same respect paid to men, as serious, successful people. When Golda Meir and Bella Abzug are asked about chicken soup instead of the affairs of state I want to punch the interviewer in the nose. Would Moshe Dayan or Jacob Javits be asked about cooking? Equally offensive is the ultimate patronizing accolade, "She thinks like a man."

The best-known menopausal woman in the United States today is television's Edith Bunker, a degrading example who is called "dingbat." This is a person who is ordered to "sit" like a dog—and she does. When the program "Maude" appeared, we were given a boost because an attractive, outspoken menopausal woman was chosen for the role. At least we were not being represented as dowdy, but Maude is a fraud because even though she openly likes sex and is assertive, she is just as locked in to the woman's role as is Edith Bunker—the man always ends up on top. Mary Hartman's mother, aged 50, is portrayed as a confused, foolish middle-aged woman who is not to be taken seriously.

The popular literature of our time is no better. Among Portnoy's complaints was the fact that his mother menstruated and used Kotex. She probably was in her menopause and had an irregular period because no Yiddisha Mama would commit the unforgivable sin of being caught without a napkin: "And once I saw her menstrual blood . . . saw it shining darkly up at me from the worn linoleum in front of the kitchen sink. Just two red drops over a quarter of a century ago, but they glow still in that icon of her that hangs, perpetually illuminated, in my Modern Museum of Gripes and Grievances (along with the box of Kotex . . .)."

I do not mean to flatter David Reuben's *Everything You Always Wanted to Know About Sex* by calling it literature. I mention it only because his book has sold so many copies (the one I read was a 21st printing in hard cover, and who knows how many editions appeared in paperback) and I yell out in rage at the number of people who read his description of the menopausal woman.

> As the estrogen is shut off, a woman comes as close as she can to being a man. Increased facial hair, deepened voice, obesity, and the decline of breasts and female genitalia [as a psychiatrist, not a gynecologist, I wonder how many he's seen] all contribute to a masculine appearance. Coarsened features, enlargement of the clitoris, and gradual baldness complete the picture. Not really a man but no longer a functional woman, these individuals live in a world of intersex . . . sex no longer interests them. [sic]

> To many women the menopause marks the end of their useful life. They see it as the onset of old age, the beginning of the end. They may be right. Having outlived their ovaries, they may have outlived their usefulness as human beings. The remaining years may be just marking time until they follow their glands into oblivion.

Can you imagine how angry vital, intelligent women in their menopause feel about such a depiction of them, such nonsense? Surely the misogynist who wrote it could not be born of a woman? Was Reuben birthed by Robert Wilson? I wonder where he has seen these masculine-looking women with enlarged clitorises? I worry about the women who read that and became afraid. I have been asked if it's true, "Do we become neuters?"

Why are we looked upon as ready for the garbage heap instead of looked upon as wise older women as the people in Turkey, the Ashanti in Africa, the Tiwi of Australia, and the Magars of Nepal look upon their post-menopausal women? Prejudiced, uninformed men have informed the culture in this way. The input is so negative, so loaded against us, that the feedback affects women's image of themselves. If your world doesn't think much of you, how can you yourself?

We want to think well of ourselves so that we can enjoy our menopause instead of hating it and enjoy our aging instead of fearing it. When I talk about loving yourself and loving your menopause, it is to overtip the scale for the affirmative to counter the negative where it has so long been. If it seems outrageous, it is, because it comes out of rage at how menopause has been viewed. My unabashed positivism is aimed at creating a balance we can live with, but in order to do so we must try to change our lives. It is not easy, for we have to do more than look into those places that are responsible for our anger. It is dangerous business. Can we become destructured in order to build our *own* new structure of awareness? Can we stand outside our previous conditioned experiences which we have accumulated? These are the challenges we must face, for without working on them as individual women, with the sympathetic ear of friends, we are culturally nonexistent. That is anger-provoking. We must be validated, not in our tradition of servitude, but in the new freedom, the new consciousness, as an individual human woman.

We have to be certain of wanting changes before we can attempt to make them. It is in a sense a kind of battle we are going into, "girding loins" and all, because those around us do *not* usually want us to change. Kenneth Burke, a brilliant scholar who is a specialist in communication, warns in *Permanence and Change* that before changes can be made, their purpose must be clarified. There can be no ambiguity on your part, because the change is up to you, the changer; that is, the change that you can execute depends upon your resolve. It is not as difficult as it sounds, for Burke explains that while many aspects of our lives can remain the same, many others can also be changing. However, he warns that "the need of a reorientation, a direct attempt to *force* the critical structure by shifts of perspective" is necessary for success. When our motive is clear to us, we make known our desire to change to those around us and communicate this through our actions and through the symbolic use of words.

It is difficult to find places to vent old accumulated anger. Some women find vigorous exercise like tennis, swimming, and bicycling helps. I have tried many methods, and they all work.

In 1972 I was in a physical consciousness-raising group for older women, organized by Lynn Laredo. We acted out our anger, our daily ones and the accumulated ones, in the form of theater games. We spoke our names with great drama and reinforced that we existed, sometimes with flamboyance, sometimes in song, in many different wonderful ways. We played children's games, women between the ages of 40 and 55. It wasn't easy, but it was necessary to allow the child in us to have space. We were all women shouldering heavy responsibilities, and we worked games around the shoulders and carrying loads.

In the winter of 1973 I attended a weekly scream class. We screamed at old angers, recent angers, current angers, and at each other. I screamed at the cruelty of my big brother, who, 40 years ago when I was 10, walked into my dark bedroom in the middle of the night with a black coat over his head. He claimed he was Dracula, come to get me. That trauma lasted 20 years, and it took me another 20 to be able to exorcise it. I screamed at the 28-year-old lover I had been with the week before who told me I looked younger after we had made love. He thought he was complimenting me.

Those three-hour sessions left me pooped.

Meanwhile, back at the job, and at home, I was trying to recognize my anger when it was building up. I wasn't always successful, and sometimes it took me as long as a week to realize I was plenty pissed at something and had let it go by. When the realization occurred to me, I'd get in touch with the person who caused it and let them know my feelings. My goal is to recognize immediately what will make me angry and speak about it. Let the person know, "No, I don't agree." There are many ways of getting rid of anger, not only by yells and screams. Speaking in a clear-cut voice can get rid of it too. I find myself using the phrase "not acceptable" in speech as well as in thought.

By letting your feelings become known, you do not build the anger and therefore do not do damage to yourself. Suppressed anger is very damaging to your health. It creates all sorts of secretions and clogs up the machine that is your body, preventing it from functioning in its proper free-flowing way. Share your anger and let the people close to you know you expect them to express their anger too. It is surprising how much less anger you feel when you express it on the spot than when you let it simmer. *Anger is like food, the longer you cook it, the less healthy it is.*

Actually one does get rid of anger: it is not the bottomless well we sometimes think. Also, there are many kinds of anger. The screaming kind had had its day for me, and by the winter of 1974 my lungs needed a break. I joined an older women's body workshop to work on the anger created in ourselves about our bodies and our aging.

Our bodies are different at 45 or 50 than they were at 25 or 30. We know that American culture tells us those wrinkles and lumps mean we're worthless and no good, so in the body workshop we worked on that and tried to turn the anger of aging into loving our bodies as they are. It's not easy to love your body at menopause when you have been critical of it all your life. Not even for me. But I did it. I began loving my body because of the support of the group, because the other women were like me. We differed only in the parts of our bodies we had been dissatisfied with. Fanny, 45, had always suffered because she was too tall; Sonya, 51, because she was too short; Linda, 49, because her breasts were too big; Tessie, 53, because her breasts were too small; Bertha, 55, because she was too thin; and Muriel, 47, because she was too fat.

Too tall, too short, too fat, too thin for what? For some absurd inhuman ideal? When I think of how we suffered as women because we were always "too" something or other, I am not angry . . . I am raging!

We also talked about the parts of our bodies we liked, because it was easier to begin loving ourselves based on a long-time positive feeling about something. Then we worked up to the other parts. We began to accept ourselves as we are, rather than be unhappy about not being the media-made ideal, which we never were and never would be. Probably only 1/10 of 1 percent of the population is.

Lately, my anger sessions are not in a group or class. My need has changed and I am working partly on prevention now, trying to keep myself centered, so that I do not become disturbed or taken off the course I have set for my life by outside influences. My weekly sessions are private massage therapy using shiatsu, the Japanese finger-pressure method. I chose my massage therapist Jan Crawford because she understands anger and shares my feelings about getting rid of it. So while she presses my energy centers, I let go of the last vestiges (I hope) of 50 years of anger, the deep, long-ago angers that are not even identifiable, and they come out in quiet cries and sobs and whimpers for all those thousands of times in my life I felt like doing that and couldn't. It's not as exhausting as the screams, maybe because I'm exhausting the anger and getting closer to the top.

The ways of getting rid of anger are myriad. Each woman can find ideas that work for her and fit into her life. It is a creative challenge and part of the adventure of menopause. I strongly recommend, dear sister, your taking up the challenge. You will live more happily, and longer.

LOVE YOURSELF GAME

After going through the blues and then anger, it's time for a game. Think of a positive word that describes you. I know you can think of plenty of negative ones, but this game demands positive ones only. OK, got one! Fine, find another and another.

I came across this idea in group therapy about ten years ago. The group was led by Dr. Leah Schaefer, author of *Women and Sex,* who suddenly asked me for such a word. I became shy (or was I anxious or embarrassed?) and couldn't think of one. She gently coaxed me, and finally, I cannot tell you how difficult it was, I came out with "warm." "I guess I'm a warm person," I said tentatively.

The idea intrigued me, and for the next few days I tried to think of more words. I typed them on a little card that fit exactly into my address book and carried that little card around for six years. I added a word from time to time. The important thing is that that little card worked for me. When I was in an anxious-making situation, I would sneak a peek at my card. If I couldn't take a look, the knowledge that it was there helped. If I was all those positives listed on the card, I couldn't be so bad. Right?

Whatever helps make you feel good about yourself in this world that is constantly telling us terrible things about ourselves is worth doing. I tried this game with many women and asked them to list words that described qualities they wanted for their identity. Then I suggested that they carry a card around with them, too. Keep adding to the list and write words you're not too sure of, because after a while you will start believing those words too. Then how can you help but love yourself if you are all of those wonderful things? It's a pretty good antidote for cultural invisibility and cultural undesirability.

The following one hundred words come from the women I talked with in workshops and in groups I addressed. They're yours for the taking. Please, help yourself.

active	frugal
alert	generous
articulate	gentle
artistic	giving
assertive	good-natured
attractive	graceful
aware	gracious
bright	growing
calm	gutsy
capable	helpful
caring	hopeful
centered	honest
charming	humorous
cheerful	independent
compassionate	innovative
competent	integrated
concerned	intelligent
confident	interested
considerate	interesting
constructive	intuitive
cooperative	just
courageous	kind
creative	knowledgeable
curious	listener
dependable	lively
determined	loving
easy-going	loyal
efficient	mature
empathetic	nondestructive
energetic	nonjudgmental
enthusiastic	open
exciting	organized
fair	outgoing
feeling	perceptive
flexible	positive
friendly	reliable

risk-taking
resourceful
responsive
self-sufficient
sensitive
sensual
sexually free
sincere
strong
supportive
sympathetic
talented
thoughtful

together
tolerant
trusting
trustworthy
truthful
understanding
unfolding
vivacious
versatile
vibrant
warm
witty
zesty

8
Move to Save Your Life

Exercise can save your life. Sitting around can kill you. Finding the right exercise for yourself is extremely important, because if it's not comfortable and pleasant and something you look forward to doing you probably won't do it regularly. The vital point with exercise is that it must be done daily or at least five times a week.

Exercise is to aging as food is to life; without it, we deteriorate. Picture in your mind an elderly person sitting in a chair, looking aimlessly at nothing in particular, and if that doesn't force you to jump out of yours, nothing will. The sedentary person is courting death.

There are no special ways to exercise, and each of us must find her own way. It can come in many shapes and doesn't only mean jogging or going to a gym class. Exercise can be as simple as walking to the store or raising your arms to touch your fingers while watching television. Music conductors live longer than the national average, and I think one of the reasons is that they move their arms and shoulders vigorously. Bear this in mind whenever you walk. If it's possible, do not carry things, even a purse, so that you are free to swing your arms. Think in terms of pockets instead of purses because I cannot overemphasize the importance of free-swinging arms. By doing so you will be strengthening and lengthening your muscles and avoiding their contraction, which is one of the things that happens with aging.

Ordinary walking is considered by medical authorities to be in the endurance exercise category and helps develop the cardiovascular system. Walking at a reasonable pace for about an hour uses more calories than jogging slowly for 10 or 15 minutes—and you won't be so tired. The heart will gradually be increasing its work, and it will be undergoing some degree of strengthening. When I asked Dr. Ida M. Golomb if she thought it was necessary to walk at a fast pace, her answer was, "It is necessary to walk. Any way you do it is fine, just be sure you do it."

Our bodies are like machines. "When an older person rests, [s]he rusts," says Dr. David Stonecypher, fellow of both the American Geriatrics Society and the Gerontological Society. A car sitting in a garage for a while doesn't have the same starting power of the car that was used yesterday. However, the human body is vastly different from any machine in that it is self-repairing. In addition, we can actually improve ourselves through using ourselves. We not only feel better after exercising, we look better, too.

Everybody knows exercise classes are healthy, swimming is super, and so is bicycle riding and tennis. Yoga is fun for some, while others prefer dance classes. All of these activities are great, but if you don't do them regularly they are meaningless. We need to think of ideas that will work for us on a day-to-day basis, that cause us to stretch our bodies throughout the day as an integral part of our lives. That is not to say weekly classes aren't great. They are, but unless you practice almost every day, or do yoga or your own exercises daily, such classes are not terribly effective. We have to find more ways that are comfortable for us without strain or pain.

The women in the workshops came up with many creative ideas that were so simple they hardly feel like exercise, yet they are. They were doing these things as a regular part of their lives. The vital point of these activities is that they work to keep your mind alert to the need for stretching and moving. Some people may even laugh at these ideas, but we're not trying to become gymnasts or enter races, we're only trying to keep our bodies stretched and strenghened. To engage in programs that don't fit into our lives, or that make us feel inadequate or uncomfortable, may cause more stress and cause more damage than good.

These are some of the things the women did: Selma, 49, has plants hanging in her windows and must stretch to water them. Minda, 62, keeps her tea on a high shelf so that she has to reach for it. Corrine, 38, moved her toothbrush holder next to the top of the mirror on the left, the toothpaste is on the top shelf on the right so she must stretch both arms. Ellen, 51, finds it is easier for her to do stretching and bending while using the vacuum, so she vacuums her house much more often than is necessary. Interestingly enough, Ellen had found that doing exercises as such was not comfortable for her, she needed the work factor added. Patti, 57, lives on the fifth floor and only uses the elevator when she's carrying packages.

Cary, 47, dances by herself for an hour after dinner. She calls it dancing "wildly" because she flings her arms about and uses a lot of energy. Another form of dancing one of the women does regularly is tap dancing. Jean, 52, bought herself a pair of tap-dance shoes—like those she had when a member of one of the original Mickey Mouse clubs—and tap dances for some 15 minutes a night. Jean keeps the shoes on longer than that, however, because while she sits doing other things, the sound of the taps on the floor stimulates her to move her feet. This is also exercise.

One can do many things while sitting. Babette, 40, sits at a desk and does toe and ankle stretches during the day. She also makes a conscious effort to get up once an hour to walk to the water fountain or pencil sharpener, merely for the act of getting up and walking, even that little.

We want to use our joints, because they "freeze" if not kept active in *all* the directions they are designed to move. If you sit and keep your legs on a box or stool so that the knees are bent more instead of your legs merely hanging down to the floor, you are flexing your knees. Andrea, 50, described many exercises she does while watching television. She massages in cream while stretching her fingers and toes. She showed us part of her ritual face exercises, such as raising eyebrows, pursing lips, and making funny faces. Theresa, 55, does knee bends while lying down and talking on the telephone, by lifting each knee and trying to touch her stomach. She showed us how she keeps the phone to her ear and raises her arms, fingers touching, moving her arms up and down in an easy way. During her work day, Louise, 44, does at least 10 head-rolls with her chin dropped, twice a day. She feels this clears her head.

Henrietta, 53, felt using her lufa sponge on her skin in her bath counts as exercise. The tiny capillaries close to the skin surface respond so that the blood flows in a different way—you can tell this because the rubbing makes the surface of the skin red for a short period. Renee, 58, felt that the additional five minutes spent rubbing her head when shampooing her hair is exercising her scalp, and of course it is.

Frances, 53, jumps rope. This can be done in or outside. Research has equated 10 minutes of vigorous rope skipping with 30 minutes of jogging in terms of cardiovascular effect. If you decide to skip rope, be certain the rope is the right length. Stand on the rope, holding the handles; the ends should reach to your armpits.

Do not think that all these exercises are too simple to be of value; on the contrary, they have great value. It is better to do a few simple movements with regularity than elaborate routines occasionally. Create your own exercises that you can incorporate into your daily life. More important, even, than the small exercise itself is the awareness of the need for it. As your exercise awareness grows, you will do more regular, small things. The vital point to remember is that no matter how small the stretch is, if it is regular and constant, it will work to strengthen your body.

LEARN TO WALK

The chief exercise that the majority of the women were most comfortable with was walking. It takes about a year to become a serious walker. Not only must the idea truly sink in (walking takes a different kind of time sense), but it also takes time to build up one's sense of distance and one's relationship to it.

Reva, 47, in an effort to become a walker, started by parking her car on the edge of the supermarket lot instead of in front of the store. For her, this was the beginning of raising her walking consciousness. Helen, 39, began to raise her consciousness by catching the bus one stop farther away from her job. Susie, 54, began by walking for the first half hour of her lunch period. The chief trick to becoming a walker is to plan to become one. And the most successful way to do this is in your own rhythm. Otherwise it won't work. If you set yourself a goal, let us say, to walk 20 blocks one way and then back but find you are tired on the return journey, or feel too strained, don't continue. Take a bus or cab. You are not a failure. If you walked 20 blocks and 5 on the way back, that is a positive achievement. Perhaps the next time you can increase the distance. As I said, it takes a building of one's walking consciousness.

Ella, 45, goes to a cheese store that is 18 blocks from her house and uses the public library that is 23 blocks from her house. For her, having goals to walk to makes more sense than simply walking. One can also do additional exercises while walking. Sarah, 47, on her walk, pulls her stomach in and out. Ethel, 52, goes through a wide range of breathing methods. Breathing deeply is also a valuable exercise because your lungs benefit and it also oxygenates your whole body.

Our exercise, like everything else about us, must be personal and fit into our total scheme of living with comfort, or else it becomes like a crash diet, unrelated to our total way of being. Eleanor, 46, traveled to work by car every day and even used her car to go to the corner store for the paper. She had to work harder than most to develop a walking consciousness. She was able to, although at first she felt uneasy because no one in her neighborhood walks. Now Eleanor has expanded her evening walk to 63 blocks.

For many people, walking is a good way to think. Some claim they work out problems that way. This can work especially when walking on well-known streets where one isn't tempted to browse. As your walking consciousness grows, so can your ability to block other things from your mind, except for the problem you want to consider. Your distance grows too.

Gertrude, 53, planned her walk so that she stopped for a cup of coffee and a muffin half way. This gave her a chance to rest. As she continued, she gave up the muffin and felt victorious when able to give up the stop altogether. This became her achievement, at her own pace and without pressure from anyone. It is a good idea, when you become a serious walker, to stretch yourself just a little. If you are comfortable with 20 blocks before a rest, try to make it 22, but do not feel like a failure if you can only manage 18. You are never a failure in this situation, because you are trying to do a positive thing for yourself. Pressure is destructive. Do not pressure yourself for speed or distance. It will come, for you are not trying to prove anything, and if you find you want to get on a bus for the return, that is OK. The fact that you have gone as far as you have is an achievement.

We are so enthusiastic about walking because that is where we have seen the greatest success for continued activity. This is undoubtedly because one can do it at one's own pace. My neighbor Florence, 84, goes to the store every day, rain or shine, because she doesn't want to let down the walking dynamic she has built up. She will shop for only one item. If the weather is inclement, she will walk only a short distance.

Maria, 54, has developed what she calls her walking wardrobe. She wears light clothes—no woolens or heavy clothes because she sweats—and adds or takes off layers as the weather changes. She prefers thermal underwear in the winter to a heavy coat because she likes the feeling of freedom when not burdened by weight. Her walking clothes all have pockets and she made an attractive red knapsack to wear on her back, if necessary, for carrying things. Maria has been a serious walker for four years and claims her health has improved enormously. Her beautiful posture is attributed, she says, to her consciousness of it while walking. It is important to stand and walk straight, not to round one's shoulders, for we want to keep our spines straight to avoid any hump and to allow the supporting muscles to do their job of toning too. Poor posture can be a cause of backaches.

Our bodies become more efficient when we walk because our blood circulation improves, natural cortisone is stimulated by the adrenals, and our bones and muscles become strengthened. Muscle makes up 40 percent of our total body weight and is the only organ of the body that is easy to rejuvenate. With conditioning exercise, we can even have stronger muscles at 50 than we had at 30. This is possible, some authorities say, because of creatine, a chemical contained in muscle and believed to be the promoter of muscle growth. Moreover, if we don't use our bones, they tend to decalcify. An arm or a leg in a cast loses calcium, and the muscles decrease. Along with the shrinkage of muscle, we lose vital hormones. Dr. Lawrence E. Lamb, who devised the medical exams for selecting astronauts, informs us that "the level of physical activity is a significant factor in maintaining optimal functions of the endocrine glands to provide life-giving hormones for continued youth and vigor." One of the reasons we feel good after a vigorous long walk is that the body has been producing hormones in a natural way.

Our nervous system is also related to patterns of muscle movements, which is why a stroke or damage to the central nervous system can result in incorrect functioning of a leg or any portion of the musculoskeletal system Physical activity influences the nervous, endocrine, and muscle-bone systems because they are all synchronized. You may find you sleep better and are less tired at the end of the day when walking regularly.

The whole body is affected by physical activity. For example, excess adrenalin and related products are stored in the brain and heart, and exercise causes them to be metabolized. This is probably another reason we feel so good after mild exercise, because it helps clear away the buildup of adrenalin products that accumulate from stress. Some say exercise increases brainpower, probably because the blood that pulses at an increased rate through exercise carries more oxygen to the brain. This produces a more alert feeling. Walking also stimulates digestion, improves bowel function, and relieves tension.

The function, circulation, and general health of the heart are best maintained through exercise which, by the way, if sudden and heavy, can also kill. Jogging or any vigorous exercise, unless begun slowly and gradually increased over time, can be dangerous. The heart and circulatory system transport oxygen to the working muscles, which means that physical activity makes the heart pump more blood. Since the heart propels the blood from the lungs to the working muscles, physical activity develops the optimal capacity of heart and circulation. If we don't use our bodies enough it becomes harder to use them if we want to.

We particularly need to use the leg muscles, as we do in walking. Using them improves blood circulation and helps lower the amount of fat particles in the blood. It also has a retarding effect on the buildup process of arteriosclerosis, which is clogging of the arteries with deposits of fatty materials.

Don't forget the most inclusive exercise of all: sex. It can prolong your life.

9
Me and My Speculum

I received the strangest present of my life for Christmas 1974: a plastic
speculum tied with red ribbons. This gift was from my daughter
Rebecca, home for the holiday vacation from Harpur College and very
excited about "self-examination." Rebecca had attended a lecture-
demonstration in gynecological self-help at school by the mother and
daughter team Lolly and Jeanne Hirsch, who travel the college circuit
with their film, slides, and plastic speculums.

"You see," Rebecca explained enthusiastically, "we're trying to learn
about our bodies, and one way is to look at them and not be afraid of
them, of the outside or the inside. When the doctors look, we don't
know what they're seeing, and we want to know what we look like."

How much I admired the Hirsch women as Rebecca described them to
me! The daughter lay on a table with a plastic speculum inside her, in
the same way one does in a doctor's examination room. The examiners,
however, were college women, filing past and taking a look at the inside
of a vagina of somone around their own age. They saw for the first time
what the walls of a vagina look like and what a cervix looks like. "It is
very different," Rebecca explained, "from any drawings or pictures in
books."

My curiosity was piqued. I wondered what I looked like inside. How
was I different from my daughters? Would thirty years make much
difference, or is being female all the same? I examined myself first and
then Rebecca. Yes, thirty years makes a difference, and no, we were not
the same. As we age, our interior color becomes lighter and goes from
deep pink to a lighter shade. However, even though the length and width
of the vagina is supposed to shorten as we age that was not discernible to

me. I could distinguish that my vaginal walls had become thinner and smoother, with less configurations on them than Rebecca's.

"You see," said Rebecca, "I knew you'd love the idea too." I loved the idea intellectually, but it took me many months to learn to use my speculum and be easy with it. Rebecca was eager to show me and help me with my exploration. She did, too, but it was a long time before I could simply insert the speculum without any fuss. I couldn't quite get the mirror and flashlight and speculum coordinated. It took a lot of trying, and one really needs the support and help of friends. Middle-aged women are not as eager as the younger generations to share this kind of experience, because we have had too many years of taboos about our vaginas.

Why look inside your vagina? What are you looking for? What do you want to see? We're looking because we're interested in ourselves. We want to see what's there. The reasons are the same as those that apply to examining your breasts. Your vagina, like your breasts, is a part of you. Nothing to fear or hide from. We examine our breasts to come to know them so that if the slightest change occurs, we can detect it quickly, very quickly. However, even more is involved with a pelvic exam. Regular examination of our vaginas will help us detect any change that may occur and to recognize cervical alterations in color, tone, or other signs. To be able to recognize the unusual and know when professional medical help is required is one of the ways of trying to control one's life. The alternative is to remain ignorant until a problem has progressed, perhaps beyond medical help.

Use of the speculum is part of the whole movement of knowing your own body, not shrinking from it, and even more—loving it. We have been taught to hate our bodies, and we are trying to unlearn that idea. By being familiar with ourselves, we have less to fear about ourselves. Learning about one's vagina is the same kind of thing as learning about one's hormones, one's menopause. By lifting the prohibition through understanding ourselves, we demystify these concealed areas. We are then less frightened by a medical aristocracy who have kept our physical functions shrouded in mystery, particularly our menopause. The vague euphemism "woman trouble," used to describe our sexual organs when they are malfunctioning, is a perfect indication of lack of knowledge, of knowing nothing specific. That vagueness about our sexual organs is why in 1975 American women were sucked into buying $80 million worth of estrogen, a drug that raises the risk of cancer.

Thousands of American women are now using plastic speculums. How did it begin? In the spring of 1971, Carol Downer inserted a speculum into her vagina and shared the view with other women at a meeting of the National Organization for Women (NOW) in Los Angeles. When she reminisced about that evening, she said, "If any woman in that room had sniggered, if any woman had looked offended, if any woman had demurred, I would have stopped." But no woman did: they responded in awe to what they saw.

The idea of vaginal self-examination fascinated women and has spread throughout the United States, but before it really got a chance to take hold, Carol Downer and Colleen Wilson were arrested in Los Angeles on September 20, 1972, for "practicing medicine without a license." Margaret Mead was quoted in the *Los Angeles Times:* "Men began taking over obstetrics and they invented a tool that allowed them to look inside women. You could call this progress, except that when women tried to look inside themselves, this was called practicing medicine without a license."

Ms. Wilson's case was settled out of court, and not until December 5, 1972, was Ms. Downer proclaimed not guilty. Upon that news Jeanne Hirsch wrote:

Now we must ask ourselves: WHAT MAN WOULD BE PUT UNDER POLICE SURVEILLANCE FOR SIX MONTHS FOR LOOKING AT HIS PENIS? What man would have to spend $20,000 and two months in court for looking at the penis of his brother? This case is a clear-cut version of the position of women in America—the lengths to which we must go and obstacles which must be overcome to be FREE. Carol Downer has given each of us a new vision for our future. WOMAN AS WINNER!

The most significant result of this case is the popularization of the use of the plastic speculum. This interest is manifest not only in feminist women's health centers in the United States and numerous countries, particularly West Germany, Switzerland, England, the Caribbean, Africa, and South America but also closer to home. On January 5, 1977, I attended a health fair in Brooklyn, New York, as facilitator of a menopause workshop. The sponsors were the Brooklyn Young Women's Christian Association (YWCA), The American Cancer Society, and The Guttman Institute— hardly feminist organizations—and the most popular workshop was on self-help examination. Women of every age filed past the examination table to look at whomever was lying on it. They were getting their first view of a woman's birth canal.

The self-help concept of vaginal self-examination is based on a sharing of experiences and knowledge in a common-sense, honest manner. Valuable preventative health care measures have evolved based on this collective knowledge. Fungus conditions, discharge, or heavy secretions are common occurrences better detected sooner than later if they are to be dealt with. These clinics teach a major learning skill: the ability to recognize what is "normal." At the meetings the women learn about their bodies and examine each other as well as themselves. This enables us to recognize the physical appearance of a healthy woman. Thus we are better skilled in recognizing what is abnormal.

When midwives delivered babies as the norm and women in families—mothers, daughters, aunts, grandmothers, sisters-in-law—got together, there existed the spirit of women helping women and giving each other support, as well as the knowledge of experience and familiarity. This was invaluable for the detection of and dealing with illnesses. Our lives are no longer structured in that way. Therefore the group experience of the self-help clinics fills that void as well. The plastic speculum is not intended to be used alone, for sharing the experience and learning from others is just as important. However, if you do not know of a group, it is better to use it alone than not to use it at all.

The self-help movement is not seeking to replace the medical establishment, just change it. The first step is for women to reclaim their own bodies; next, to remove fear through information. An informed medical consumer is a more dignified one. She will not accept the hocus-pocus of "There, there, honey, I'll take care of everything," from a doctor. She wants concrete information because she has learned she has the ability to understand her body. An informed woman will be patronized only once and will not return to a doctor who is still involved with the role structure of me-God-the father, you-child-helpless. Because their consciousnesses have been raised, informed women will no longer enter into that unconscious collusion.

This is not to say we aren't scared of disease. Who wouldn't be, when we know that in 1976 33,000 women died from breast cancer, that 89,000 new cases were diagnosed, and that there are over 225,000 women in the United States walking around now with "unexpressed breast cancer." It is most frightening to be aware of the recent rise of uterine cancer when we know that 27,000 American women had such tumors in the hormone-sensitive tissue of the endometrium, the lining of the uterus, in 1975; 3,300 of them were fatalities. This knowledge is coupled with the alarming fact that lung cancer in women is on the increase. Another significant figure that reflects the value of self-help and self-knowledge is that after menopause, over 30 percent of American women have hysterectomies. Could this figure be lowered through self-help? Possibly. Yes, there is plenty of reason for concern, particularly since we hear about iatrogenic (doctor-caused illnesses) disasters every day. However, bridging the gap between informed interest and fear and trembling when face-to-face with a proprietary physician will require our efforts and discipline.

Many women fear touching or inspecting their vulvas, let alone looking inside themselves. Remember that looking alone gives us a lot of information about our bodies. It is most enlightening to look in a mirror and discover how you are made. Touch, also, and really explore your clitoris by pulling the hood back to make it visible. A source of such pleasure should hardly remain a mystery.

If the whole idea of using the plastic speculum interests you but you don't know where to begin, here are a few suggestions. If there is an active women's group in your town, they will very likely know where a self-help clinic exists. There are many of them throughout the country. If you're lucky enough to live in Los Angeles, Santa Ana, or Oakland, California, each has a superactive one. Salt Lake City, Utah; Detroit, Michigan; Boston, Massachusetts; and Tallahasse, Florida, also have very active women's health centers. If you live near a college campus which has a women's center active in self-help, I'm sure they would welcome you because you're interested.

If you are not in contact with any women where you can get information and you want your own equipment, send $2.00 for a speculum to New Moon, Box 3488 Ridgeway Station, Stamford, Connecticut 06905. This group publishes *The Monthly Extract, An Irregular Periodical,* which reports on women's health issues. This communications network on the global gynecological self-help clinics constantly has new information coming from women's own experience. They will send instructions on how to hold the mirror and direct the light. You will find it easier to use a stand-up mirror (called a shaving mirror in stores) because the two round wires which create the stand free your hand. I have found that propping pillows against a wall and leaning against them is the easiest and most comfortable position for using the speculum. Also, a gooseneck lamp is preferable to a flashlight. The lamp's light will reflect off the mirror into your vagina so that you can view your cervix in the mirror. Do not be discouraged if you are not successful the first time you try. The speculum may have to be moved a little before the cervix comes into view. It is much easier if someone is with you to tell you when the cervix is visible.

If you do not see your cervix the first time, keep trying. You will be successful—every woman who tries is. Make it a regular thing in your life, and look once a month at least. It is only by becoming familiar with yourself that you will be able to recognize any change.

VAGINAL ECOLOGY

Our chief concern throughout this book has been health—before, during, and after menopause—with particular emphasis on the prevention of illness. As we try in our maturity to examine those areas of our lives which have been traditionally hidden or uncomfortable to look at straight on, so, too, we try to do the same with our vaginas. That is why we are learning to look into them ourselves. As we try to love ourselves, we don't skip over any parts, even if we have been taught that our most important female place is smelly, dirty, shameful.

A group of women in Portland, Oregon, made a concentrated study of vaginal ecology which was printed in a four-part series. Their conclusion is that "gynecological disturbances are often an expression of negative concepts about ourselves as women." They are right. Our female history of health and sex testify to that. However, there is much for us to learn from another group of American women who held the opposite view, a positive view, about their sexuality, but who have been tragically ignored as the important contributors that they were to this culture. I am talking about Black women who sang the Blues (which are not always sad) in the 1920s and 1930s (these women are the subject of my next book). Their view of their femaleness and their sexuality was very different from the prevailing White-Anglo-Saxon-Protestant one, which was to hide feeling and hide sexuality. The roaring 1920s roared about gin, money, and locomotion, not sex. These Black women celebrated their sexuality in their songs, which many of them wrote: "I've Got the Sweetest Cabbage [euphemism for vagina] in Town" or "I've Got What It Takes" or "Shake That Thing" or "Organ Grinder Blues." Ethel Waters recorded the latter in 1928—she wasn't singing about the joys of a Wurlitzer but the organ that is the subject of this chapter.

Our way of going about loving ourselves is to learn to know ourselves. In what way does the fact of our menopause affect our vaginas? Is there a relationship between our estrogen production and our vaginal climate, so to speak? Yes, there is, and it's kind of complicated because a healthy vagina has a natural flora of microorganisms: bacteria, protozoa, and fungi. The cells of the vaginal walls and the cervical secretions contain a lot of glucose. Lactobacilli, an acidophilus bacteria (which ferments yogurt) is crucial to a healthy vagina. We also need the common infection-causing organisms such as Trichomonas, different species of yeast (either monilia or candida; yeast is also referred to as fungus), and Haemophilus. If these organisms multiply more rapidly than usual and a greater concentration develops, we get infections.

If the opposite happens, and not enough develop—which can occur in some menopausal women due to a decrease in cervical secretions—organisms causing infection can thrive more easily. This is true in the case of a decrease in the Lactobacilli in the vagina, because without enough Lactobacilli to digest the glucose, the glucose is eaten by harmful organisms, which multiply.

Sugar rears its ugly head again. It is bad news for your vagina. The more we eat of it, the more glucose we have in the cells of the vagina and cervix. Some is normal, too much is no good. We need a healthy balance. Too much glucose creates a vaginal discharge with a high pH (alkaline). Under normal conditions, lactic acid keeps the pH of the vagina low enough (acid enough) so that infection-causing organisms cannot thrive.

Sugar and hormones don't mix. We have seen that the women who ate little man-refined sugar had milder flashes. Natural estrogen, which we manufacture in our bodies, and synthetic estrogen such as that used in estrogen replacement therapy stimulate numerous minute cervical glands into secreting an alkaline mucus which is sticky, thin, and clear. This discharge passes through the vagina. As it does, it collects the outer cells of the vaginal walls which are constantly being sloughed off and replaced. These cells are the primary storehouse of glucose; thus, as these outer cells disintegrate, the sugar is released into the vagina. What does this mean? Again, it means supplemental estrogen is dangerous because it increases the amount of sugar and the alkalinity of the vagina, making a high pH which encourages infection. Diabetics must be careful because yeast fungus thrives on the excess sugar in the system.

An infection is usually felt by itching and irritation. However, the same symptoms can be felt without infection and can be the result of the changes taking place as a result of maturing. When some older women do not engage in any form of sex—and I include masturbation—their vaginal tissues may become quite tender and even thinner than usual, as well as less elastic, all of which can cause itching and irritation and painful intercourse, if the latter should happen. Therefore, the women in the workshops feel safest using only yogurt for dealing with vaginal infections, for to exacerbate the condition with douches or drugs seems risky. You will find instructions on yogurt therapy in chapter 17. In addition, one must be careful with cleansing. Stay away from chemical douches and vaginal deodorants. They can cause irritations and infections from the propellant, alcohol, perfume, talc, and hexachlorophene. Many women use cranberry juice to restore the acidity of the vagina. It is the perfect food to drink for that.

Altogether, I have noticed that the women who take vitamins regularly have less problems. Remember, the soft tissues of the mouth and vagina are healthier when there is enough niacin (vitamin B₃) in the diet. Vaginal infections have been associated with vitamin B deficiencies. Brewers' yeast is the cheapest source of the B vitamins. Vitamin C should not be overlooked for fighting infections, too; it is necessary for maintaining the health of mucous membranes.

Many women have noticed that they are more susceptible to vaginal infections when they are emotionally upset. Which only proves again what we have been seeing all along: everything in us and about us is related. The best prevention against vaginal problems is that which applies for the whole body: plenty of rest and a healthy diet with a lot of B vitamins (which work for stress too).

10
The Language of Menopause

The word *menopause* is being brought out of the closet. It is no longer the dirty word it used to be. Although it is not yet as common as the word *abortion,* it is on the way to emerging into spoken language as itself instead of being covered up by its euphemisms: "change of life," "going through the change," "the change," or "climacteric." The cover-ups for menopause make it sound less ominous. That is the function of euphemisms, to substitute a more agreeable or inoffensive expression for one that is unpleasant or distasteful. The word *menopause* offended people; it embarrassed them in the same way that a woman's pregnant body used to at the turn of the century.

The word as well as the concept of menopause has been shoved under the rug for too long. It means more than merely the cessation of menstrual periods. It has come to mean, as Gertrude Stein put it, "middle living," viewing oneself in relation to the past and the future, as well as where and how we fit. The culture, through silence, pretended menopause didn't exist. But it does, it is our truth, and we see nothing wrong with it. We don't hide from it but embrace it to better understand it.

One may wonder, if menopause has not been much discussed, can there be a language of menopause? Although it has not been discussed openly, it has been talked about behind closed doors. My goal is to put a spotlight on the semantic environment of menopause by focusing on the words and phrases that are used and misused. The intention is to show how destructive and undermining the language is; how anti-woman it is; how this has created a negative status for us who are involved with menopause. We must change that polluted environment. We must enhance menopause, for our emotional and social survival are at stake.

We think of scientists as being objective, unprejudiced. When it comes to women's bodies, however, and especially at menopause, we find a bias we cannot ignore. I kept wondering, are they talking about me, about what is happening to my body? I had to know, for by knowing what is taking place physiologically, I could stand on firm ground and not be afraid. Understanding gives one a sense of power. Ignorance and confusion make one feel helpless. I wasn't experiencing the physical and mental feelings described about menopause, and as I interviewed women and facilitated the menopause workshops I came to realize that the words I was reading were a distortion. They were deleterious, in fact, and were highly injurious and creating harmful effects on women. Many of the phrases were linguistic conveniences derived from a narrow scientific conception imposed on our experience by people who are observing it, prejudicially, from a distance.

For fun, at first, I began to jot down words and phrases that jolted me. And as the list grew, it was no longer funny. It became offensive as I realized the irreparable damage that was being done. Why should the idea of menopause be so repugnant? Why indeed are all women's bodily functions so repulsive that menstrual periods become "the curse" or "falling off the roof," and the worst thing short of death that can happen to a woman is to let a bodily function show, such as a red blood stain on her white pants?

It would seem to follow, then, that if a woman's bodily functions are revolting, when a woman stops menstruating she should be less revolting, no? But a seemingly worse thing happens to the menopausal woman. By not menstruating, she's worthless, she cannot bear children. She becomes, in the language of misogynists, barren, and to be barren is the quintessential female crime.

TWINGE LIST

From my reading I collected the following "twinge list" of words and phrases used to describe menopause and the menopausal woman.

a state of mind
abrupt crisis
anguish
   mental anguish
   physical anguish
   unbearable anguish
atrophic mucosal surfaces
atrophic vaginitis
barren
breasts atrophy

breasts shrink
castration
cessation of the sex impulse
change
   change of life
   degenerative changes
   going through the change
   the changes
chemical castration
clitoral hypertrophy

completely desexualized
damaged body
despairing years
destruction of personality
disease
  crippling disease
  curable disease
  deficiency disease
  painful disease
  serious disease
dowager's hump
dreaded time
dreaded years
dyspareunia (painful intercourse)
emotional agitation
emotionally marooned
empty nest
end of useful life
entire genital system dries up
estrogen deficiency
estrogen replacement
estrogen starvation
eunuch
extreme suffering
fateful dilemma
femininity abridged
genital atrophy
her body betrays her
her decline
hormonal deficiency
hormonal deprivation
hormone replacement therapy
  intensive hormone decay
  missing hormones
horror of living decay
incapacity
involution
involutional melancholia
irrational anxieties
irritability
lacking female hormones
life crisis
loss of good health
melancholia

menopause
  cure of menopause
  elimination of menopause
  menopausal castration
  menopause is curable
  menopause is preventable
  menopause prevention
  menopause therapy
  opposite—feminine forever
  pathology of menopause
  physical barrier of menopause
  suffer menopause
  threat of menopause
  tragedy of menopause
  treatment of menopause
nervous disposition
neuter
osteoporosis—grotesquely dramatic
  disease
ovarian dysfunction
ovaries fail
ovaries petrify
ovaries stop
painful aging process
prematurely aging castrate
prolonged crisis
psychosexual stress of rapid physical
  decline
senile ovaries
senile thinning of vaginal walls
serious crisis
sexual neuters
shrunken hag
steroid protection
steroid starved
stoppage of female sexual function
suffer disruption and disabilities
tissues dry out
unspoken fear
vagina shrivels
womanhood, death of
womanhood, disruption of
womanhood, loss of
womanhood, waning of

I could not include all of the variations for it would have been too long a list. For instance, the frequently used phrase "vaginal atrophy" is missing.

If I believed the words in this list I would have to kill myself. Yet these absurd descriptions of us are a functioning part of the literature of menopause. By exploring the language of menopause we learn about how we, as menopausal women, are viewed, for language is one of the major methods of communication and it mirrors the culture. In communicating meaning, the question of *whose meaning* presents itself. Certainly not mine, for this impoverished use of the language to describe menopause is not the way I conceive or perceive it.

Language takes a long time to develop; it is an integral part of cultural thought. Constant usage confirms and reaffirms my lack of value as a menopausal woman because the negative ideas communicate negative messages. Am I then a negative? These negative concepts become amplified and reinforced so that whoever uses these phrases is negating us while putting themselves in a superior position. Why superior? Because they do not claim this list of negatives for themselves, they only lay them on us. The actual fact is *the current menopause language is incorrect.*

Bear with me please. This is important precisely because it is subtle. The users of such negative language think they are superior because they are *not* menopausal. It is inherent in their use of the word *menopausal* that it is bad. You see, a relationship has developed, however fleeting, by merely using these phrases. One person is on top (the speaker) and the other (the menopausal woman) is on the bottom. These phrases are coming from the speaker's unconscious thought, from a complicated system of the speaker's reality. That reality has meaning for the speaker and certainly for me, for if I am viewed negatively I must respond to that. We perceive and define ourselves through words. How do I respond? I can accept this language, internalize it, and hate myself, or I can try to reject it—not an easy thing to do, especially if the language is the common currency of communicating about menopause.

I have read in a hundred places that menopause is a disease. If we analyze "disease" carefully in this context we are compelled to recognize that it does not make any sense. The medical dictionary says a disease is a "definite morbid process having a characteristic train of symptoms." But I don't feel morbid or diseased. And no two women have the same train of symptoms. Around 50 percent have hot flashes in some degree, but we do not look upon those as illness or disease. The namers of our condition and the users of the cruel words are well-established people, with medical degrees and connections with the "best" hospitals. Who am I to question them? I'm a middle-aged menopausal woman trying to define my reality, trying to understand my natural process, and I reject the way those men have defined my menopause. Such people have put all kinds of appalling static between me and the facts, which is a reflection on them, not me. These are men who are not sympathetic to menopausal women, men who must despise us, for if they didn't they wouldn't think up such a dreadful vocabulary to describe us.

When men name their own menopausal condition they do not employ the same vocabulary. Therefore we do not have "testicular insufficiency" to match "ovarian insufficiency," or "senile scrotum" to match "senile ovaries." In *The Merck Manual of Diagnosis and Therapy,* the common physician's handbook, in describing premature menopause, specific medical directions are given for the "preservation of a serviceable vagina." Do you think there is equal discussion for "serviceable penis?" You're right! Of course there isn't! When a doctor injects testosterone in a man, it is not for the purpose of preserving or creating a "serviceable penis." No way. Men do not serve. Women do. The purpose is to increase his libido, to raise his hormone level. The purpose of an erect penis is not to serve a woman but to prove a man's prowess.

You will not find horrid phrases to describe male menopause—a condition which we accept as existing, despite the protests to call it "male climacteric." Impotence and dysfunction have no rococo elaborations; they are what they are, with minimum rhetoric to define them. Susan Brownmiller claims that "cultural sexism is a conscious form of female degradation designed to boost the male ego by offering 'proof' of his native superiority (and of female inferiority) everywhere he looks." Why, then, should "he" exclude menopause from his sexist attitudes?

The kind of probing used in this chapter is imperative, for as we explore the subconscious meanings and look at the general principles underlying them, we will reach a better understanding of our menopause, as well as sharpen our sensitivity as we uncover the relationship between language and thought and language and logic.

ATROPHIC VAGINITIS OR VENERABLE VAGINA

Let's examine an objectionable phrase like "atrophic vaginitis," which has probably scared more women than any other pair of words. "Does it mean my vagina will atrophy?" many ask. The phrase was arbitrarily chosen to describe the condition of aging in the human female as it manifests itself in the vagina. Let's look realistically at what the condition is: a thinning of the cells of the walls of the vagina, a loss of thickness of the mucosal membranes. The vagina shortens and becomes narrower and less elastic. In addition, vaginal secretions lose some of their acidity, and there is a possible increasing susceptibility to vaginal infections. The tissues of the external sex organs also lose some of their fat. None of this need be negative; it is merely different from a younger vagina. We learned that regular sex, which includes masturbation, makes these changes hardly noticeable.

Let *me* name this condition and it becomes "venerable vagina." If anyone insists on medical jargon we can call it "venerablic vaginitis." One namer admires and respects menopausal women and the other hates them.

We celebrate Masters and Johnson's contribution to correcting Freud's mistake about the source of our pleasure. However, their commitment to medical jargon is infuriating and shows them to be most insensitive to older women. They speak of "senile women" when they mean "aging women." Insensitive is an understatement, particularly since in the vernacular, "senile" is a heavily loaded word. There is no excuse for the phrase, "senile pelvic involution." Medically it means the shriveling of organs in an aged person, but it sounds atrocious. How simple to speak of the natural aging pelvis, which diminishes in size. Or their use of "atrophic mucosal surfaces" instead of thinning walls of the vagina. This following extract is a pip. The italics are mine. I have rewritten the same information in the second extract, changing it from repellent, frightening material to realistic and factual information:

As the human female experiences *endocrine starvation* during her *involutionary years,* the cervix and the uterus respond to the *deprivation* of sex-steroid stimulation by shrinking in size.

Mine:

In the normal aging process of the human female, her estrogen supply changes. The ovaries supply a lesser amount and more estrogen comes from the adrenals and from the extraglandular source, although not as high a level as in the premenopausal years. In the normal aging process the cervix and uterus get smaller.

You might say I took more words to explain the same things, but we are writing books, not telegrams. These are explanations to communicate information that we hope reflects the older woman's reality. The term "endocrine starvation" is a biased, nonsense term because it is implying that our endocrine glands are not supplying what we are supposed to be getting. This is a false assumption. At 50, one's endocrine system functions differently than it did at 25. Using the 25-year-old body as a criterion is inaccurate, for what is *normal* at 50 is not "deprivation" or "starvation." "Steroid-starved" belongs in the same category. It is an irresponsible, glib term. A healthy 50-year-old endocrine system is the only standard acceptable for discussion in comparison.

Webster's dictionary has, under the listing *involution,* "decline marked by a decrease of bodily vigor and in women by the menopause." It is not entirely Masters and Johnson's fault, because they are using the existing language, but one hopes for more from them since they were unwilling to use Freud's existing concept about our sexual pleasure, an erroneous concept that had been accepted for 50 years.

Aldous Huxley reminds us of the power of words and how they mold our thinking. "Conduct and character are largely determined by the nature of the words we currently use to discuss ourselves and the world around us." Menopausal women are beginning to choose to discuss themselves in a positive way.

If I am accused of being oversensitive to language, I'm the first to agree that is the case. Is the medical profession aware that the negative labels they have attached to our menopause have affected our identity? Perhaps they cannot understand why menopausal women resent being called "deficient" or "diseased." However, to point out the oppressive nature of medical menopausal language to doctors is not enough. The American Medical Association must be persuaded that such language is dangerous and has far-reaching implications involving inconsiderate treatment of middle-aged women. Middle-aged men are not so maligned. For example, it is normal in the aging male for his prostate to increase in size, the opposite of what happens to our ovaries. Nowhere in the literature do we find this biological fact embroidered with negative language nonsense. The male condition is stated plainly. We need a revision of this vicious language so that medical dictionaries, texts, and manuals can be freshly written with redefinitions more in keeping with the times and our wishes. And our wishes should start being respected, because we give the medical profession more than 50 percent of their business.

Our experience of menopause, which is our reality, is comprised of our own personal physical and emotional feelings, as well as the collective cultural representations of menopause which are reflected in the language. Theologian Dr. Mary Daly, in *Beyond God the Father,* insists that women have had the power of naming stolen from them. "We have not been free to use our own power to name ourselves." She is all for our taking it into our own hands. "Feminist naming is a deliberate confrontation with language structures of our heritage . . . it is a break out of the deafening noise of sexist language that has kept us from hearing our own word."

Dr. Haig A. Bosmajian of the University of Washington also reminds us that ours is a "male supremist language" characterized by the use of male as generic, by the "firstness of men" when listed with women (rarely do we see women and men), by the ritual of women adopting the name of their husbands upon marriage. He, too, speaks of the power men have in defining through naming and argues that the liberation of women "will have to be accompanied with a conscious effort on the part of women to allow themselves to be defined by men no longer."

We are looking for a clear, concise way to describe the healthy condition of middle age, without insults and degradation. We want to detect inadequacies, correct the errors, amass fresh unbiased information, and generate new concepts about menopause, concepts closer to the truth with, perhaps, added sensitivity. Since language is the symbolic representation of concepts, we must confront the language that is used to describe us. To make change, we must dig deep and interpret the meaning of words, for words make assumptions.

We start out with a sexist language in the United States. Therefore the language about and surrounding menopause is inevitably sexist. The clearest example of the menopause stereotype we have in the United States is Edith Bunker of television's "All In the Family." She is a woman who is scatterbrained, characterized by triviality, and views herself as unimportant. This is someone dependent upon others for self-definition, male-identified, living only through her role as wife and mother, always putting herself down because she is perpetually being put down by her husband, Archie. He calls her a "dingbat" and tells her to "Sit," (like an animal) and be quiet or "stifle yourself," so that he will not be interrupted, since his opinions are more important than hers. Why?

Ethel Strainchamps, a linguist, says females serve as an example to developing males of what they must not become. "The deleterious effect this has on the status of women is shown most unarguably in our national language, the most masculine branch of English, itself the most masculine of languages." What is sexist language? It is "any language that expresses stereotyped attitudes and expectations or assumes the inherent superiority of one sex over the other." Another feminist linguist calls it "Manglish," which is defined as the "process of the degradation of women in language."

Shall we take a look at the "empty nest" idea? It is a phrase that otherwise sensitive people use about menopausal women without the faintest notion it is derogatory. Even though it dehumanizes, people who should know better—whom I believe do not have evil intent—have expanded on it so we have "empty-nest syndrome." There is also "empty-nest blues," an attempt at currency, but where is the father? It is as though the children belong only to the mother in this lonely picture. If he were in the nest with her, it wouldn't be empty. Has he disappeared because she "henpecked" him? Look how sly this is. You see, she is too old to be attractive for sex, while the assumption is that he is not. That is why he is not with the "old hen"; he is out with a "young chick." We do not like "chick" because besides being inhuman it is an unimportant person. A man who refers to a "chick" is clearly making himself more important. Therefore the accolade "a groovy chick" has little meaning even though it has a positive ring, for how important can a "groovy" unimportant person be? The poultry metaphor is all tied up with sex.

The "old hen" is a "chick" grown up and not very valuable in the scheme of things, for an "old hen" cannot lay eggs any more. As a hen, "cooped up" with her "brood," she filled a necessary function. She is *personified* by her egg-laying ability. What good is she, except to cluck or cackle foolishly with others like herself at a hen party? A woman whose "feathers are ruffled" can turn into a "feisty hen." That would make her a spunky, frisky person who would fight back. A "tough egg" is a person who's insulated with a thick shell from getting "broken-up." In England, females are "birds," but that, with "ducky" (supposedly a term of affection), never caught on in the United States. Generally when animals are used as masculine metaphors it is to exalt male sexual prowess. Such as, "Who rules the roost?" The rooster, of course. When he can't sexually (sex is power), Spanish people have a saying, "The rooster doesn't sing anymore." It is interesting that an "old crow" is an old woman, but one never hears of an "old cock," because "cocks" do not age. They are seemingly always "cocksure" in spite of the talk about middle-aged impotence. We do not have "cock dysfunction."

Although "stud" is dehumanizing, for it reduces a man to his sexual capability, it implies success in that area. As does "cat," more particularly, a "cool cat," who is an independent, free male on the prowl with implications of irresponsibility and lack of attachment, altogether insinuating a positive sexual image. Peter Farb in his book *Word Play* points out sets of words have male and female connotations. Males roar, bellow, and growl; females squeal, shriek, and purr.

Before we leave the animals, I want to point out that those hen parties are proving to be something more wonderful than merely clucking and cackling, for women are learning from each other that they are not worthless, that their sexuality has great value even though they are no longer reproductive. I can't resist adding that, when making mother's medicine, chicken soup, a hen makes a much richer, more flavorful broth than does a spring chicken.

How about a middle-aged woman who has never married? She is an old maid. This is a reference to her sexuality—the epithet "old maid" means an old maiden, maiden being a young virgin, old maid being an old virgin, or she's a spinster, also implying virgin. But when we say an unmarried man, a bachelor, this does not imply anything about his sexuality. An aging woman becomes a crone, hag, dowager. There are no male counterparts to these words. An aging man may become a "dirty old man," which, if anything, has taken on a positive connotation because the implication is that he is sexually vigorous and can still "get it up."

WOMAN'S LANGUAGE

The following experts, all linguists, offer these views on language. Robin Lakoff, writing in *Ms. Magazine,* claims the existence of a "woman's language." She contends that women are taught to use it, and it is later used against them. This manifests itself in the way that women speak, without precision or force. Do women and men really speak differently? Are there sex differences in language? Mary Ritchie Key thinks so. She claims there are differences in intonation patterns, in syntax used, and in the semantic component. Cheris Kramer, writing in the *Quarterly Journal of Speech*, hypothesizes that "women's speech reflects the stereotyped roles of male and female in our society, i.e., women in a subservient, nurturing position in a male-dominated world." The English linguist, Otto Jespersen, says women are more euphemistic than men, "instinctively avoiding the coarseness of male speech." He claims that the vocabulary of women is more given to hyperbole, to adverbs of intensity, because of "the greater rapidity of female thought," and the "superior readiness of the speech of women."

In the menopause workshops, many women did not use powerful language to express anger, but some, the freer ones, used expletives to express theirs. Those who couldn't be forceful used food as metaphor, as in "I'm fed up," usually accompanied by a hand gesture, going across the face, always above the mouth. The implication: I have been forced to ingest or take in more than I want of something I don't want. I am overfull. In this case it does not mean nurturing at all but, figuratively, "shit." A similar phrase used to express this idea, also accompanied by the hand movement, is "I've had it up to here." These statements imply a feeling of discomfort, a feeling of having to contain and absorb more than one wants. The ways of release are to evacuate or to vomit. In the workshops, some women did figuratively "throw up" that which they couldn't "stomach" about their lives. A few articulated this idea with more cogency, as in "I won't eat shit any more." It is curious that many men have tried to protect women from strong language like "shit," but they have not acted to protect women from cleaning it up. Cleaning it up is woman's work, but saying it is man's privilege.

The concept of nurturing was expressed also but in the opposite way from the expected. Nurturing was a galling experience as expressed in, "I'm tired of being sucked on" or "they (or he) sucks off me" or as in "suck my life." These were metaphors for feeling used, of feeling "deplenished" from giving sustenance to others without enough return. Also the women spoke of others who "feed off me," and "I need to be fed." So that it was not unusual to hear, "I'm sick of feeding others"; "who will feed me?"

As attitudes about menopause change, so will the language of menopause change and so will the language used by menopausal women. A new and greater awareness is taking place. The old sense of loyalty to the oppressor is disappearing. "The new circumstances under which we are placed," wrote

Thomas Jefferson in 1813, "call for new words, new phrases, and for the transfer of old words to new objects." This applies now as well. As the language of menopause becomes less impoverished, richer with positive expressions, there will be more open talk, and more talk means viewing from more perspectives, thereby adding more dimensions. Instead of being oversimplified by our ovaries and hormones, we will actively add input, expanding the menopause experience so that it more correctly mirrors a time of life with respect for its complexity.

Edwin Newman in his book about language, *A Civil Tongue,* was not referring to my twinge list, but what he said certainly applies: "The use of language that is at bottom nonsense leads, as might be expected, to the advocacy of nonsensical ideas and, by the law of averages alone, to the adoption of nonsensical ideas. At the least, the language and the ideas go hand in hand." His point is most sensible when you look at the phrase "feminine forever," for it is at bottom nonsense. We have seen how destructive the nonsensical ideas that have stemmed from it have proven to be, particularly the idea of estrogen replacement therapy, which is to begin around the age of 40 and is taken for the rest of one's life.

Or look at the words on the list coupled with womanhood—"death of," "disruption of," "loss of," "waning of." Such nonsense belongs in the medical wastebasket with archaic ideas like the "toxicity" of menstrual blood or the "vice" of masturbation. We must get rid of this monumental legacy of negativism about menopause and there is only one way to do it. Bitch! Complain every time you hear menopause demeaned.

The book *Women and Social Policy* by Constantina Safilios-Rothschild goes even further than speaking up, for the author gives specific instructions on how to work effectively at eradicating sexism. She delineates strategies and laws and even calls for the passage of a legislative act so that we can sue mass media or leading figures or experts for using sexist rhetoric.

Although it is difficult, language can and does change. Many middle-aged women have reported that when they are referred to at their jobs as "girl"—for instance, a boss saying on the phone, "My girl will send it to you,"—they have stated their objection with dignity. The boss, who didn't mean to be offensive, has in fact changed. He would probably not have changed voluntarily, but when asked to, did. Curiously, other changes occur. The woman who makes the request automatically gains respect and consideration, and consequently her status changes.

Generally, people take language for granted and don't think much about being precise or sloppy. That is why insidious and undermining ideas remain as regular parlance. It is dangerous business. Dr. Haig A. Bosmajian argues in *Language of Oppression*:

The implications of all this is that if we can minimize the use of the language of oppression we can reduce the degradation and subjugation of human beings. If the nature of our language is oppressive and deceptive then our character and conduct will be different from that which would ensue from humane and honest use of language.

All of this leads us to the big one, the main word of our concern: *menopause*. Is it used humanely and honestly? What does the word mean, to you, to me, to others who use it, to the writers of the books and articles, to your friends and relatives and lovers? Let's probe around, and we'll find it has many meanings, some positive, but mostly negative ones. Words can be magical symbols that can carry strange powers. The power comes not only from the word itself but from the speaker of the word. We know this, for a word in one mouth can be beautiful and in another it can be poison, because the user's intent is also a part of communicating.

When a foolish statesman objects to a middle-aged woman holding office because she is in her menopause and publicly refers to the danger of her "raging hormones," meaning that the woman in question cannot be responsible, you know the intent behind his use of *the* word is to malign, to denigrate, to make the woman appear incompetent. It is as though his, the speaker's, hormones are on a constant level. You will find that this is certainly not so when you read chapter 21, "Male Menopause."

When I speak of menopause, you know it is a positive state of being. By the fifth session the women in the workshops used the word *menopause* differently. The meaning of the word had changed from the first session. It became a word spoken without fear or shame. It was, in fact, a joyous word. To be free of the worry of having a tampon or sanitary napkin at hand in case one gets caught with a menstrual period, especially since menstruation has become irregular. To be free from staining underwear and sheets and the nuisance of washing out those stains. If you experienced cramps with menstruation, to be free of them. To be liberated from conception; not to worry about birth control; to be able, at any time one feels like it (if it's convenient) to be sexual, with no concern or preparations. To enter upon a new cycle of life, while one is still vigorous, and yet have the benefit of experience; and for many women, to confront death, to realize time is limited and to value it to the point of allowing no room for deception. These are positive feelings about menopause.

Look at the 14 items on the twinge list under the word *menopause* and you will have an entirely different impression. The intent behind those listings is different from mine. The words coupled with menopause do indeed sound like a disease: *cure of, elimination of, suffer, prevention, threat, tragedy, pathology, treatment.* We are certain women did not name those conditions of menopause, because the words are too hateful.

For many women without the knowledge of the actual physical facts, the word *menopause* is frightening because there has been a frightening vocabulary surrounding it. Many women who are in their menopause today did not discuss their mother's menopause with her, but they are discussing theirs with their daughters, which means their daughters will be informed, and thereby have an easier time than if they were ignorant.

Adrienne Rich, co-winner of the American National Book Award for poetry, sums up this chapter exquisitely with some lines from her poem "The Stranger":

> I am the living mind you fail to
>   describe
> in your dead language
> the lost noun, the verb surviving
> only in the infinitive . . .

11
Masturbation

Mothers and grandmothers masturbate. So do daughters and wives and aunts and sisters and sisters-in-law. It is a healthy thing to do, especially for women over 40, because it may help postpone "atrophic vaginitis" or "genital atrophy," the woman-hating terms used by the medical profession to describe our vaginas when they age. There is a thinning of the mucous membranes and a loss of elasticity of the walls of the vagina, which can cause an uncomfortable feeling of dryness. This condition, preferably referred to as a mature vagina, is currently considered to be one of only two "legitimate" symptoms of menopause other than the cessation of menstrual periods. Hot flashes is the No. 1 characteristic.

The trend among more forward looking gynecologists is to question the cause of all other symptoms that used to be attributed to menopause. However, just as many women are not troubled by hot flashes, so many women never have any problem with their vaginas. Although the condition is labeled menopausal, it usually doesn't show itself until after menopause, when a number of changes take place in the vaginal area.

I believe that sex is the chief factor affecting this condition. When the mucous glands just inside the vaginal walls are activated by sexual stimulation, they secrete a natural healthy lubrication in the vagina. Any woman over 40 who is engaging in regular sexual activity once or twice a week with a partner probably doesn't have to masturbate for health, only for fun. But we know that most people have individual sexual rhythms which do not always coincide with their partner's rhythms, especially as we age. We also know there may be a difference in sexual energy and desire. Also, people are changing partners more than they used to. This makes chances for continued regular sex over the long haul, say for the next 30 or 40 years, possibly irregular.

There are 35 million women in America over age 45. A considerable percentage of them are without partners some or most of the time, which means a lot of women are having to depend upon themselves for their sexual gratification. To masturbate is to engage in sex and that creates lubrication which is good for you. It is pleasurable, generally uncomplicated, brings quick release of tension—both physical and emotional—and altogether has healing effects. Your body, after all, doesn't know who's on the other side of the action: husband, lover, or yourself.

Masturbation is an easy source of orgasm for most women, contrary to the stereotype about female sexuality that women need a lot of time to become aroused. According to *The Hite Report,* which is the most recent information compiled on female sexuality (it was published in 1976), of the 3,000 women ages 14 to 78 who responded to Shere Hite's questionnaire, 82 percent said they had masturbated. And 95 percent of them said they "could orgasm easily and regularly whenever they wanted."

An atmosphere of guilt surrounds masturbation. Though it is a hereditary instinct, it has been overloaded with shame and fear. The subject has been largely hidden from speech as well as literature, but that is changing. Masters and Johnson in *The Pleasure Bond* tell us "children have absorbed from the adult world the idea that the human body is indecent. . . . Don't touch yourself, it's naughty; don't touch her, that's nasty; don't touch him, nice girls don't do such things—the specific prohibitions may vary, depending on the situation, the age of the children and a family's values, but the message is clear."

Most of us have grown up with the idea that we were not to touch our "female parts," certainly not to explore "down there" for there was something not quite "clean" about it. This negative image of the female genitals is due largely to the fact that the blood of menstruation and childbirth comes from that place. There seems to be an unspoken agreement that men masturbate and women don't. It is true, little girls do not share masturbation in the way little boys do, who seem not to be as shy about the experience in front of each other. The reason for this is the male sexual organ, unlike the female one, is visible and it erects, making the whole business more concrete. It is even treated as a competitive sport: whose is bigger or smaller, harder or softer, who can shoot farther.

One need only to look at the No. 1 synonym for masturbation to get the full impact of the general attitude toward it: *self-abuse.* Why not *self-pleasure?* Or look at the slang term, *to jerk off.* Crude, right? Hardiy self-loving. *Onanism,* another word for masturbation, refers only to men and comes from the Bible. Onan, the farmer, feared that if he masturbated and his seed fell to the ground, the earth would get the idea of waste and not be fertile. The land not yielding a harvest was also his punishment for doing what is "unnatural."

We have all heard of the foolish things foolish people tell children such as, it'll drive you crazy or give you pimples or some other disaster. The communication is that masturbation is not normal and that it is not right to have pleasure with yourself. Sexual pleasure alone is suspect. Something is wrong with people who "play with themselves." A delightfully contrary view is held by Dr. David Stonecypher, who considers sex a healthy sign of enthusiasm for life. In his book *Getting Older and Staying Young,* he says, "Masturbation is not childish, abnormal or evil."

Our bodies are like machines: "to rest is to rust." If we don't use them, the unused parts tend to stiffen and dry. Just as we keep our sewing machines and automobiles oiled, so, too, we must keep our bodies lubricated for prime functioning. The idea is that if you stop having sex with a partner for a time, it is wise to keep your body in good working condition in order to avoid problems when and if you resume the activity. This can be so whether your partner is a man or a woman. For all practical purposes the crude phrase "use it or lose it" refers to more than desire. After a period of abstinence from any kind of sex, including masturbation, there can be pain caused by the dryness resulting from lack of natural lubrication.

True, creams, oils, and jellies can be applied before any kind of insertion (including your own finger) but when the vaginal walls become really thin, the synthetic lubricants may not be adequate. The pain during and after sex can last for a few days, and the walls can easily be torn, even with the gentlest precautions. I don't want to sound like an alarmist, but I have interviewed too many women who have told me their stories of pain, "even after I used K-Y jelly," or when "it was only six months since I had intercourse last." Very frequently, women in their late fifties are not aware that there is any problem at all until they engage in sex—any variety, even masturbation—and discover a condition of dryness they didn't know existed.

This is not something that is easily talked about. Usually only gynecologists hear these complaints, and they prescribe regular use of estrogen cream, which does help. Since we are interested in prevention, however, and don't like using hormones anyhow, it's a good idea to be aware of the possibility of the condition. There are women in their late fifties and sixties who suffer from this dryness who do not engage in any form of sex, nor do they have any interest in it either; yet the condition can become so uncomfortable that they seek medical help to alleviate the pain from dryness which may cause itching, burning, or discomfort upon urination. Does it not, after all, make more sense then to stimulate your own hormonal secretions than insert prescribed ones? There are other health benefits from masturbating, too, such as exercising your uterus and vagina because of their contractions (every part of our bodies need exercise); it is also a superb way to release tension.

We can take the example of the three cultures—the mountain people of the Andes, the Hunzas of the Himalayas, and the Azerbiajans of the Georgian USSR—where people live to be a hundred or more. One of the elements these peoples have in common is that they enjoy regular sex. This is thought to be a contributing factor in their longevity. If you do not have a partner regularly, masturbating is a good thing to do, and it may work to help you live longer.

Female masturbation is not a new idea; it has always existed. There are sculptures of dildos from ancient Babylon and India. Havelock Ellis long ago reported "the use of an artificial penis in solitary sexual gratification may be traced down from classic times, and doubtless prevailed in the very earliest human civilization."

I remember reading, some twenty years ago, about one of the pleasures of Chinese aristocratic women in antiquity: use of gold balls for masturbation. A small ball was inserted into the vagina first and then a large one as a stop; the women would swing on a swing and giggle while the smaller ball would roll back and forth. They sound similar to the gold-plated Ben-Wa balls, the size of large marbles, which women keep in place by inserting a tampon.

Nineteenth-century America was full of fear over women's sexual "voraciousness" and used surgical intervention in the form of excision of the clitoris and removal of the ovaries to cure that appetite. Ehrenreich and English, authors of *Complaints and Disorders*, explain:

> Masturbation was seen as a particularly vicious character defect that led to physical damage, and although this was believed to be true for both men and women, doctors seemed more alarmed by female masturbation. They warned that "The Vice" could lead to menstrual dysfunction, uterine disease, and lesions on the genitals. Masturbation was one form of "hypersexuality," which was said to lead to consumption.

Freud taught us "vaginal orgasms" were healthy and any other kind were suspect, and clitoral orgasms required psychiatric consultation. Psychoanalyst Wilhelm Stekel referred to women who enjoyed them as harboring an unconscious "will to displeasure," the refusal to enjoy intercourse. Alfred Adler explains it through his "masculine-protest theory." Other psychoanalysts have called it the "renunciation of womanhood" or "denial of the role of the vagina" theory. The "sex expert" of the 1950s, Dr. Frank Caprio, warned that "masturbation plays an important role in the development of frigidity among women. . . . Wives who are sexually unsatisfied are apt to masturbate as a substitute form of sex gratification." I say, "Right on," but they called it sick because "substitute" is not the "real thing."

Luckily, these views are reversing. Shere Hite, who conducted the nationwide study of female sexuality, says:

> Surprisingly, most researchers have not shown much interest in masturbation. . . . To assume intercourse is the basic expression of female sexuality, during which women should orgasm, and then to analyze women's "responses" to intercourse—is to look at the issue backwards. . . . Researchers must stop telling women what they *should* feel sexually, and start asking them what they *do* feel sexually. . . . Sharing our hidden sexuality by telling how we masturbate is a first step toward bringing our sexuality into the world and toward redefining sex and physical relations as we know them.

She then proceeds to give about fifty pages of women's testimony on *how* they masturbate.

The authors of *Our Bodies, Ourselves,* written by The Boston Women's Health Book Collective, also positively advise it. "Masturbation is not something to do just when you don't have a partner. . . . It's a way to find out what feels good, with how much pressure, at what tempo, and how often. . . . The more you know about your body, the easier it is to show someone else what gives you pleasure. *It is different from, not inferior to, sex for two.*"

Practical Sex Information by Marjorie Hackmann discusses masturbation, too. She says it "can be a useful part of a person's sexual development" and goes on to reassure the reader not to worry if you never feel like masturbating, for that too is "in the range of normal human experience."

NOT "SECOND-RATE" SEX

The best-known authority and also the first person to write on the subject of masturbation is Betty Dodson, sometimes called the masturbation maven. The first time I saw and heard her was in June 1973 at the NOW Women's Sexuality Conference, whose stated purpose was "to explore, define and celebrate our sexuality." Individual women spoke to an audience of more than 1,000 women, from the stage of a large public school auditorium in New York City about their sexual feelings and experiences. Ms. Dodson dropped a bomb. Her subject was masturbation. We had never heard the word spoken in public before, nor has anyone ever been so bold, so honest. Her talk was totally disarming and delightfully humorous about enjoying oneself. She believes masturbation for women is a powerful force and source of energy and is not "second-rate" sex.

Ms. Dodson's booklet, *Liberating Masturbation, A Meditation on Self Love,* has numerous drawings (she's an artist) of different vulvas showing their wide variety and how very unalike they can be. She calls them "portraits of women." We have seen the male organ illustrated much more than we have our own. She outlines the sexual double standard of our society, men having "the social approval to be aggressive-independent and sexually polygamous—but that women should be non-aggressive-dependent and sexually monogamous." She was the first to "go public" with the idea by lecturing, writing, and running masturbation workshops. It is practically a religious experience for her, the way she describes her involvement and her work with groups. One of her most liberating experiences was when she was able to masturbate to orgasm with her lover. She describes how difficult it was for her to share masturbation for the first time, and as preparation she watched herself alone in a mirror. This reassured her for "I didn't look funny or awful," she says. This was the beginning of her freedom from the romanticized image of sex—a Sexual Independence Day.

> There is a vast range of sexual and sensual pleasure available to everyone if we simply get more openminded about what sex and pleasure are about. The romantic image of sex creates a ritualized genital sex that leaves no room for sexual play or growth. We must let go of the idea that there is a "right" or "best" way to have sex and orgasms.

One of her students, Jane Wallace, was so much "helped by Betty Dodson's book" that she also wrote one. It is called *Masturbation: A Women's Handbook*. Ms. Wallace does not masturbate as meditation, but she too shares her experiences as well as those of about a dozen friends. Hers is a practical "how to do it" book. She warns it is important to enjoy what you're doing rather than be concerned with whether you will or won't have an orgasm. Ms. Wallace also believes in the concept of self-love, as do I, and when she refers to the female genitals she is forceful. "It is not a dirty thing, a hole, a smelly area, an emptiness, a gap, a void, a gash. It is a beautiful, pleasure-giving body part."

Her enthusism never wanes. "It's a woman's right to masturbate, her right to have orgasm after orgasm if she wants." There are some women who feel that to be able to satisfy themselves sexually makes them more able to enjoy the ultimate independence. It seems, however, that what is operating here is an emphasis on the problems involved when two people intimately relate to each other, for I cannot believe anyone would not prefer another human's warmth and touch some of the time if it were easy and comfortable.

There is concern among some that masturbation may replace the need for sex with a partner, but I think this is foolish because nothing could do that. The laying on of hands has been and always will be a most healing element, and sharing affection and getting another person's response could hardly be replaced.

If you are considering giving yourself some relaxed pleasure, a good way to begin is by taking a long luxurious herb bath. After that, anoint your body with a fine light oil such as apricot kernel or safflower or sesame to which you have added some herb or floral essence or cologne. Oil is good for our bodies because our skin loses moisture as we age. Apply it all over your body. Self-massage is healing and is a good way to "get into" masturbation. When you oil your body, be sure to do your breasts and your vaginal area. Don't skip those because this whole business is about touching yourself and accepting yourself and loving yourself. It is also a good way to introduce you to the idea of oiling your partner's body, including the genitals. Handling them after they have been oiled makes the experience even more erotic. Don't worry about the sheets. You can always wash them, but if it bothers you, place a large towel on the bed before you use the oil.

The women's movement is adding some new twists which derive from the self-help health movement. Really get acquainted with your vagina by looking at it in a stand-up mirror using a good light. Be sure you have plenty of time. This is nothing to do in a hurry. Self-examination is one of the first steps in removing fear. Move the folds of your vulva, the external genitals, and look and see how you're made. Look at the outer labia, and then the inner labia. Find your clitoris. You will be surprised to find you are really not fragile but very strong. Open the inner labia and look as far inside the walls of your vagina as you can, and get to know its color. Our color changes as we age, from maroon to rosy around 50, going toward light pink in the later years. The configuration of the walls also changes— they become smoother. If you want to have a really good view of your sexual self get a plastic speculum and look further inside. It is amazingly interesting, and when this discovery is new it is most revealing in spite of how unsure you may be. Remember, this is all part of the revolution of demystification, of getting to know your body and loving yourself and seeing how you're made. You won't hurt yourself. Rather, you will be doing yourself good by not being a stranger to yourself. Contrary to Benjamin Franklin and other sexist men, we are not all the same in the dark. We are unique, and each one of us is different from the other.

Don't be impatient. Masturbation takes time, and the first rule is to relax. This is your experience, and it needs the tender, loving care you have so long given to others. Now is the time to give it to yourself. You deserve it.

Eventually some may want to share masturbation with the person they are close to. Choose a time when you are making love, when you are intimate and caressing each other, and ask your partner if they masturbate and let them know that you do. This will make it more comfortable later to ask your partner for something you may want, which may be communicated in a nonverbal way, such as moving the other person's hand half an inch one way or another. Your asking, incidentally, will most likely give your partner pleasure as well. The best road to success is to let it be known when you are being pleased; if it is difficult for you to tell the person, indicate it by showing pleasure. Deep breathing, sighs, and inarticulate sounds communicate volumes. Let your sounds go—pleasure is good for you. You're entitled to it and have everything to gain. It is the best "turn-on" in the world for both of you to be aware of positive results.

Mutual masturbation can be foreplay, the second act, or the whole play. I don't think it is necessary to define what people do, for whatever is pleasing is pleasing, and to oe pleased is to enjoy and to enjoy oneself is also giving pleasure to one's partner. There are plenty of books written about women giving men pleasure; now we're concentrating on getting it. As Jane Wallace advises, "Remember to take it easy, but take it!"

"Making love" to some people means whatever two people do together. To call a partner's manual stimulation of the clitoris masturbation embarrasses many. Some women think masturbation is only what they themselves do. The word itself implies a negative, particularly as it relates to another person's presence. Physical manipulation of a clitoris by another person changes from masturbation to the more acceptable "making love." It becomes a linguistic problem. If a partner "plays with you" and does to you what you might do to yourself, is that person masturbating you? Does the activity become "legitimized" because someone else is doing it to you? Then what is cunnilingus, oral sex? Is it a person masturbating you or is it "making love?" By the old definitions only penile insertion counts, and we know that's been proven foolish. These are definitions for out-dated books, not beds.

If the idea of masturbating is one you have to warm up to, or if doing it with your lover is scary and you don't know how to begin but you are tempted, then look at the best-selling *Joy of Sex* and its sequel *More Joy* by Dr. Alex Comfort. They are to the bedroom what the *Joy of Cooking* is to the kitchen. Look at them by yourself first, and then perhaps you may want to share them with your partner. The drawings are sensitive, so don't worry about pornography. These have been best sellers for years and can be found in any bookstore. If you want to go further for yourself, look at the two booklets on masturbation I mentioned or the masturbation chapter in *The Hite Report*. (You can order the booklets from Eve's Garden, 246 East 51st Street, New York, NY 10022, whose catalog notes, "We grow pleasurable things for women.")

ANY WAY IS OK

Masturbation fantasies fill a function for us. They correct many of the distorted relationships we see around us and on television and help us to soften the corners on our own relationships by putting them more in our own control. They discharge an energy which, if it was left hidden and forbidden, might emerge in a harmful way, physically or psychologically. It is unbelievable, but as recently as 1973 Dr. Allen Fromme said in a popular magazine, "Women do not have sexual fantasies. . . . How do we know? Ask a woman, and she will usually reply, No. The reason for this is obvious: women haven't been brought up to enjoy sex . . . women are by and large destitute of sexual fantasy.'' What woman would tell *him* anything?

If you want a little help with fantasies you can find plenty of them in Nancy Friday's books, which are now in paperback; large bookstores carry them: *My Secret Garden* and its sequel *Forbidden Flowers,* which goes even further in frankness. Some of the fantasies are bizarre, but as a group they work to liberate one's imagination. If it would embarrass you to buy them you can order these by mail, too.

The more I talked to women about masturbation, the more inventive I learned they are. Running water seems to be a big "turn-on," either under the faucet in the bathtub (by focusing the water on the genitals, which usually requires legs up), or with the shower on strong. One woman told me that when she waters her garden with the hose on a sunny day she waters her own watering place.

The old masturbating standbys which used to be inserted, like candles, bananas, carrots, cucumbers, and zucchini cut to size, are being replaced by machines which are used to stimulate the clitoral area: the electric tooth-brush (the smooth back, not the bristles or brush) and vibrators, partic-ularly Prelude 3, which is designed especially for women—but men are using it, too! Its shape is nothing like the battery operated imitation penis, for it is plugged into an electric outlet and has five attachments, designed to be used for massage all over the body as well as the exterior genitals. Its illustrated booklet shows a woman and man using it together. It costs around $25.00 and is also available from Eve's Garden.

Masters and Johnson have voiced concern over the fact that vibrators can bcome addicting, but I do not share their consternation, for I believe humans have more power than machines. I do not believe masturbation is a substitute for making love with another person, rather a complement to it. Barbara Seaman, author of *Free and Female,* suggests, "While it is true that vibrators have become very popular, there is little imminent danger that they will replace sexual intercourse. In one recent survey of vibrator users only four women out of several hundred came to prefer these gadgets to their human partners."

Although Masters and Johnson are cautious about vibrators, they are gung-ho on touching. *"Touch is an end in itself.* It is a primary form of communication. . . . Touching is sensual pleasure, exploring the texture of skin, the suppleness of muscle, the contours of the body, with no further goal than enjoyment of tactile perception."

If you are interested in your aging health, but the whole idea of sex turns you off and you don't want to masturbate, I suggest you indulge your mind anyhow. When you watch people you like in the movies or on television maybe your vaginal walls will lubricate from thinking—it can happen. Did you know that some women can turn themselves on just sitting in a chair? They tighten their vaginal and anal muscles and release them.

The most common way women masturbate is lying on their back and touching their genital area. They touch to the left or the right or above or below the clitoris and sometimes very gently on it. Some women insert one or more fingers at the same time. Others turn over and face down while masturbating, while some prefer lying on a side. Whatever works for you is fine. Soft cloths are used by some to create friction or a towel or blanket or pillow between the legs while lying face down instead of using the hands.

Dildos, once made of rubber in the shape of a penis, are now made of plastic that is firm, but not rigid. They come in various sizes, and fortunately one doesn't have to go to a sex shop for them because Eve's Garden sells them through the mail. Some women look at themselves in a mirror as a way to begin.

The more we learn about what other women who do not seem "bad" or "crazy" do, the more we will be able to please ourselves, and the easier it will be to expand what we do comfortably. Try any way you can think of that appeals to you. Don't be shy with yourself. If setting the scene in fact or in your imagination will help, then by all means do it.

When we talked about masturbation in the workshops, some of the women chose not to participate in the discussions. At least one in every group said she did not masturbate and could not identify with it. They merely listened. The following are some of the methods that were discussed:

Lenore, 51: When I masturbate, I feel like I'm taking care of myself. Maybe it might be better to have someone else take care of me that way, I'm not sure. Since I don't have the choice these days, doing it for myself feels right.

Bella, 43: When I masturbate regularly the orgasms are better. Sometimes I don't masturbate for a few weeks, and then I have to build up to them. It takes time to build them up where they last longer and are more intense.

Donna, 53: I didn't really learn how to masturbate until I was 41, after my husband and I separated. I learned there was more to sex than I had known. Now I can tell my lover what I want. It makes all the difference.

Florence, 49: After enjoying a wonderful orgasm through masturbating, I'm amazed and angry that I was made to feel that this pleasure was forbidden.

Jeanne, 54: Sure, masturbation is great. I love it, but I'd rather not have to do it. I'd rather have a person there doing it for and with me.

Clara, 44: My best masturbation comes after I've smoked a joint. I'm more relaxed and can enjoy it more.

Vivian, 48: I really give myself to myself when I masturbate. I know I need a lot of time for my fantasies, at least an hour, and I give it to myself. The best part is, I always end up a winner, getting what I want.

Anna, 50: You may think this is crazy, but on some levels I prefer masturbating to being with someone because then I don't have to share anything. I'm totally in control and I can decide in my mind exactly how the story will go. It's more personal, more private.

Miriam, 52: My orgasms from masturbating are different from the ones I get from fucking. I like them but they are not as deep. I don't get the reverberations throughout my body. I mean that the masturbating orgasm is more localized.

Julia, 45: Since I discovered I was not "hurting myself" to masturbate, it has freed me to have better sex with a partner. I can relax and let it happen instead of being anxious about coming, because I know I can make it happen myself.

Ilene, 49: My husband and I went to a couple's consciousness-raising workshop. After we heard what other people do, even though we had read a number of things, we became freer with each other. It has changed our lives because we are now telling each other our fantasies and sometimes even play them out instead of only thinking about them individually. It's marvelous. It's more fun to spend the weekends at home than to go anywhere.

Roz, 55: My sexuality comes in waves. I'm not interested at all or else I'm totally turned on for a period and then I masturbate between having sex with my lover. I'm just very interested in it in every way when I'm on the crest of one of those waves. Everything I do becomes sexual, like taking a shower or even moving my bowels. It's nutty, I know, but I can even get a sexual thrill from urinating too. I think my whole lower body becomes more sensitive.

Lillian, 51: It embarrasses me to hear you say the word [masturbation]. I'm having a hard time now, and I'm trying by talking to get over it, because I want to get over it.

Maxine, 46: After I really got into masturbating five years ago, I began to understand my body better so that sex with my husband got better. I know more about what works for me. It made me less shy as a lover.

Perry, 56: My problem is I can't get over my shyness. My friend encourages me to, but somehow when it comes to telling him exactly what, I can't speak. I think hearing all of you tonight will help.

Jennie, 57: I like it physically, but emotionally it makes me feel like a failure because I don't have a man to have sex with.

Helen, 42: Since I became a lesbian, my lover has taught me things I never knew before about my body, and it has changed the way I masturbate. I take more time now.

Abigail, 49: When I finally let my masturbation fantasies have free rein and no longer worried about being depraved, I was able to ask for more variety during sex with my husband.

Patti, 51: No matter how much I know it's OK to masturbate, I still put the cat out of the room and lock the door of my bedroom. You know I live alone.

Minna, 50: Once I discovered I could have any kind of fantasy I choose when I masturbate—that is, when I finally learned the fantasies were not really suppressed desires that I wanted in reality—I became freer with creating them, and then I was able to talk about them with my partner. He shared his with me too and that made our sex more exciting, even though we both knew we wouldn't live them any further than our talk.

Lila, 47: the most wonderful thing about masturbating is that I never feel used.

It is difficult for most people to talk about masturbation. When we discuss it with other women it is easier. Doctors are usually the last ones anybody would speak with, because usually they are not helpful. Bessie, 52, told us an experience she had with one doctor. She had a fat globule removed from the back of her neck. It required anesthetic and a short hospital stay. While convalescing at home she vividly remembered the first time she masturbated after the operation because it scared her so much she thought she was dying:

When I reached orgasm, the blood in my head felt like it had no place to go and was going to burst open. I tried it again a few days later to test it and, as I was building to orgasm, the same feeling started to return so I stopped immediately. When I went to see the doctor I told him about it, because I was afraid something may have gone wrong with the operation. His response was, "Don't you have a husband? That's not a good thing to do." I wanted medical information, not his morality. It never occurred to me that a mature physician these days would question my sex life.

It has been said that the best masturbators make the best lovers, and women who have practiced masturbation do know how to come to orgasm. Dr. Mary Jane Sherfey, author of *The Nature and Evolution of Female Sexuality,* underlines the point: "The more orgasms a woman has, the stronger they become; the more orgasms she has, the more she *can* have." Masters and Johnson discovered a fact that is still shocking people, that a clitorally induced orgasm by automanipulation can be more intense than a vaginal orgasm during intercourse. However, no one is arguing that this fact makes masturbation superior; it only proves that it's a positive pleasure.

Most middle-aged women masturbate because they like it rather than because it is good for their health. Many do it because they don't have partners. Those who do have partners masturbate because they aren't getting as much or the kind of sex they want.

Our high priestess Simone de Beauvoir was very realistic about such matters when she wrote *The Second Sex,* and that was more than 25 years ago. She says that "even when sexual love exists before the marriage or awakens during the honeymoon, it very rarely persists through the long years to come . . . and the magic of eroticism spontaneously evaporates rather rapidly." And when speaking about sex between female and male for people who are along in years, she put it plain and straight: "Coition is a far more complex and difficult undertaking than masturbation, since it constitutes a relationship with a second person."

Some women don't have partners because they have become more discriminating than they were when they were younger. Women who have lived through a relationship (and most had) and who work for a living (this was true of all the women who attended the workshops) are less likely to "settle" for spending an evening with someone in whom they're not really interested, even though it will lead to sex later. They say, "I'd rather masturbate." They want more than sex; they want friendship, too. Many are reluctant to enter relationships with men because they are finding that the men around their age are still thinking along the old lines of male and female roles of 20 and 30 years ago, and the women are looking for more equality. Those who have brought up children speak about not wanting to "take care of anyone anymore." Among the women who are married, the changing roles are creating sexual friction. The married men are more reluctant to change.

It is considered inappropriate for a middle-aged woman to show her sexual desire. Thus, when sex may be available, she may not know how to avail herself of it. Another reason could be true fear and lack of trust in oneself and in the possibility of a relationship.

There are many other reasons why a lot of women around the age of 50 don't have male partners. Statistically there are more women than men. About 200,000 more men than women die annually. An historical fact frequently overlooked is that over 545,000 possible American male partners for menopausal women today were killed or reported missing in World War II. This automatically creates a shortage of men in that age group. Furthermore, the divorce rate keeps rising. Divorce statistics in 1975 soared over the one million mark for the first time in US history. The result of this is that men who remarry or take new lovers usually choose younger women.

I believe there is yet another historical reason for the kind of sex practiced by men in this age group: these men are more prone to anxiety than younger ones. They were coming of age in the 1930s and were trying to make their start in life during America's Great Depression. I think the state of the country and each family's concern about a living, school, jobs, and the future weighed heavily on them, and as a sociological group they were affected by this. To have been frustrated and poor as a "normal" phenomenon of the time must have had a profound effect on their personalities and left some with permanent problems. I feel that this element, which operated in the masculine formative adult years, spilled over into other areas of behavior, including the sexual one. Women's experience seems to prove this point, too, for they claim there is a decided difference in the sexual behavior of men under 40.

Another reason for the shortage of male partners for menopausal women is the difference in sexual rhythm and interest of men and women in this age group. Gail Sheehy, who has written extensively about this difference in *Passages,* says, "Many modern women exhibit their erotic potential most boldly at just about the time their husbands' sexual incentive is diminishing. For men, the very *thought* of this can be disastrous." Hiding behind headaches used to be a woman's excuse in Victorian times, but it has been taken over by middle-aged men. Watching television instead of going to bed is also common. Sex researchers tell us midlife "impotence" results in most cases from a combination of ignorance and male sexual anxiety. Masters and Johnson have actually noted that it is almost unbelievable how susceptible the human male is to the power of suggestion when it comes to his sexual prowess. This means that even though the men may be around, they are not necessarily available for or interested in sex. Many who are are so concerned with their fear and trembling that all kinds of problems arise, none of which makes for successful sex for either person. It's a big problem.

When we discussed this in the workshops, the women concluded that the best way to take the pressure off a middle-aged man is to let him know you can bring yourself to orgasm by masturbation, and therefore orgasm is not a problem for you—meaning it needn't be a problem for him. Also, let your partner known that touching and cuddling and snuggling is of great value to you. Explain that his ability to be tender and loving and to masturbate with you is desirable. By helping men take the pressure of performance off themselves, the women help themselves, too, because the total sexual ambiance changes. It becomes a more equal experience, for the man then is not making love *to* the woman but *with* her.

Until the situation is clarified, trouble is likely to remain. Communicating this easier approach to sexuality is a delicate matter. The women talked about finding ways to do this without embarrassing themselves or their partners. Some men, because of their vulnerability, may look upon their female partner as wanting to take over. We decided, however, the only way to deal with this sensitive situation is to take the risk of talking about it and making it clearly known that the bed is not a battleground and this is the one game everybody wins. There are no losers.

Let me say again, masturbation is a natural, healthy activity that may prolong your life. It is a healing pleasure that is available to you, yours to take and enjoy unless you yield to the old-fashioned restrictions. Besides, with so much sex all around us, it seems a waste to be frustrated, especially when relief is in your own hands. Take it. Enjoy yourself.

*Sexual activities have a plurality of
ends. . . . It is unusual for this quest for
pleasure to be reduced to the simple exercise of
a function: generally speaking it is an
adventure in which each partner realizes his
own being and the other's in a unique
manner. . . .*

Simone de Beauvoir

12
Sex Is Better
When You're Older

The question is no longer whether there is sex after 40, 50, 60, 70, 80, or 90, but how to get it, on your terms. Sex is all around us, but it is rarely visible as part of the life of older women. What is older, anyhow? When do you become an older woman? Masters and Johnson place women over 40 in "The Aging Female" section. Their aging male starts at 51, however. Old feels like somebody else, somebody older than yourself usually, if you are feeling healthy and well.

The title of this chapter comes from the women, from their empirical experience. Why is sex better when one is older? What makes it better? It's better because all female sexuality is better since Masters and Johnson corrected Freud's biological mistake and clinically confirmed what all women know, that the source of their greatest sexual pleasure is the clitoris, not the vagina. "The clitoris is a woman's sexually most sensitive organ, equivalent to a man's penis." It, not the vagina, is the primary female sex organ. It is amazing to learn that the small clitoris contains the same number of nerves as the penis. Those women who have only recently discovered their clitoris can hardly be blamed, considering the conspiracy of centuries to hide it. It is not pictured on anatomical charts and although most tampons and birth control devices carry diagrams of the female genital anatomy, the clitoris is rarely illustrated.

What has been thought to be vaginal orgasm was due to a misunderstanding of the role of the clitoris during intercourse. At the highest peak of arousal, the whole vaginal area is congested. The clitoris is engorged to twice its unaroused size and is automatically stimulated during intercourse because the hood that covers it is pulled over the clitoris each time a thrust in the vagina is made. The case for the clitoris has been most eloquently described in Ann Koedt's *The Myth of the Vaginal Orgasm.*

Sex is better because women in the women's movement started talking about faking orgasms and talking about women's rights in the bedroom as well as on the job—equal sexual pleasure and maybe a little extra thrown in for reparations. The women say sex is better mainly because they are freer than they were when they were younger. Older women are enjoying masturbation more because they have lost or are losing their guilt about it. Indeed, Masters and Johnson claim that older women need regular sex for lubrication more than when they were younger, and they are enthusiastic about masturbation because it serves so many functions at once. The women who are enjoying sex claim to have more sex drive. They are also more eager to have experiences count for more; and if they don't, they know why they don't. The women are less confused.

All older women are not engaging in sexual activity. The main reason for this is that they want to enjoy it more than they did; they want to have it closer to their terms or not at all.

Some doctors do not agree with the idea that sex is better when you're older. A prominent gynecologist on the faculty of New York University's School of Medicine and the author of a book on menopause, Dr. Sherwin A. Kaufman, says:

> I disagree with the claim that sex is "better than ever" when a woman reaches menopause . . . and I've met few women who were pleased that their reproductive function was over, even though they did not expect to use it. As far as sexual spontaneity is concerned, if they have never been spontaneous before, chances are the menopause will not make them so.

I guess Dr. Kaufman will not agree with most of the ideas in this book either, but one wonders how closely he talked to all those menopausal women he saw, or rather, how closely he *listened* to what they had to say. My guess is that they listened to him and then talked to the nurse outside his office or to no one at all until they found a woman with a sympathetic ear.

It is no wonder we read more about the negative side of menopausal sex. Most of the books are written by doctors and they don't know about the good part. If a woman is having good sex, her doctor is the last to know. If she's hurting, however, the doctor will be the first. This means doctors have a generally distorted picture of our sexuality. So that is why we read so much about "atrophic vaginitis" in their books and so little about increased sex drive. Who goes to a doctor for that? A very few do, and only if it scares them. The emphasis that is given to thinning walls of the vagina in most books on menopause would lead readers to believe that most women suffer because of it. That's not true. The walls do become thinner, but most women are not aware of it. Some women have the problem of dryness of the vagina, but not all. Just as all women don't get hot flashes, even less are troubled with dryness.

In the 1970s a great deal has been written surmising that as women age their response to stimulation is likely to be slower. This needs much more research because I'm not sure it is correct. According to the women I talked with, many variables exist. There is no question at all that women who masturbate have a much more active response to stimulation; and many report that they need less time to be ready than when they were younger. It seems that when women are engaging in regular sex, they become responsive more easily than when they are not so engaged, no matter what the age. There is an ambiguity here that needs clarification.

I think the sex researchers are interpreting their scant data on older women incorrectly. I think they are confusing allowing entry with being ready. When the women are interested in sex, they say they get ready in terms of lubrication in a flash. However, that is not synonymous with being ready to permit penetration. Most women want more foreplay, and when they are older are more likely not to allow entry until they are ready for it psychologically. This is not to be confused with physical lubrication.

Women are now on guard about theories about us because we have learned the biological imposition, namely, that the vagina is the source of our pleasure, was inflicted on us and documented, verified, and discussed as fact in scholarly books and journals for over half a century, yet it was false. Therefore, when new ideas about older women's sexuality are presented without numerous studies verifying them, and when it is contrary to many older women's experience, we hesitate to accept them.

The nutty thing about being an older woman as far as sex is concerned is that most women don't feel old when it comes to sex. It's like swimming. Are you ever too old to swim, especially if you've been swimming right along? It's very important to remember older women are only recently starting to talk about sex. It hasn't been culturally acceptable, not even to doctors—they get embarrassed! They're not trained to talk to menopausal women about sex (as though one needs anything but interest) except for dry vaginas, and you know they'll give you estrogen instead of telling you to masturbate to create your own secretions.

The talking about sex that is going on now is mostly among older women themselves, with each other. It got underway during consciousness-raising when younger women in groups started to talk. The feeling among older women was it was "disloyal" to speak against your husband or lover. But when a woman hears another in a group say in anger, "He gets his and then turns over," she is witness to another woman's release from that old loyalty. She is also witnessing a very important change in that the woman is putting herself first instead of the relationship as a couple first. There is nothing subtle operating; it is wide open. This is making claim for one's own life; not being a "miss goody-two-shoes," as we have been taught. Not "covering up," as we have been taught. Not "blaming yourself," as we have been taught.

When one of my daughters read this, she asked, "Ma, didn't two close sisters talk about sex, or two close friends?" My answer was, "They talked, but they didn't say anything, never details. After years of marriage, one might say, 'He's not so hot,' nothing more." If women did talk to each other, it was rare, not usual. And if it did happen, it was certainly not open, in front of a group.

Sex for the mature woman is not only orgasm. It is everything that surrounds an orgasm. The before and after and in-between and the yesterday and tomorrow, too. It is also the thinking about it 20 years later and the feelings about it two weeks and two months later, the feelings of joy and anticipation or the feelings of anxiety and fear.

For many middle-aged women there is concern about "measuring up." Our female collective unconscious seems to fail us sometimes, when we allow ourselves to be swayed by the perpetual onslaught of propaganda that tells us how we don't measure up. Can one fulfill another's expectations? Would the partner prefer to be with somebody else? A younger person perhaps? Is my body too old? Do my wrinkles show? Do my bumps and lumps make a difference? Does having less pubic hair seem strange? Are my cold feet alarming? If I ask for this or that will I appear selfish? These are only some of the elements surrounding older women's sexuality that bring anxiety.

How is this sex different from the sex of 20, 25, or 30 years ago? The complexity of older woman's sexuality is only beginning to be explored. Until we learn more about what actually takes place, not only in the bed but in her head, we will not know about an area of woman's experience that is rich and valuable and important. It must become known, for all women will be strengthened from this knowledge, and it will correct many misconceptions. We hope that it will also make everyone more understanding, more generous, and more lovable.

Please remember that many of the women found it difficult to discuss the sexual details of their lives, and I felt privileged to hear them. Every woman was absolutely ensured of anonymity, and all names have been changed. The testimony that appears later in this chapter comes from two sources. They are from the menopause workshops and from the personal interviews on a one-to-one basis in my house over a meal or a snack, over a three-year period.

I cannot stress the importance of talking with other women enough, and listening, particularly in groups. That is why I made the menopause workshops a series of five sessions each. I knew the real lowdown would not come out until the fourth or fifth session; not until trust was established and it was clear that judgments would not be made. The dynamic that develops in such a situation is especially valuable because it is truly liberating. It offers the opportunity to voice the unspoken without fear and the opportunity to listen and learn from other women like yourself. There is no authority figure, no leader, no boss, no teacher, no one with whom to ingratiate yourself. Rather it is women learning from each other through sharing experiences. It's the most mature idea for communicating that I know.

HOW IS IT DIFFERENT?

We hear about some women not wanting to participate in sex with their partners after menopause. What exactly is operating here? Has their sex drive disappeared? Do they feel "too old" for sex, as some say? Why are they turned off? Upon further questioning, we learn that those women have not enjoyed sex, that it has not been a pleasurable experience for them. For a variety of reasons they have not been able to work it out so it gave them satisfaction. For many women it was duty; sex could be only one way, his way.

Menopause creates a sense of freedom. Although it is primarily freedom from menstruation, there is fallout in other areas of experience, and one of those is not wanting to "do your duty" when that has been unpleasant. There is tragedy here, largely unspoken until recently, and it is doubly tragic for women currently in that position because all around them they're hearing about the joy of sex and they are feeling cheated.

Women who say they aren't interested in sex mean they are not interested in the kind of sex they know, or the kind that is available to them. In other areas in their lives, areas that they don't identify as sexually related to themselves, their libido is lively in spite of their denials. It manifests itself in the romantic films and television programs they watch and in the books they read. When these women are given the space for conjecture, given time and interest in their thoughts, it turns out that they would be sexual under the right circumstances, and those are not demanding ones. I found this to be true for women in their seventies, too. Many would happily become active if they could be sure their partners would be sensitive and gentle. In fact, that seems to be the criterion at every age.

There is much fear surrounding sex at all ages. As I wrote at the beginning of this chapter, it's the terms that count, particularly for middle-aged women who are experiencing new plateaus of desire (when they are not suppressing it) in a cultural atmosphere that represses middle-aged sex. It is not easy. Vivian Gornick, the brilliant feminist journalist, lays it on the line in no uncertain terms: "The terror of felt sexuality is the terror of our lives, the very essence of our existence."

A woman's opportunities for sexual experiences, adventures if you will, are quite limited to the milieu she finds herself in. She cannot move about as easily or as casually as can a man. For example, let us picture two people, a 50-year-old man and a 50-year-old woman, both interested in meeting someone, in exploration. It is socially acceptable for him to do this, but not for her. Let us say they both meet in a restaurant. If he expressed interest in her, that would be fine; if she expressed sexual interest in him, he might be shocked. Even though he may be interested, her aggressiveness might be disturbing to him. Her problem is different from his because she will require another kind of strength and purpose to proceed. She may find resistance even in a man who had been thinking earlier in the evening he would like to "run into someone." Without his even thinking this through, the subconscious principle operating is that *he* should make the move. If she does, it's not quite correct.

This restrictiveness imposed on women makes it difficult to proceed without the support of other women. These ideas are discussed in groups, and when we learn what other women do, it expands our options. For example, Rachel, 49, told about an experience she had had. She met a man at a party, they enjoyed each other's conversation, and they found many areas of mutual interest. They exchanged phone numbers. She called him the next day and asked him plainly, "When are you coming over?" "Whenever you say," was his reply. He came over that evening and they had a terrific time. He probably would have called her, but what a feeling of being in control Rachel got from making the call when she was moved to do so. She removed herself from her old way of wishing, wanting, hoping he'd call, of being a telephone victim. The women discussed the possibility of rejection when one reaches out. Rachel said, "It's easier for me to take rejection than it is for me to be passive. If my friend couldn't or didn't want to make it, then I'm better off knowing that than wasting energy on a futile possibility. I thought I was reading the signs right. I'm not certain about that sort of thing yet, but I felt sure enough to call."

The biggest problem is where to find partners. There are no places, no ways, no tricks. The first requirement is to make a conscious decision that you want one. That fact is basic, and when it is clearly established in your mind you will be surprised how you can let it be known, in appropriate ways, without doing anything tasteless or gross, that you are available for friendship. It used to be inappropriate to respond, but as we become stronger we can keep our eyes and ears open, for we have nothing to fear, because we know we can always say no, too.

Sitting alone at home is not the place to find partners. But going about doing whatever you like to do, is. Wherever people gather, there are potential partners. Florence, 51, told us she met a new friend while standing in a long line at the bank. Cynthia, 50, met one while buying broccoli in the supermarket. Helen, 52, has a new lover. He's the man who came to inspect the new intercom system at her office. People are all over, and when you get over being self-conscious you'll be amazed at the response you'll get. You give off those vibes. One hit is worth 50 misses. In general, the women didn't care for singles bars or resorts, but no one knocked them either, for each woman has to find her own way, the way that is most comfortable for her.

The experts are in unanimous agreement that continued sexual activity until late life depends almost entirely upon two factors: health and attitude. Some women showed concern about their sexual vigor and enthusiasm. Jill, 48, was afraid that her appetite was "unnatural," because she was experiencing more desire than she ever had before. She was worried about feeling like "a bottomless well." Nature has set no fixed limitations on sexual capacity. Some women bloom, so to speak, in their thirties, some in their forties, and some in their fifties. Dr. Mary Jane Sherfey tells us:

> The popular idea that a woman should have one intense orgasm which should bring "full satisfaction," act as a strong sedative, and alleviate sexual tension for several days to come is simply fallacious. It should be stressed that the intensities of the multiple orgasms do not abate until fatigue of the responding muscles has set in. Each orgasm is followed promptly by refilling of the venous erectile chambers, distention creates engorgement and edema, which create more tissue tension, etc. The supply of blood and edema fluid to the pelvis is inexhaustible.

Once and for all, Sherfey makes clear and establishes the absurdity of the idea that women are or ought to be satisfied with sex that gives them anything other than full satisfaction.

> The nearly universal sentiment, still very prevalent in our Hebrew-Christian culture, that the female of the species does not, need not, or should not require orgasmic release can now be said to be biologically unthinkable. . . . That the female could have the same orgasmic anatomy and not be expected to use it simply defies the very nature of the biological properties of evolutionary and morphogenetic processes.

Kinsey was important, no doubt, but his questions about sex were biased and based upon a man's view of enjoyment. Masters and Johnson's sex studies were based mostly on committed couples. *The Hite Report* is to date the only large public study in which older women's sexuality is considered for itself. Shere Hite has done a superb job, but in a 438-page book on female sexuality, only 14 pages are on the older woman. We're grateful for those and for her being the first to break the ground. It is our hope that many books on the subject will appear soon. I am not ignoring the excellent articles that have appeared in feminist publications, but there have been all too few of those.

You might ask, well, aren't older women women? Aren't they included in all female sexuality? Yes and no. Older women have lived longer, and a woman around 50 has had around 30 years of sexual experience. Experience is everything; it counts and cannot be denied. A menopausal woman today was a 20-year-old during the dark 1950s, when successful life in America for a woman was to be married and have children and find her identity through them. Pleasure, too, was then vicarious. Translated to the bedroom this means that his pleasure becomes yours. Carried to the logical next step, his pleasure then is more important than yours. That is why many women faked orgasms—to make men feel successful.

Living this role for many years has affected older women of today. My three daughters, who are in their early twenties, have very different ideas about sex from the ideas I had when I was their age. They consider themselves as equal human beings. I'm having to learn that in my gut, even though I know it in my head. It doesn't come naturally to me as it does to them. The more negative conditioning about sex one has had, the harder it is to get rid of it. This is the big difference between us.

The menopause literature as it relates to sex is mostly outdated and distorted. It's obsolete because it's written with the assumption that every woman in her menopause is in a monogamous marriage and suffering from not enough to do. Volunteer work and hobbies are the major outlets suggested for curing boredom as well as being the advice for widows— meaning a way to keep busy when you don't have sex.

If you stop to think about it, there are very few models of older women's sexuality to look at in any kind of literature. It's not a popular theme. The sexuality of middle-aged men is plentifully covered; they are usually coupled with younger women. After hearing the women speak about middle-aged men in reality, we know we have been reading the fantasies of middle-aged men, rather than their every-day sexual experience. How old was Molly Bloom or Lady Chatterly? They were mature, but they don't count because they were Joyce's idea and Lawrence's idea, men telling us what women are feeling—and they don't know. They don't ask the women, and they don't listen to the women.

Women's orgasms have been described by men in literature, but they are extremely limited descriptions because they are men's ideas of what makes men feel successful. Many women do not yell and scream in ecstacy but remain quiet, making neither move nor sound. The silent movement of interior contractions is effortless. When the women describe their orgasms, they cover as wide a range as there are women. The Ernest Hemingway depiction of female orgasm has had a deleterious effect on many women because the women didn't experience their "earth move"; thus they felt they weren't living up to their potential.

The truth of the matter is that many women have release that is gentle and flowing and sometimes keeps going for longer than most men can imagine. Because it is not big and fast—like the male orgasm—and not enough is written or discussed about this reaction, some women think that kind of orgasm doesn't count, that it's not the real thing. It's real, all right, because it feels good while it's happening and when it's over.

Edith Wharton could have told us but she was ashamed; middle-aged women's sex wasn't anything a writer became explicit about, but her hints held plenty of promise. However, she did find the challenge of erotic writing irresistible and her recent biography by R. W. B. Lewis has a sample of her unpublished sexual writing, discovered after her death. It's stupendous, exquisite, a key to indicate what she could have done. How deeply sad I am because we don't have her sexual work to turn to, or George Eliot's, who was a brilliant, passionate woman who could write rings around any man when it came to women's feelings. She couldn't have done it for us because things were so hard for women in the 1800s that she had to take a man's name to be able to publish at all.

Even decent male writers have not been encouraged to write about middle-aged women's sex. Daniel Defoe's *Moll Flanders,* for example, who was sexually vigorous far into middle age, is an embarrassment to the English. Defoe is known for *Robinson Crusoe,* a book about a man, not for his magnificent, even distinguished book about an independent woman. Descriptions of mature, independent women might have been the line for all writers, male and female, to follow.

There can be very deep feelings and profound communication connected with sex in maturity. It's an important part of life, and to have that part of woman's experience remain a vacuum is unforgivable. If women have the opportunity to live many years and cultivate those feelings, that is something worth knowing about. Younger women can learn from older ones, but it must be put down in writing. It is essential that this part of the human experience become known. Doris Lessing and June Arnold are two women who are working at this task; we are happy about it and wish there were more.

There is a marvelous plea by a French writer, Helene Cixous, at the University of Paris, for more mature women writers to write about their sexuality:

Woman must put herself into the text—as into the world and into history . . . what strikes me is the infinite richness of their individual constitutions; you can't talk about *a* female sexuality, uniform, hemogeneous, classifiable into codes . . . women's imaginary is inexhaustible . . . their stream of phantasms is incredible . . . I wished that woman would write and proclaim this unique empire so that other women, other unacknowledged sovereigns, might explain: I, too, overflow; my desires have invented new desires, my body knows unheard-of songs. Time and again I, too, have felt so full of luminous torrents that I could burst. . . .

What's the meaning of these waves, these floods, these outbursts? Where is the ebullient, infinite woman who, immersed as she was in her naivete, kept in the dark about herself, led into self-disdain by the great arm of parental-conjugal phallocentrism, hasn't been ashamed of her strength? Who, surprised and horrified by the fantastic tumult of her drives (for she was made to believe that a well-adjusted normal woman has a divine composure), hasn't accused herself of being a monster? . . .

Now women return from afar, from always: from "without," from the heath where witches are kept alive; from below, from beyond "culture . . ."

She believes, and I agree with her, that mature female sexual writing will have to be different from the male writing we know.

For what they have said so far . . . stems from the power relation between a fantasized obligatory virility meant to invade, to colonize, and the consequential phantasm of woman as a "dark continent" to penetrate and to "pacify. . . ." One can understand how man, confusing himself with his penis and rushing in for the attack, might feel resentment and fear of being "taken" by the woman, of being lost in her, absorbed, or alone.

There is so much to be said by women for a better understanding of women. The womanly strength that we know exists has too long been suppressed so that women themselves have not given themselves access to their own sexual depths. And for good reasons, because we have been living under a shroud of fear and guilt. Guilt because we're too motherly or not motherly enough. (How often I have worried about appearing like a Yiddisha Mama because I showed loving concern for a lover, or worried that I was not showing enough concern because I wanted to be served.) How many women have not been afraid that they didn't know how to move, how to be sexy enough, or the reverse—afraid to be too sexy, thinking they'll scare their partner and he'll think she's an insatiatiable demon?

All of these feelings must be given voice, and that voice can only come from the women who have experienced these things . . . and that is every woman. Putting things down on paper adds dimensions that memory alone cannot serve; nuances of feeling are forgotten without written words. By writing these feelings out, we come closer to understanding them. If every woman kept a notebook, we would suddenly be flooded with marvelous texts giving us a look into this netherworld. Men would learn a new way to love. They would discover an infinite complexity about female sexuality they have only feared. They would expand their own eroticization. They would be able to venture into new adventures, enter new zones of feeling perhaps timorously, but emerge forthright eager to return. But to do this, the old censors, the old codes, the old man-on-top concept must be smashed, for this is a place where only equals can dwell and harvest the fruits.

One hopes middle-aged men will be able to take this trip and travel to this wonderful world. It is probably an easier thing for younger men to do, for they have already given some hints of their readiness. I am thinking of their use of language toward the woman they love. They refer to her as their "old lady." It wasn't until I came to understand the meaning this term has for them that I was not offended, for it is not derogatory, it is in fact complimentary. An old lady has wisdom from experience and can be trusted and relied on.

Interestingly, the prejudice against older women is not the same in the black community as it is among whites. Among blacks, middle-aged women, particularly in their forties and fifties, are not looked upon as older in the same sense as in the white Anglo-Saxon culture. It is more a matter of being "wiser" than "older." Therefore, to be an older woman is to be a mature, serious, not flighty person. It is related to the same idea as "She's a mean woman." This, too, is complimentary, for it means this person will not put up with nonsense. This is not a person to trifle with or to take lightly. It is a most positive view of a woman because it gives her the regard she should have as one who will not passively accept unjust or unkind treatment. In the black culture, it is an accepted fact that middle-aged women can teach younger men a lot about sex. And they do.

We have been victims of the system of sexual roles, but we are now awake and learning to assert ourselves in many areas including the bedroom. However, the bedroom seems to be the most delicate place to execute this transition, for middle-aged men are not used to assertive women in bed. When women take the initiative, they may find themselves being accused of not being feminine (meaning passive) or of being aggressive or of causing impotence. That's a hell of a risk for a 50-year-old woman to take. He may put on his pants and run. Some do.

But what about all the talk? Does the new sexuality count for anything when you really get down to it? Sure it counts, but some are slower to come around to it than others. On balance, middle-aged women prefer middle-aged men as lovers because they are more comfortable with them and because they, too, have developed a pacing and appreciation of time. True sensuality demands time. Men must understand this because women of all ages are coming around to this thinking.

As women, we have been brought up to understand that men know more about sex than we do and will take the initiative. Therefore we have been conditioned to wait to respond. Ideas like "fast," "cheap," "not nice," are connected with reaching out and making sexual feelings known. If you were in high school in the 1930s, 1940s, or 1950s, this is the kind of early culture overlay you got. "Nice girls don't," and "Men don't marry that kind" are heavily loaded concepts.

"Good girl" becomes "good woman," which is the way everyone wants to be thought of. In sexual terms, a good woman is a passive woman, one who does not make sexual demands. For instance, if she has discovered what her clitoris can do for her, she'll try to ease it into position but will not always succeed. A good woman is busy fulfilling her cultural functions as wife and mother. She is not thought of as a sexual being in her own right for her own pleasure. That's not a good woman, that's a whore, a slut, a bitch, an irresponsible, selfish self-centered woman. Notice, however, that whenever a great man is described, his sexual expression is considered an ornament to his person, a natural thing. A wholesome man is a sexual man, a successful man is also a sexual man—but a successful woman is not thought of in those terms. It is considered healthy for a man to be sexual. A sexual woman is somehow not quite so wholesome. She is questionable.

The women who are enjoying sex more are the women who are accepting themselves more. Accept yourself, accept all of your parts, which especially means your body. I emphasize this because we have been taught to dislike our bodies and that there is always something wrong with them. Our breasts are too big or too small, we're too fat or too thin. There is danger all around us, all the time, as we age, for middle-aged women are rarely shown as sexual beings in the media, particularly in the popular women's magazines, and this can have a deleterious effect which must be combatted.

When older women's sexuality is discussed, there are insidious overtones that can be dangerous if you are not on guard and realize they are foolish. For example, an article titled, "Sex Begins At Forty" in Harper's Bazaar sounds good, right? But they don't simply proceed to tell you to go ahead and enjoy yourself. No, they get their double pronged instruments sharpened first to prick us with: you might enjoy it *if you fix yourself up.* It is presumed things are wrong with us because we are older, and, of course, they can supply the remedy. They tell us instead of thinking about menopause as "the last grasp" (who would if they didn't suggest the idea?), we could correct all of our sexual problems because they most coyly have the answer in the form of a little magic pill:

Estrogen replacement therapy has come seductively to the fore. And what a little girl-Friday hormone it has turned out to be. There doesn't seem to be a sexy thing estrogen can't and won't do to keep you flirtatiously feminine for the rest of your days—and nights. It restores a feeling of confidence and well-being, makes your skin smooth and resilient, bounces up your hair, firms your breasts, sparks your interest in sex—a real package deal that spruces up your vagina, uterus and clitoris. In no time at all, everything is exactly as it should be: your whole body is primed for sex.

You see what I mean about being on guard because of their insidious language? "Everything is exactly as it should be" if you take the pill. The implication is that you're not OK on your own, as you are. To insult us further, they use slick terms like "the over 40 crowd"—meaning of course, they, the magazine, the writer, are not—and then presume to tell us what to do to enjoy sex.

Let's look at the person who is called oversexed. When such a word is used for a young man, 18 or 19, when he is experiencing his highest sexual potential (for re-erection) in terms of his libido, it is found amusing. A boys-will-be-boys attitude prevails. The same goes for the concept of the dirty old man. In fact, that is really a compliment, because the implication is he's active and robust. Isaac Asimov, who knows better, wrote a funny book about the idea, only I didn't find it funny. And to be a Don Juan is to love them and leave them. This is not necessarily considered a negative concept either. Transfer oversexed to women and you get nymphomania. There is no way oversexed (an absurd word) is even funny when applied to women.

What if we were lucky enough to have women senators (it's disgraceful that we don't) and they carried on with young lovers; they would be thrown out of office no matter what their political record of good works. It would be intolerable for 50- and 60-year-old women to be cavorting with younger men in the public eye. It would be disgraceful, disgusting, unladylike and they couldn't get away with it. Have you ever heard of a man losing his job because he was very sexual? The middle-aged and older senators who were using public funds for their amorous adventures were merely chastised for using the taxpayer's money, not for having sexual relations with young women.

YOUR SEX DRIVE—SATISFACTION AND SATIATION

A woman authority whose analysis of our sexual biology we trust, Dr. Mary Jane Sherfey, tells us, "To all intents and purposes, *the human female is sexually insatiable in the presence of the highest degrees of sexual satisfaction.*" Dr. Sherfey has only begun to think about the far-reaching implications of this understanding of women's paradoxical orgasmic potentiality and will discuss it in her next book. She stresses the distinction between satisfaction and satiation. This is an important point because it does not mean a woman is always consciously unsatisfied. Her hypothesis is the woman usually wills herself to be satisfied because she is not aware of her orgasmic capacity.

Helen Kaplan explores this idea, too, in her book *The New Sex Therapy* and points out the difference between men and women after orgasm. The male returns to his pre-aroused resting state, both physically and psychically, rather quickly, but the woman returns to the nonsexual state much more slowly. The resolution stage for the woman not only lasts much longer but it can bring profound and prolonged sensuous pleasure, and she "can be brought to orgasm again at any point during this period, if she is open to this." The women in the workshops had a lot to say about this resolution stage. Many of them experienced additional smaller orgasms without their partner's or their own stimulation, just from simply being. Most of the women felt this stage of pleasure increased with age and was foreign to male partners. The second orgasm, and any other additional ones were, they said, very much easier to achieve without much effort during this period.

Shere Hite reports that the women in her study were not very much acquainted with this information, but she qualifies that statement with the possibility that the phrasing of her questions about one orgasm being satisfying did not include the possibility that many women have more than one. Ms. Hite's conjecture is that many women are unaware of how many orgasms they may be capable of having.

Older women generally seem to have grasped their potential for multiple orgasms. They understood the step from one to two orgasms is minute compared to the leap to get from zero to one. The women agreed that they generally have more than one orgasm when they masturbate alone.

Which brings us back to middle-aged women's sex drive. In chapter 13, "Our Hormones," you will learn that estrogen cannot and does not have any effect on it. If the level of estrogen in a woman's body is not related to her sex drive, are there any sex hormones that are? Dr. Estelle R. Ramey (another woman whom we admire and trust), from the Department of Physiology and Biophysics at Georgetown University School of Medicine, believes:

> There is good evidence that androgens tend to increase libido in both men and women. Both women and men secrete the entire spectrum of steroid hormones. Males have higher androgens and lower estrogens than females, but both require androgens for normal sex drive. The adrenal cortex of the female secretes androgens, and the adrenal cortex of the female tends to be larger than in the male.

Can it be, then, that women who are more sexual are producing more androgens than their sisters who are not feeling very sexual? I wonder, then, if when our libido is demanding attention is it because our body is producing more androgens at that time? I don't know the answers, but I'm certain the complexity cannot be denied. Further thought only brings more questions: if, when our sex drive is more apparent, and if it is because we are producing more androgens, why are we producing more at that time? Why didn't we produce them the day before or the week before?

Women do wonder about their sex drive. It seems to vary quite a bit, and they are beginning to talk about enjoying sex a lot, engaging in it a lot, and wanting a lot of it. However, I have never seriously thought of that as a problem for which one would visit a doctor. It would seem that if a woman doesn't have a partner or partners whose capacity matches hers, masturbation could either serve as a supplement or serve in lieu of a partner for sexual release. Going tó a doctor puts you in danger of being given a drug to make you "normal." And the doctors do prescribe medication routinely even if you may be in a cycle they don't understand. The libido is not static;

it grows, diminishes, and shifts in response to a myriad of stimuli. It is no accident that people are more sexual when they are on vacation. Removed from the stress of their everyday lives they have the opportunity to become fully rested and relaxed.

Gynecologist Dr. Sherwin A. Kaufman, discussing being oversexed in menopause, informs us that "progesterone is the one [drug] that can have the most effect in lessening such feelings. Usually rather high doses are necessary." He tells about a woman, 49, who complained of feeling "oversexed," and who was "considerably bothered by heightened libido." He treated her for her ailment. "It was progesterone that succeeded in alleviating what she considered her oversexed emotions." He tells us, "Occasionally it is desirable to *decrease* female libido, for example in an elderly woman who is bothered by erotic dreams. The use of the hormone progesterone will usually accomplish this" (sic).

If your problem is the reverse, not feeling sexy enough, that, too, can be fixed with hormones. Dr. Kaufman says, "The male hormone, testosterone, will frequently increase the sex desires of those women who previously had a good response." This idea worries me because fooling with our hormones is dangerous. It seems that poor response indicates the need to change partners or unleash one's imagination for fantasy, less dangerous surely than tampering with the endocrine system. There is so much we don't know, but we do know that sex hormones given to menopausal and post-menopausal women increase their cancer risk.

"Frigidity," with its connotation of icy coldness, used to be the word used to describe female sexual dysfunction. The word has been so misused and abused it really hasn't much meaning anymore, especially since it was also commonly used to mean not being able to reach orgasm vaginally, only clitorally. The word is still used, however, to describe women who are unable to achieve orgasm even though they can become sexually stimulated. Thanks to the work of Masters and Johnson, women who have learned to masturbate can correct that condition for themselves. A very fine book on the subject is *For Yourself,* by Lonnie Garfield Barbach, a University of California therapist.

Jane E. Brody, my favorite *New York Times* reporter, describes orgasm as a double-decker phenomenon involving mind and body:

> Orgasm, for women as for men, is a natural reflex response, and varying amounts of stimulation may elicit it in different women and in the same woman at different times. But orgasm is also very much in the mind. Guilt, fear or anger can inhibit it completely, and sexual fantasies can stimulate it.

We get another perspective on mature sexuality from Simone de Beauvoir in *The Coming Of Age.* She says it is not "a mere collection of reflexes that beget a pattern of sensations and images," but much more than that.

"It is an intentionality that the body experiences, lives through, an intentionality that exists in relation to other bodies and that conforms to the general rhythm of life. It takes form in relation to a world which it provides with an erotic dimension."

As much as we value our independence, we are happy to give it up momentarily when sexually engaged with someone who is giving us pleasure. Please do not misunderstand. I'm not talking about the old doormat idea, but something entirely different, something very subtle. Simone says it beautifully. She has been talking about the quest for pleasure:

Generally speaking it is an adventure in which each partner realizes his [or her] own being and the other's in a unique manner: in the turmoil and desire of sexual activity the consciousness and the body become as one in order to reach the other as a body and in such a way as to enthrall and possess him; there is a twofold reciprocal embodiment, a transformation of the world, now a world of desire. The attempt at possession necessarily fails, since the other remains a subject; but before it reaches its end, the drama of reciprocity is experienced in the act of love in one of its most extreme and revealing forms.

We often learn more from poets than from scientists, and since poets are traditionally the writers about love, I asked one, Edward Field, who is my age, what his thoughts were about the problems of middle-aged sex. "People confuse sex with friction," he said. "Men especially, must learn more about tenderness."

We have all heard sex is good for your health. Is this really true? Maybe because it's a pleasant experience one feels better for it. According to Dr. Abraham I. Friedman, a specialist in human metabolism for over 25 years, frequent sex is extremely beneficial from a purely physiological standpoint. It lowers the cholesterol level of your blood, and "sexual activity helps to get rid of excess fat deposits because it results in an increased production of fat-destroying hormones, such as pituitary growth hormone, epinephrine, and thyroid." He considers it the perfect exercise, because during the height of sexual activity the pulse, blood pressure, and respiration of the participants approach those of an athlete during maximum effort. During sexual intercourse there are considerable voluntary and involuntary contractions of many muscles throughout the body, from head to toe. And wouldn't you know it, Dr. Friedman says that the person on top has an additional "advantage as far as exercise is concerned, since the pelvic and gluteal [buttocks] thrusting is unimpeded." For those who care about numbers, 200 calories are spent in 15 minutes of sexual activity, and for women who experience multiple orgasms, additional calories are burned up.

It is not uncommon for some postmenopausal women to complain of burning on urination shortly after intercourse, especially if the engagement extended for some time or if it was the first time after a period of abstinence. The burning may last for a couple of hours or as long as a couple of days. This condition comes from mechanical irritation of the urethra and the bladder, which is the result of the so-called "normal thrusting movement of the penis." In our discussions of this phenomenon, many women said they had found that by telling their partners not to penetrate too deeply, this condition was either greatly improved or avoided.

The lining of the vagina becomes thinner as we age, and we do not have the same thickness of interior skin that we once had. This seems to be related to our ability to absorb the mechanical irritation of active intercourse. The texture of the walls of the vagina changes, too, becoming smoother with less ridges, bumps and little points, and the color changes from deep pink to lighter pink. However, we have learned that dryness in the vagina changes, too. That is, some women experienced dryness occasionally but not necessarily always, and that it may come and go. Even though the vaginal cells are thin, there are many other factors involved in feeling discomfort or not. Women who engaged in regular masturbation as opposed to haphazard masturbation reported increased lubrication with a partner and the disappearance of vaginal pain due to dryness. Thinness of vaginal walls does not automatically mean pain during intercourse.

Lubrication is pertinent. Some of the women said that the way they felt about their partner affected the amount and speed in appearance of lubrication. The length and width of the vagina is reduced a little as we age, but it is amazing how elastic the vagina is. Women who do not have sex, which includes masturbation, lose more elasticity.

As we age, many sexual anatomic responses remain the same as they have always been. For example, uterine contractions continue during orgasm, and the nipples and the clitoris both erect and increase in diameter, but not all women continue to have increase in breast size during sexual stimulation. Those who do follow the pattern of their youth, with an increase in size of one quarter to one fifth. There is less tension during voluntary muscle contraction unless a woman has been regularly responding to sexual stimuli. Interestingly, over 50 percent of males also have vascular congestion in the nipples of their breasts during arousal, some erect fully, others partially.

Among other changes that occur is a lessening of automatic muscular tension during the orgasmic stage. This can be felt, for example, in the greater or lesser contraction of the rectal sphincter. The more intense the orgasmic response, the greater the contraction in the anus. The vaginal lips, the major and minor labia, lose fatty tissue as we age and eventually lose some, but not all, of their capacity for vascular congestion that causes the puffy, expanded feeling that makes it seem as though the entrance to the vaginal area has grown in size.

Uterine contractions during orgasm can be painful according to Masters and Johnson, but I did not have a single such report from any woman. Masters and Johnson say, "While these uterine contractions occur in women of all ages experiencing orgasmic response, younger women rarely have accompanying physical discomfort that reaches a level of clinical distress." Their recommendation for relief from this pain is estrogen and progesterone.

Their interest in ERT as a conjunct to female sexual capacity is as unfortunate as the terms they employ, such as "endocrine starvation" and "steroid starvation," which they say "has an indirect influence upon female sexual drive." They have clearly been proven to be unrelated. The sex hormonal level of women decreases after menopause, but the libido or sex drive increases in most women unless they suppress it.

THE WOMEN SPEAK

Sex generally brings problems and conflicts. The women who attended the workshops, as well as those I interviewed, talked about these situations. These women are feeling more in control of their lives than they did when they were younger. Since we're tired of people telling us what we're feeling when they don't know, it seems wise to listen to only the people who have had the experience. The following come from my notes and tapes and are selections of what the women are saying about sex. They know better than anyone else and can certainly speak for themselves, sometimes quite poetically, when asked. I asked, and this is a sample of what I heard.

Toni, 46: I want to be alive and creative, and the only way I have been able to be that is when I have been having regular sex. I hate myself because I'm dependent on it. I've got to learn not to be and be alive and creative by myself for myself.

Julia, 64: He comes over twice a week, and he's been doing that for 28 years; it's always a party. Our sex keeps expanding into new areas. I couldn't stand to have him around all the time.

Sherry, 42: My sex drive only emerges when there is someone there to stimulate it.

Elaine, 54: I thought I was dead forever that way until I met Tom, [38], and I was surprised how alive I was.

Claudine, 57: After a few tries with people I didn't really like and finding it painful in every way, I decided it wasn't worth it. But if I liked a person, I'd give it another try.

Esther, 49: I haven't had sex with anyone for a few years because I haven't come across anyone I liked, but if I did I would suggest it even though I never have before.

Dorothy, 48: I just never got over my embarrassment about being older even though I loved the sex. I think that's why I stopped seeing him.

Ethel, 50: When a big man with a big dick is on top of me, his weight validates me; then I know I'm there.

Tracy, 47: Once I learned I had a clitoris, and what it was for, I became sexual. And that was only five years ago.

Hilary, 51: Since I started relating to other women sexually, sex has become a different story. It's freer. I can be myself without being afraid.

Jill, 53: When [the orgasm] is super, the special kind, I feel in touch with the whole cosmos. It's as if I'm floating in space and related to every woman all through time.

Bobbie, 52: My lover is five years younger than I am. It didn't seem to bother him, but it did me. I had to talk about it. He said, "I don't love your age, I love you, the whole person that you are, your enthusiasms and the way you move and enjoy sex and everything about you." It was a relief.

Eva, 36: The most annoying kind of lover is the one who thinks you've come because he has.

Gloria, 42: Soft warm breasts turn me on more than a cock does.

Gina, 47: I'm into oil massage—that's the biggest turn-on for me these days. I love hands all over my body and then concentrating on my genitals. My fantasy is to have more than one pair of hands doing it.

Patricia, 49: By calling things games we do a lot of kooky things. Like I'll pretend I'm not going to let him have any and he begs and makes promises. I love it. I never thought I could do such a thing. It sounds like cheap porn but it's enormously erotic.

Laurel, 50: Since I decided if I don't tell him, he may not know, I tell. Life is too short to waste wondering.

Sondra, 48: Five years ago I had a lover who was chairman of the board of directors of a big conglomerate, and his cock collapsed just as he attempted entry, every time. It became frustrating because he wouldn't go down on me, though he wanted me to go down on him, which I did. I got a kick out of the irony, his being such a big shot and all in the rest of his life, but he was no big shot with me. That's when I turned to women. At least I could do things with a woman and not end up hanging.

Daryl, 46: I love a lover at my breast. I love to hold and cradle the person I care for. There's something in the nurturing experience that's delicious. When I want it, you understand.

Matina, 43: I had a lover two years ago who was into S & M [sadism and masochism]. He tied me to the bed with my ex-husband's ties, my legs and arms to the posts. I was high and grooved with it then, but it taught me an important lesson. It was the peak of my masochism, and I realized I have been emotionally violated by men all my life. It was good because it lifted me right out of that place. Never will I let anyone hurt me again.

Audre, 57: "Come for me," he says. I could kill him. I come for myself.

Katie, 55: I used to get out of bed to turn the record over or to get some more wine, but I don't anymore. I tell my lover to do it. It only took me a hundred years to learn to do that.

Maud, 40: When I ask him if he's come, he's so surprised. I tell him I've been too busy following my own progress to be concerned about his. They get over the shock and settle down finally being pleased that you're into your own pleasure. It also relieves them that you can take care of yourself.

Elana, 58: I used to need plenty of time to get wet but that has changed. I enjoy the fact that practically as soon as I decide to masturbate or play with my lover, I'm all slippery and sticky.

Martha, 51: I've been reading about such a variety of things people do together, but I haven't got the courage to initiate them and my husband is so predictably boring. Maybe if he read those things too, he'd get some ideas. Since I've been coming here [to the workshops] I'm building up courage to give him the things to read, and let him find out how dull he is.

Karen, 46: This wonderful new lover looks at my vagina, explores my genitals, moves the folds of skin. It embarrasses me a little that someone could be that interested in how I look, but it excites me too.

Audrey, 41: Women are more gentle than men, and you don't have to massage their egos.

Deborah, 56: When I was younger, I used to feel that eventually we'll get used to each other, which meant I let him do what he wanted—but I don't anymore. The first encounter has got to count. I'm not living in the future but now, and I've developed my rap. I say, "Be gentle," at the start and I repeat the word "gentle." If they don't oblige, there's nothing to get used to, that's it for me.

Constance, 48: We start out with the vibrator on shoulders and legs, doing each other, then we get very relaxed but geared up too. It stretches the sex.

Eda, 46: When I very slowly caress a lover, man or woman, with only the very tips of my fingers, a thing I love to do, all over the whole body, it drives them wild. It's such a pleasurable and easy thing to do, I can't figure out why it's always news to people.

Phyllis, 44: One night we were kidding around, and my lover asked me, "What do you want?" He was already pleasing me so I reached for what I thought was a joke. "Kiss my left big toe." He did. It became extraordinarily exciting after the initial shock of his doing it. What amazing things our bodies are. I really got into it and sometimes we do that, kiss and suck each other's toes. It's a kick to find all the new places there are.

Caroline, 50: It's best when you sleep the night together because the second round is so much better. The initial hunger, so to speak, has been taken care of, and then you can be more sensual, take a lot of time. My orgasms are longer the second time around.

Inge, 62: I love to get up in the middle of the night and suck his cock gently and feel it grow in my mouth as he awakens. I also like to be quietly awakened by his sucking me. Yummy!

Caroline, 39: "Let me know what you like," I say, because I really want to tell them what I like. But I start it that way. Then I feel easy about saying, "Yes, I like that, too," or being specific about something else. I'm happy to give them what they want because I want to get what I want.

Suzanne, 42: I haven't met a man yet who didn't hop on too soon and off too soon.

Gabrielle, 52: I am only beginning to learn not to be afraid of my passion. I used to keep it hidden because I found it overwhelmed most lovers. Now, to hell with it. If they can't handle it, they can't get it. I'm not living fragments any more. I want to experience everything in life, especially my own sexuality to its fullest. Yes, I do have more than one regular lover.

Marin, 56: My new lover is an engineer, so I typed a page of what and how I like because I was feeling like a nag always reminding him exactly *how* I want it.

Ella, 54: They don't listen. They have to listen with their bodies, as well as their ears. There is a whole language of sex men are not sensitized to. When I move his hand one quarter of an inch lower or higher I am telling him something very important to me. Women listen to this language. That is why it is easier to make love with a woman.

Selma, 44: I love my nipples pinched and bitten.

Cary, 38: I like the whole palm on my nipples. I hate to have them tweaked or bitten.

Dale, 42: The fuckers don't remember what you tell them about how you prefer them to touch you. They just do their own Pavlovian thing they're used to.

Renee, 58: The trouble with most men in bed is they come at you too fast, instead of two people meeting there on equal ground, and they set the pace. I think I mind that more than anything. I want to set the rhythm of how to proceed and have to fight hard for that.

Susan, 56: My orgasms have changed over the years. From 42 to 52 they were much quieter; they were not so intense or as long as they were in my thirties. Around 52 they started building again. I think it may be because my masturbating fantasies have expanded and that has freed me in other ways.

Arlene, 37: I hate a silent fuck. Without the sounds it's almost like nothing's going on.

Sally, 52: I had a relationship for six years with a man I cared a lot for, and early in it, when I was enjoying him very much, I said, "I love your cock." Six years later, when we separated, he told me no one had ever said that to him before, and he valued it more than anything else.

Georgette, 46: I don't want to be celibate, but I'm tired of priming up their cocks and egos. I'd like to be with a woman, but it scares me. I might like it too much.

Rachel, 60: The difference beween being 60 and 30 is you *know* the orgasm is going to take over; you don't have to hope so or try to make it happen. You're sure.

Anna, 44: I find sucking and being sucked terribly exciting, especially the anal area because it symbolizes total acceptance of yourself and the other person. It makes everything about both of you acceptable.

Coleen, 50: I only had sex with another couple once. These friends were over and we were drinking and enjoying ourselves and it happened very naturally. It was a beautiful experience and freed me in a new way. I'm glad I had it. No, I don't care to repeat it, but if it should flow from a pleasant evening again, I wouldn't try to avoid it.

Gloria, 37: I hate it when a man puts his hand on the back of your neck and pushes you to go down on him. Why doesn't he ask, or say, "Would you mind," or "Please," or "I'd like that?" I love to do that, but I refuse if it isn't requested gently.

Pat, 38: I don't know how to tell my husband things I would like. It's weird, because I know him better than anyone else, but I'm afraid it'll hurt him if I suggest things. It might make him feel like I'm criticizing him, not that he can't use some.

Maggie, 49: Once I decided the rest of my life is for me, I was shocked how easy it became to get what I want. There's hardly a thing I can think of sexually that I want to experience that I can't. I'm amazed and wonder why it took me so long not to be afraid to ask.

Molly, 52: When I became 50 I realized I was too old to be a prostitute, not that I ever was one (except probably covertly), but like many American women (I discussed this with many friends at the time), I carried that fantasy in the back of my mind, in case the going ever got too rough. It was a shock to have to give up that fantasy, and it remained very much on my mind. The insanity of it, me, this middle-aged responsible mother.

I have a friend from my home town, from childhood, who comes to New York on business a few times a year and calls me. I went to his hotel room in midtown a few times, and one night, as I stood to flag a cab, I felt like a hooker, only not as smart. He got his, I didn't get satisfaction, and at least a call girl would have gotten paid. Where was I? Being a good kid again. It struck me as crazy. He'd pay someone else—why not me? I could use the dough. Besides, there must be an exchange in a relationship.

It took me a couple of years before I could build up the courage to act on this idea. In the meantime, when he called, we were friendly but didn't meet. When he was in last time and called to ask me to have a drink with him, I put my feelings to him, half as a joke. "How much do you give a call girl?" I asked. "A hundred dollars," he said, "and ten extra. Why, do you want me to give it to you?" he asked in surprise. "That's not enough," I said. What had I to lose? "You've liked me for over 35 years, you're comfortable with me, this is the way I see it." Being in business I knew he'd like me to itemize. "One hundred and ten dollars, plus fifty you'd spend if we went to dinner (which we never did) makes a hundred and sixty, and the balance is for some of the other times, that makes two bills." "You got a deal," he said.

I went to his hotel and felt very free. Everything was clear. I was neither coy nor wondering. I asked him to tell me what he wanted, and I gave it to him. It was much better than when I did the same thing for nothing. This time I knew what I was doing, what would happen, and I was in control. You see, even though he's a pig, I like him. It's complicated, because it's almost like incest.

Nancy, 46: My eyes are sensitive to sex. When I am releasing tension, my eyes tear. It's not crying, it's tearing. It happens after the climax when I keep getting the extra dividends.

Catherine, 48: I used to enjoy the special occasion kind of sex when I was with the same man—putting on a long, thin, black thing. But since the woman's movement I haven't been comfortable doing that. I'm ready for it again if I liked and trusted someone enough.

Jo, 50: I always tell my partner when I'm having an orgasm. I like to share it.

Joyce, 44: Sometimes I don't want him to know when I'm building up to a climax because I want it all for myself.

Ruth, 56: When the sex is super good, I get a feeling of numbness, especially in my face. It feels as if all my tensions evaporate. I become my unadulterated self.

Rita, 52: I love the smell of sex sweat when it's fresh. And I love the hot slippery sweat of both our bodies when the sweat matches. You know, some people sweat cold, and that's clammy. I don't like that kind.

Mary Ellen, 39: The most best [laughter] sex comes after a full night, and then the morning and then the afternoon again when I am so tired that I just let it happen without hardly doing anything. Then my body takes over and my head is out to lunch.

Carole, 51: Last year, for a few months, I had three lovers. That's the best situation to be in. One was an old friend from college who comes to town once a month, one was my regular man I was seeing a couple of times a week, and one was a dear woman who I've known for many years and we have lunch sometimes. I loved them all in different ways. They're still my friends, but I don't have sex with them anymore.

Lisa, 46: My dear friend was over and we were having a wonderfully intimate time talking and sex with women came up. Neither of us had tried it before and did. It was very sweet and lovely, and although we have never done it again I think it acted to make our friendship closer.

Alice, 49: I like to speak and be spoken to while enjoying sex. I don't mean conversations but talking about the action such as, "I'm enjoying your hand where it is" or "You're doing exactly what I like." It gets me more excited.

Jeanne, 55: I don't care if it's a man or a woman, the person has to be interesting to me first. Also I have to be able to trust the person before I would expose my vulnerability.

Genevieve, 59: There is such a fuss about orgasms today. Just to hold and snuggle is so delicious. If young people wouldn't worry so much, they would learn that things happen naturally if you just take it easy and let them.

Becky, 66: I never believed when I was 21 I could have such a good time with sex at my age. It never ceases to make me wonder that there can be so many new things to discover.

Henrietta, 41: The trouble with good sex is you keep wanting it. It's not that I'm not satisfied—that's the old nymphomaniac idea. I'm very satisfied, but after plenty of rest I want some more and it takes so much time. I have sex for at least an hour, usually more, about five times a week and this has been going on for four years. It's not only the time during the sex but the time I spend thinking about it.

June, 62: Oh, my second husband was big and powerful. He wanted it all the time, but he was so damned crude. I had to leave him.

Edna, 53: After 30 years with the same man, I wouldn't dare try another, but I've figured out how to make it—the sex—work. I think of someone else.

Yvette, 42: I have a few hairs on my nipples and never thought about it while I was married, but since my separation it worries me with a new lover.

Grace, 56: I apply the estrogen cream for a few days before I have a date and it [the vaginal walls] becomes soft and puffy. Then I know everything will be fine. It won't hurt.

Elaine, 49: My husband's always been a lousy lover, quick dick, you know. I can't wait for my menopause then I won't let him bother me anymore. What can I do? I envy the women who enjoy sex. I never did. Move out? I haven't any money.

Eleanor, 43: He goes down on me but I won't on him. I don't like him enough. But that's what I've got now. I'm not young anymore and am too tired to find another man.

Rose, 52: Something happens to my body after fucking that makes it feel so good. It's like everything's been shaken up and put back together better.

Selma, 47: My problem is I get the ritual mixed up with the romance. When a lover is coming, I get excited about the preparations too—the bath, the getting dressed, the cooking dinner. It all turns me on. I wonder if that is immature?

Judith, 46: My criteria for going to bed with someone have changed as I've gotten older. It's not romance I want, it's a reasonable human being who is gentle and considerate and who is interested in the things I'm interested in. They're not easy to find.

Marcia, 55: A concrete cock is like nothing else. When I haven't had one for a few months, oh, how I miss it.

Nellie, 44: I had one of the biggest thrills in my sexual life yesterday. Someone who had rejected me changed his mind and called me up. I was in bed with someone else at the time and did that feel good.

Beth, 38: I know I can go to bed with someone when it feels easy and comfortable. Those other feelings—like shy and self-conscious—get in the way. When it feels like that, I don't do it because then it doesn't work, and I avoid that. Saves me from a lot of rotten sex.

Lorraine, 54: Older men are better lovers because they know how to control coming. When they get it up, they know what to do with it.

Millie, 42: I wish there was some way to let men know that sweetness counts more than anything else.

Bess, 46: I've noticed that the times when I don't have regular sex, I put weight on.

Robin, 51: I love all the other things, but there is something about the vigorous thrusting, when my body gets numb, that really makes me feel like I've been fucked. I get mileage from that for a week.

Trudi, 39: I used to think coming has something to do with caring for a person. I find it does, only the person is me because I come so easily now that I've learned it's up to me and caring for someone else has nothing to do with it.

Kathy, 50: My new lover says, "Whatever you say," when I tell him something in bed. Why, why, didn't I have the sense to *say* for 30 years? A decent person is glad to know what you want.

Mae, 54: For 20 years, every morning when he got up, he wanted it. I didn't all the time and resented it a lot, but now that he's dead I miss it.

Dorothy, 46: I love using and hearing dirty words. It's such a turn-on. I've been doing it now for a year. I never dared before.

Ruth, 39: I used to think he gave me the orgasm and would get so frustrated when he'd change position. Now I know that isn't so. If he moves, I move him back.

Ellen, 56: I want somebody to be good and sweet, no macho shit. I couldn't hack that any more. If I can't get it good, I don't want it. And probably won't get it either.

Eudora, 45: It seems hopeless to me that I could encounter somebody as forceful as me.

Alma, 53: I need romance—and I'm afraid I'm not going to get it.

Bertha, 47: Sex would have to be part of a total relationship which would be more liberating than restricting. It wouldn't be without responsibility.

Muriel, 44: Yes, I'd like to have a relationship, but not a possessive one. I don't want to be circumscribed in any way.

Marion, 40: I can't accept sex for sex itself. I wish I could. Then sex would be satisfying and I wouldn't lay all the other things on it.

Tessie, 57: I'm most fearful of sex because if it doesn't work, the parting is full of guilt and conflicts and pain.

Bessie, 48: Sure I'd like a lover, but only if he wouldn't betray me emotionally and wouldn't try to make me feel inferior. If he would be considerate of me, if I could trust him.

Dorothy, 46: Since I stopped taking the birth control pills, I'm lubricating more and that has made the sex better.

Ida, 62: I married at 21 and was a virgin. My husband died last year, and after 40 years of regular sex with one man it is very strange to find yourself nonsexual. I guess I'll have to learn to masturbate.

Shirley, 50: When I don't have sex, it's like I'm not healthy. It's like my body isn't being fully utilized.

Marjory, 38: When the sex is good and when it's building, there's a soft melting feeling, as though my body is changing form.

Paula, 46: I feel freer now, and I want to live. I want to do a lot of the things I've heard about, to try them at least once.

Shirley, 50: It's strange, now that I'm plumper, I'm less ashamed of my body. I guess I've come to accept it more.

Geraldine, 45: My orgasms are different now that I'm older. The first one doesn't last as long as it used to, but the orgasm period lasts longer. I get more of the follow-up ones—they just keep coming every couple of minutes, sometimes five or six of the smaller ones.

Bessie, 63: Even though my genitals are thinner, when I have sex they get fatter than they ever did and that feeling remains longer.

Ellen, 51: Not worrying about getting pregnant—that did it for me, that turned everything around. The same sex is different, it's better.

Kate, 60: I hear so much about the problem of lubrication, but since I'm enjoying sex more and having it more I'm lubricating more.

Lucy, 47: Since I learned to masturbate it liberated my sex with my husband because I'm no longer worried about going after the orgasm. I know I can always get it and I do, without trying anymore.

Emma, 49: I used to have big orgasms. You know, "shooting sky-rockets" kind. They're not like that anymore, but they are not less delicious, they're gentler. I don't know how to describe it because they have plenty of power.

Maxine, 50: I've always been sexual and have masturbated as long as I can remember, so I never thought I'd stop being sexual at menopause.

Tillie, 52: My desire is clearer to me. I never wonder *should I or shouldn't I* anymore, I always know that now.

Nell, 44: My sex is a more beautiful part of my life now because that's the way I want it to be. I finally learned I can call the tune, too.

Louise, 51: It took me until I was 49 to be able to ask for a finger in my anus—which I find very erotic.

Grace, 53: When I was 37 my vagina was dry with my husband, and I was worried about getting old. Since we separated I haven't had that problem.

Joy, 51: If I could only find the way to tell my daughters not to worry when they don't have lovers, not to move too fast when the hunger builds, because the rotten experiences are not worth the trouble, and the good experiences are easy and comfortable.

Lily, 48: I'm pissed at the fact that now that I'm more sexy my husband is less.

Joanna, 55: I get all mixed up with my old training to please the man, and my new thinking, please myself, and it gets in the way during sex. I've got to figure it all out better.

Diane, 38: Every man wants to put it in too soon. I tell them, "No, not yet, not until I let you know."

Mary, 49: When I care for somebody very much, when I am loving them, the orgasm is the closest I have ever come to a religious experience—the feeling of my engorged genitals surrounding his engorged penis so I don't know where I begin and end and can't separate him from myself and don't want to. The orgasm is like waves through my whole body. Then I feel I'm only middle, that my body has become five times enlarged from my waist to my knees. My eyes tear at that time, too. Then I need a lot of recovery time after that because it's as if I've been away on a journey.

Freda, 54: There are times when before and during coming I feel like a mountain and he is the sky, surrounding me and penetrating me.

Molly, 52: I know before it happens when it's going to be a block-buster because I can tell from the buildup. I suppose in a way I plan it, because I fix a special meal and light the candles. When we're eating dinner and I'm feeling very close to him, the feelings well up in me so that I can hardly eat. We take plenty of time and drag out the meal and listen to music and drink wine and smoke a little pot. Then when we do get in bed, after about an hour of loving each other, he enters me and there is no way I can describe that feeling, because even though I've known for hours it will happen, it still comes as an amazing shock. There is something about that initial entry that is so magical because it transforms me from being myself to becoming a whole circle. It's not that I lose myself, it's more like I've taken him into myself.

Isabel, 45: When I was younger, I couldn't just lie there and let him *do* me without feeling guilt, you know, just sheer enjoyment, but it is very easy for me now. I love it. He knows I love it from my breathing. My breathing turns him on.

Mary Jane, 51: I thought of a game two years ago and I play it often, as fun, fooling around. I tell my lover I want him to be my slave and then I will be his. I ask for what I want, and he asks for what he wants. We give it to each other, and because the idea is jocular we are freed from embarrassment.

Madeline, 44: At my age, if a man doesn't know what to do with a woman's clitoris, I don't want to know him, let alone fuck him. Pity you can't find out unless you try him out.

Leah, 42: If they don't make sounds to let me know they're coming, I don't know it; they think because they feel it I do. I don't.

*What comes out is what I feel . . . I have to
change a tune to my own way of doing it.*
                                    Billie Holiday

13
Our Hormones

Our bodies have many kinds of hormones, and they are all related to each other. Even though these sex hormones, estrogen and testosterone, are decidedly female and male and are responsible for our secondary sex characteristics, everyone has some of each hormone. Nature put a balancing agent in all of us.

The word *hormone* means to urge or arouse or set in motion. Although Hippocrates used the word in the fourth century, it wasn't until early in this century that the word came to be used commonly in medical circles to denote the then newly discovered inner body secretions. They are substances produced by a gland that affects another part of the body. Hormones are secreted by the endocrine glands. One of the first hormones understood was thyroid, produced by the thyroid gland. It was initially extracted from animal sources for treatment of human metabolic illnesses. Then came the discovery of insulin, the hormone secreted from the islets of the pancreas that regulates the way the body handles sugar. This knowledge made the treatment and control of diabetes possible. Cortisone, discovered later, is one of the hormones produced by the adrenal glands.

The sex hormones are classed in a group sometimes called sex steroids or steroid hormones. There are more than a hundred of them, but we are mostly concerned with estrogen, progesterone, and androgen (testosterone).

It is no wonder we are always searching for harmony in our lives: we come by it naturally, for our bodies are constantly working to maintain a healthy balance. Dr. Katharina Dalton, the British authority on female hormones, says, "There is not a day in a woman's life when she is not subject to the ebb and flow of these hormones." She is not making a judgment, merely stating a fact which we accept; we neither embrace it nor hide from it. The old cliche, "You can have too much of a good thing," absolutely applies to our bodies. For example, too much estrogen or too much cortisone could cause our body enormous stress as it tries to regulate itself.

The sex hormones are manufactured mostly in the gonads—ovaries in women and testes in men—until menopause, when their production increases in the adrenal glands and in what is sometimes called an unidentified or extraglandular source. This third supplier seems to be diffused through many parts of the body because the fat in the body makes estrogen, too.

I want to make it absolutely clear: our bodies do not suddenly stop producing estrogen, our chief female hormone. When the ovaries are surgically removed, it takes the other sources a little time to learn their new jobs. The long and gradual slowing down process has been going on in our ovaries since our middle twenties. Anyone who tells us our "ovaries fail" at menopause does not know what he is talking about. Fail to do what? Fail to respond to the pituitary? Fail to make babies? Is it a failure if ovaries are 50 years old instead of 25? No one has yet found out if the ovaries stop producing estrogen entirely and if they do stop, when that is.

The imbalance that some of us feel at menopause is because the body is trying to regulate itself while it finds the new level of decreased estrogen output from the ovaries. In its miraculous way of balancing itself, our body manufactures more estrogen in the adrenals and the extraglandular source. I repeat, our ovaries do not stop producing estrogen—as many of us have been incorrectly told. They do not release eggs anymore because we no longer have any, but that does not mean the ovaries die. The ovaries continue to make some estrogen. In fact, there are healthy women in their seventies and eighties whose urine shows their bodies manufacture estrogen, but the source has not been clearly identified.

We are born with half a million unripened eggs, and each time we ovulate an egg is released from an ovary. In a menstruating lifetime, we discharge about 400 mature eggs—the others have gradually been disintegrating all along—and then we no longer ovulate. Our ovaries, like other parts of our body (the brain, for instance) get smaller as we age. Our bodies are not suddenly deprived of estrogen as some would have us believe. Rather, the lesser amount produced by the ovaries is the natural, normal way for our bodies to function at an age when we are no longer desirous of bearing children. To change that by supplying estrogen from the outside is to disrupt our natural process, for all the endocrine glands in the body are interrelated. The healthy functioning of one depends on all the others.

Women who take the combination estrogen and progesterone may continue to menstruate beyond their natural stopping point, but it is a useless, artificial bleeding. It fills no natural function since there are no eggs and we are infertile. The disquieting side effects such as sore or tender breasts, weight gain, nausea, vomiting, breakthrough bleeding, bloating, cramps, increased cervical secretions, and nervous tension are not the effects that are advertised.

Since we are all individual, no one knows the correct doses. Therefore each woman forms a one-of-a-kind experiment. Moreover, taking these hormones is dangerous because it causes the body to become sluggish about producing its own estrogen, because once the hormone is brought into the bloodstream from an outside source, why would the body have to work to produce it?

The *Merck Manual of Diagnosis and Therapy* warns that "it is important to remember the limitations of endocrine therapy. Hormones merely alter the rate of existing biochemical reactions being superimposed on other, fixed-rate regulating factors." Which means that fooling with hormones is pretty tricky business. They say, "Because of the interdependence of the endocrine glands, administration of hormonal substances of a particular gland may not only produce their primary replacement effect, but also secondarily stimulate or depress other endocrine glands."

Estrogens must be broken down in the body. That is the job of the liver, which must create a specific agent for that purpose. Estrogen also stimulates fibroids to grow. That is why doctors usually postpone operations to remove fibroids in women past 35, whose natural level of ovarian estrogen will decrease and diminish the fibroids along with it.

While we were menstruating, the ovaries also produced the hormone progesterone during the second half of the menstrual cycle. Progesterone has two functions in the body. First, it builds up the lining of the uterus, creating an engorged preparation for the fertilized egg, which no longer applies to menopausal women. Second, it forms a base from which other adrenal hormones are manufactured. It is the lack of progesterone in the body which is responsible for the end of menstrual periods.

Some women during menopause have quite a bit of estrogen in their bodies but very little progesterone, which is the reason they have the uncomfortable feeling of heavy and sore breasts and water retention for many days. This feels like premenstrual symptoms, which were swiftly and dramatically relieved at the onset of full menstruation. But when there is not enough progesterone to create the sloughing off of the lining of the uterus, the condition can sometimes persist for over a week at a time. I have discovered, from talking to such women, that this is particularly so among dark-skinned, large-breasted women. However, I have not seen this phenomenon much noted in my reading.

Our adrenal glands are miraculous, for they secrete more than 40 substances in addition to their main function of supplying adrenalin. Some of these substances are hormones and others are precursors, the building blocks of hormones. Adrenalin is also the hormone which is involved with our defense mechanisms of flight, fight, and fear. The menopausal woman's adrenals are also supplying more estrogen than they once did. The outside part of the adrenals produce many hormones known as *corticosteroids,* which control the body's water and salt regulation, the sugar metabolism, the natural defense mechanisms against disease, injury, and stress and are also partially responsible for the secondary sex characteristics. Aldosterone is the corticosteroid hormone which regulates the water and salt content in the body. Water retention, for example, is a result of the body producing excess aldosterone or not enough aldosterone-antagonist.

Hormones are a crucial factor in regulating body chemistry, for the hormones maintain a most intricate interrelationship, both in the amounts circulating in the blood at any one time and in their actions on the body's metabolism. London University's Dr. John Yudkin says, "It seems to be always true that an increase in the amount of one hormone results in an increase or a decrease of several of the other hormones." In his book *Sweet and Dangerous,* he warns against the effect man-refined sugar can produce on the hormones. For example, it can cause "a striking increase in the level of adrenal cortical hormone." One of the first questions I always ask a woman who tells me about her hot flashes is "Do you eat much sugar?" Sugar is all around us and often added to foods where one would hardly expect to find it. Women who do not eat man-refined sugar seem to have fewer and milder flashes. "A high sugar diet can slow the rate of transport of hormonal chemicals by as much as two-thirds *even in one week.*"

It has been proven for many years that women's sex drive is unrelated to our estrogen supply, contrary to the very old propaganda that the amount of estrogen our ovaries release is in direct proportion to our sex drive. It has been established that most women around 50 are more sexual than they have been, even though they are manufacturing less sex hormones in the ovaries. Middle-aged men are also making less hormones in their testes, but while most middle-aged men's sex drive lessens, women's increases.

Doctors disagree as to the cause of our symptoms. Many think it is "the disturbance of the equilibrium between the hypothalamus and autonomic nervous systems." A standard textbook, *Obstetrics and Gynecology* by J. R. Willson, *et al,* does not describe flashes and sweats as coming from decreased estrogen but "rather, to some unknown factors operating to produce vasomotor symptoms. One of these might be the hyperactivity of other glands involved in the endocrine upheaval of the climacteric." I favor this position, because that would explain women getting hot flashes 10 and 20 years past menopause when they are in stress situations. Such flashes are not likely to be due to fluctuating hormones, for the level of estrogen has long become relatively stabilized.

IT IS NOT ONLY ESTROGEN

I have been feeling for some time that entirely too much emphasis has been placed on the estrogen level, for the more I read about the endocrine system the more I began to see how important the interrelationship of the whole glandular system is. It is difficult for me to understand how trained physicians have for years oversimplified and overemphasized estrogen at the same time.

Some writers refer to how our hormones work by comparing them to an orchestra. The pituitary is the conductor or the leader who directs the players (the other glands) to play louder or softer or perhaps remain quiet for a while, depending on what is needed by the body to function smoothly. However, the pituitary or leader of the band is in turn also affected by what the other glands (the members of the orchestra) have been doing (or playing).

Let me carry this a little further if I may, because it is important. Take the Duke Ellington orchestra, the best example we have of improvisation and change while still keeping its own particular identity. The personality of that group, like our body, is recognizable, but it is always changing. It has always amazed me how the band would play their standard tunes like "Satin Doll" and "Caravan" yet they were always different. That is because the leader, like our pituitary, is responding to elements in the environment. So do our bodies, too, respond to the environment, not only to the glands alone but to outside influences such as stress.

To carry the metaphor further (thank you for your indulgence), when the orchestra is playing and it is time for Johnny Hodges to take his solo on the alto saxophone (estrogen) he might just need more time to express his idea. In that case, Ellington (the pituitary) has to change something, perhaps even deprive another player of time for his solo in order to get the whole tune to end in the allotted time. Why Duke Ellington is such a perfect example of the pituitary is that he listened to the other players (the organs—no musical pun), and related the feedback he got from them to how he, the leader, would proceed. The pituitary respects what the other glands have to do, even to the point of letting them have the space to blow a little extra if need be. Then it jumps in quickly to correct the situation so it all comes out to be "your sound," even if it's a little different this year from last year. It is still your music, your glands, your personality.

Behind the pituitary, there is another even greater power called the hypothalamus, which is situated at the base of the brain and which controls many vital life processes. It is the trigger that causes the pituitary to go through its number as leader of the orchestra. The nerves emanating from the hypothalamus are known as the autonomic nervous system.

Sometimes the music gets mixed up and we have cacophony, which is what hot flashes and sweats are all about. During our fertile years, the pituitary gland and the ovaries worked together to maintain a delicate balance. By menopause, the ovaries have done their hard work and don't respond to the pituitary the way they used to. Therefore the signals from the pituitary are not carried out smoothly by the glands. For example, as the ovaries slow down in their production of estrogen, the pituitary frequently doesn't get the message and keeps ordering the ovary to produce hormones, but the ovary is not responding to those directions. Until the pituitary gets the message not to make that demand on the ovary, the glandular balance is upset while the adjustment is made. Unless we're anesthetized or out of touch with our bodies, we will feel this activity. It may or may not create discomfort. One may even view menopausal symptoms as due to too much pituitary hormones.

The hypothalamus is vital in contributing to our feeling comfortable, as well as being responsible for keeping our bodies in a healthy balance. The work of the hypothalamus is believed to be one of the most important aspects of aging in women. Even though it is part of the brain, it is most often referred to as itself. It is connected by nerve routes to the cerebral cortex on one side and to the pituitary gland on the other side. It is so important to us because it is related to many areas of our life such as our sex drive, sleep, and appetite, as well as body temperature.

EXTRAGLANDULAR ESTROGEN

The unidentified estrogen source in the menopausal and postmenopausal woman is extremely important in proving that the propaganda we have been fed—that we are "steroid starved," suffering from "estrogen starvation" or "hormonal deprivation" or "hormonal deficiency"—is a lot of nonsense. Those ideas have served women in the true American tradition of selling us something we don't need: estrogen replacement.

I have had the feeling all along that women do not fall apart when they stop menstruating because their estrogen is "cut off." I knew there was estrogen in our bodies. I also knew there must be sane doctors who are closer to my feelings than the ones pushing estrogen for everything. And, among the sane ones, some must be checking it out in the laboratory. It saddens me that more doctors who seem to be concerned with menopause don't bother to take the time to ask healthy women what and how they are feeling in order to obtain a rounded picture.

My search for information became an adventure. I hunted hard and found that it has only recently been definitively discovered that the ovaries and the adrenals are not the only sources of estrogen in the body. Some distinguished researchers said, "Numerous studies in postmenopausal and oophorectomized [removed ovaries] women demonstrated that such individuals continue to excrete measurable amounts of urinary estrogens." If it comes out in the urine, it must be in the body. The authors of this statement, Dr. Pentti K. Siiteri and Dr. Paul C. MacDonald of the Departments of Biochemistry and Obstetrics and Gynecology at the University of Texas Southwestern Medical School in Dallas have been working for over 13 years on discovering where the estrogen comes from after menopause. The answer has become known: "The major source of estrogen in the postmenopausal female is peripheral formation of estrone,'' an estrogenic hormone converted from one of the male sex hormones in the blood and "not ovarian or adrenal secretion." It is called extraglandular estrogen and is responsible for the rise of estrogen in the urine after menopause. "The exact tissue site(s) in which this process occurs is presently unknown." Other researchers have also reported a steady rise in urinary estrogens following the menopause.

This third source of estrogen does not suddenly appear. It is functioning in the body before menopause and is at its peak production in the premenopausal woman during the time of menstruation. Say Siiteri and MacDonald,

In normal premenopausal women, the extraglandular production of estrone [one of the estrogenic hormones] from circulating androstenedione [a male sex hormone] at the extremes of the menstrual cycle may account for 50% or more of total estrogen production, whereas at midcycle, during the follicular surge in estradiol, another estrogenic hormone secretion by the ovary, extraglandular estrone may account for only 10% of total estrogen production.

This idea of a change within the body of one kind of sex hormone into a hormone of the other sex (how androgynous it makes us all) has been known since 1934 when the researcher Bernhardt Zondeck published his findings. He says, "I believe that the female hormone which is regularly present in the male organism represents a normal physiological product of the metabolism of sex hormones, especially since—due to our present chemical knowledge—a conversion of the male hormone into the female one appears to be quite possible." It is this conversion that takes place in the body which makes it understandable that males and females have characteristics of both sexes. In fact, it shatters the concept that more estrogen from outside sources makes for greater femininity because the natural estrogen produced during and after menopause is manufactured from our male hormone precursors.

"The increased incidence of human female breast and endometrial cancer after the menopause, at a time when estrogen production is assumed to be decreasing or to have ceased," states an editorial in the *New England Journal of Medicine,* "also confounds a cancer-inducing role for endogenous [created in the body] estrogens." This information presents a paradox, for it has been assumed that estrogen levels drop after menopause, yet here we have evidence of new production. The chief difference in estrogen production after menopause is that the major source of estrogen is no longer the ovaries but an extraglandular source. Also, there is no longer the old cyclicity of estrogen levels, and progesterone production is no longer necessary since we don't ovulate and are not preparing the womb for a possible pregnancy. Too much estrogen, whether it comes from one's own body or is taken from an outside source, seems to be the chief factor in causing diseases of the uterus, such as overgrowth of the lining of the uterus and postmenopausal uterine bleeding, because there is not the moderating and "perhaps protective effects of progesterone."

Dr. Saul B. Gusberg, chairman of the Department of Obstetrics and Gynecology at Mount Sinai School of Medicine of The City University of New York, has been working with the problems of estrogen overstimulation in women under conditions "where estrogen may be elevated for a prolonged period." His findings indicate that the association "of abnormal and elevated estrogens and abnormalities of the endometrium is very suggestive" of elevated estrogen levels being the cause of cancer.

Siiteri and MacDonald believe that unknown changes occurring during menopause and excessive weight may lead to increased extraglandular estrogen. The estrogens are produced in body fat from adrenal and ovarian male hormone precursors, which are forerunners of the material that makes the estrogen during the menopausal years. This clarifies where the estrogen comes from. "This peripheral estrogen production increases after the menopause, and the amount produced is proportional to body weight, paralleling the association of increased risk of endometrial cancer with age and obesity. In fact, increased conversion of androgen to estrone has been reported in patients with endometrial cancer."

Even though we do not have the ovarian cycle anymore, which gave a kind of regularity to our irregularity, the estrogen level has not become stabilized. "The postmenopause cannot be considered as a time of quiescence with respect to estrogen production." The mechanisms involved in this production of extraglandular estrogen are not static; therefore the output alters widely. The processes operating show a variety of metabolic patterns which influence the quantity of estrogen produced. These patterns are different from those involved with ovarian hormone production. The true physiological and pathophysiological roles of extraglandular estrogen production are yet to be defined.

There are tests that are supposed to be able to measure the amount of estrogen in a woman's blood, but they are not reliable. As we have learned, the estrogen level varies not only from day to day but from hour to hour. For example, stress from a job or from lack of sleep can change the estrogen level. We are, as I have stressed before, individual and unique and no amount of standardization is going to encompass all of us.

One test that has received quite a bit of attention is the vaginal cytogram, which measures estrogen function indirectly by measuring, as in a Pap smear, the percentage of cells in the vagina that show the effects of estrogenic stimulation. An estrogen deficiency is indicated if less than 10 percent of the vaginal cells show a "good" estrogenic effect. The vaginal cytogram is not an accurate guide to the need for treatment. Another test measures the levels of pituitary gonadotrophin in a 24-hour urine sample and is the common method used for diagnosing menopause.

The fact that the level of our hormones is normally variable is often used against us, although it is hardly a reliable guide to anything. When we hear pejorative terms like "raging hormones," the implication is that the man using the phrase is always as calm as a cucumber, as though only women's hormones have cycles. Men have fluctuating hormones, too, and also have cycles that influence them. Some guess that Thomas Jefferson's periodic migraine headaches and Abraham Lincoln's periodic depressions may have been related to their hormonal cycles. Dr. Estelle Ramey says, "The potential women leaders of this country have cycles, as all living things have to varying degrees, but women do not have the encouragement to mitigate and work around their cycles. Women's chains have been forged by men, not by anatomy."

*The modern era of steroid metabolic
technology has offered us new evidence of the
hormone sensitivity of cancer in target organs.*
Saul B. Gusberg, M.D.

14
Hormones and Cancer

Breast cancer is the No. 1 cause of cancer deaths among women in America. It's the leading cause of death for all women between the ages of 37 and 55. About 33,000 women died from it in 1976 and 89,000 new cases were diagnosed in that year. Over 225,000 women in America alone are walking around with "unexpressed breast cancer."

Cancer is essentially a wild, uncontrolled growth of abnormal cells. The most common forms of cancer for women are those of the breast, cervix, and uterus. They generally appear in women in their forties and fifties. Cancer authorities believe that most, if not all, cancers require years or even decades before an identifiable tumor appears. There is usually a long time, called a latent period, between the first existence of altered cells and the final development of a full-blown cancer.

Cancer of the breast is a malignant tumor that starts either in the milk glands or in the ducts that carry the milk to the nipple. The cancer tends to spread to the lymph nodes in the armpit and to the nodes behind the breast bone.

Until 1976, the evidence linking breast cancer to the use of post-menopausal estrogens had not been definitively established (although in 1975 data had been published clearly linking postmenopausal estrogens with uterine cancer). But in August 1976, a research report that left little doubt was published in the *New England Journal of Medicine.* The study, of 1,891 women in Louisville, Kentucky, who took estrogen drugs after menopause, indicates that in ten years or more after women begin using estrogens, the risk of developing breast cancer clearly increases. The study was conducted by medical researchers at Harvard University, the University of Louisville, and the National Cancer Institute. The authors say estrogens "raise this risk as a definite possibility, and indicate that a thorough evaluation is necessary." They do not show that estrogens cause breast cancer but that they do "raise this risk." The study found estrogen use was associated with 30 percent more breast cancer cases than expected, and 15 years after beginning estrogen therapy, breast cancers developed at twice the expected rate. The study suggests there is a somewhat lower risk among women who started taking the drug less than five years earlier. The risk started rising after five years, reaching twice the expected risk 15 or more years after the start of estrogen therapy. The findings also suggest the strength and schedule of the dose may be important factors.

Most of the women in the study received a small dose—0.3 and 0.625 milligrams daily. The usual daily dose prescribed in the United States is 1.25 or 2.5 milligrams. When the dose was larger or when it was used intermittently, the researchers concluded those women had a higher breast cancer risk.

When women have had children, there is a relative protection against breast cancer, but the authors of the Louisville study found that estrogen replacement therapy seemed to negate that natural protection. ERT also removes the protection from women who have had their ovaries removed before menopause.

Women who have benign breast diseases normally face twice the usual risk of developing breast cancer later. The researchers found, however, that if benign breast disease developed after starting ERT, the risk of getting breast cancer was seven times higher than average. However, there is good news in the fact that statistically the rate of increase in breast cancer declines after menopause.

Dr. Alan E. Nourse, explaining the connection between hormones and cancer, says:

The female hormones have no significant role in the first development of breast cancer, but they *can* actively influence the progress of the disease once it has actually started. It is known, for example, that the spread of breast cancer in certain patients can be slowed down remarkably by removing all sources of estrogen from the patient's body. Thus removal of the ovaries sometimes leads to prolonged improvement in a patient with advanced breast cancer. When the disease becomes active again, removal of the adrenal glands, another source of estrogens, sometimes helps. Still later, removal of the pituitary gland, the source of hormones that stimulate estrogen production elsewhere in the body, often proves helpful. Similar temporary improvement sometimes occurs when the patient is treated with androgens—male sex hormones—which seem capable of neutralizing or blocking estrogen activity.

However, this is by no means a cure for breast cancer; rather it is a desperate attempt to slow the spread of the disease for a few months or years.

Other evidence exists linking estrogen and breast cancer. Cases of cancer of the breast have developed among men given estrogen for prostate cancer. At the major conference held on menopause in 1971 it was reported that it occurred in "men treated with estrogens for prostatic carcinoma, in transexuals given estrogens and in Bantu men with gynecomastia" (breast development). Since the occurrence of breast cancer in men is normally very low, it is highly suggestive that the development is the result of the estrogen.

In case you are using or have used estrogen and wonder about its composition, you may be interested to know that it is prescribed sometimes by itself, or in combination with progesterone, testosterone (a male sex hormone), Miltown, vitamins, or methamphetamine (speed). It may come as a tablet, capsule, or liquid; the latter may contain alcohol.

The Breast Cancer Profile below is a guideline adapted from a report by Dr. H. P. Leis, Jr., of New York Medical College. His study determined that women in the following categories run a greater risk of developing breast cancer than women in general.

If you are the daughter of a breast cancer victim, you run twice the risk.

If you are a sister of a victim, you run two-and-a-half times the risk.

If you are infertile, you run one-and-a-half times the risk of a fertile woman.

If your first full-term pregnancy came after 25, you run twice the risk of women who got pregnant sooner; after 31, three times the risk of women pregnant before they were 21.

If you began menstruating very early and have been menstruating for a long time, you run twice the risk.

If you have been taking the drug reserpine for hypertension, you may be running two to three times the risk.

Your risk is also somewhat greater if you eat large amounts of fat, have earwax that's wet rather than dry, have a hypothyroid (underfunctioning thyroid) condition, live in a cold climate, or have a relatively high socioeconomic status.

One wonders about the previous studies of the possible relationship between breast cancer and estrogen compounds. Dr. Robert N. Hoover, head of the environmental studies section of the National Cancer Institute, discounts them, for he notes that previous studies were "meaningless because they had been used to show that the substances protected women who took them from breast cancer."

Birth control pills also contain estrogen hormones, but there is no known association between the use of the pill and breast cancer, yet. Up to this time, some studies have suggested that "the pill" may protect against this disease. However, we have heard this before when we were reassured there was no possible cancer risk for menopausal and postmenopausal women who took estrogen. Unfortunately, time is a necessary requirement before cancer shows up.

As much as 15 or 20 years may elapse between the first appearance of abnormal cells in the cervix, which is sometimes called the neck or the mouth of the uterus where it joins the vagina, and the point at which a fully developed cancer begins to invade deeper layers of cells. Cancer of the cervix is one of the easiest to detect early with the aid of Pap smears.

The sharp rise in uterine cancer in women who were taking estrogen replacement therapy was reported in two studies published in the *New England Journal of Medicine* in December 1975. The studies showed that ERT is associated with an increase of 5 to 14 times in a woman's chances of developing cancer of the endometrium, the lining of the uterus. It was the first time definitive studies that clearly linked estrogen with cancer were published and subsequent studies have confirmed that link. Before that "there had been no carefully conducted studies comparing estrogen use among patients with endometrial cancer and controls."

Cancer of the uterus, as distinguished from cancer of the cervix, involves the endometrium, the glands that line the uterus. It is known as either uterine cancer or endometrial cancer and consists of a tumor arising in a hormone-sensitive tissue. It struck 27,000 American women in 1975, killing 3,300 of them.

In the two studies, patients with endometrial cancer were matched with similar groups of women without that cancer or with another kind of cancer. The different groups were then examined for prior use of menopausal estrogens. One of the studies, conducted in Los Angeles by Drs. Harry K. Ziel and William D. Finkle, investigated 282 women patients at the Kaiser Permanente Medical Center. Endometrial cancer was diagnosed in 94 of these women. They were then compared with control subjects who belonged to the same health plan and also matched for age and residential area with two women who were cancer-free. The researchers found "that the incidence rate of the development of endometrial cancer for women at risk (those with an intact uterus) has increased dramatically during the past decade." They use the term "intact uterus" because one cannot develop cancer of the uterus if it has been surgically removed.

It is interesting to note that recent national survey data show continued increase in the rate of hysterectomy. By 1968, the rate of hysterectomy performed on American women by the age of 60 years was 31 percent. One shudders at the thought of how many of those were unnecessary. I have discussed with various women the appalling choice they have been offered for treatment of excessive bleeding (one symptom of possible uterine cancer). It was a choice between two vastly different operations: one doctor recommending a simple D & C (dilation and curettage, which is scraping of the uterine lining), the other doctor suggesting a hysterectomy.

Hysterectomies are taken all too lightly by some doctors. In 1975, an estimated 1,700 died of the 787,000 women who had hysterectomies, according to figures from the Commission on Professional and Hospital Activities, a nonprofit research organization sponsored by professional medical groups. Yet, according to Jane Brody, medical writer for the *New York Times,* "studies have indicated this operation is often done when more conservative and less dangerous treatments could have produced the desired result. . . . Some doctors have been accused by others in the profession of performing 'hip-pocket hysterectomies,' where the only beneficiary is the doctor's wallet. In England and Wales where doctors are salaried, the rate of hysterectomies is only 40% that of the United States, where most surgeons are paid by the operation."

A hysterectomy is a surgical operation which removes the uterus either through the abdominal wall or through the vagina. It is a "total" or "complete" hysterectomy when the cervix is also removed. A hysterectomy by itself does not create menopausal symptoms other than the end of periods. It is the ovaries which are the key. If they are left intact, if even a part of one remains, the menopausal symptoms will show themselves at the same time they would appear without the surgery. *Oophorectomy* is the term used for the removal of the ovaries and it is when they, not the uterus, are removed that we get "surgical menopause." A woman whose uterus is removed is still making some estrogen from her ovaries, and if they are removed too, her adrenals and extraglandular source will both supply some.

But back to the Los Angeles study. It also indicated that women in whom endometrial cancer develops have a higher rate of conversion of the male hormone precursor to a higher level of estrone. Researchers confirmed the discovery that adipose (fat) tissue of patients with this cancer converted the male hormone precursor four times as fast as those subjects without cancer.

In the other study, Dr. Donald C. Smith and others at the University of Washington investigated 634 women patients, 48 years of age or older, in Seattle hospitals. Of these patients, 317 had endometrial cancer and the other 317 were controls, i.e., patients with other gynecological cancers. They found "the risk of endometrial cancer was 4.5 times greater among women exposed to estrogen therapy," as compared to those not receiving estrogen.

Because cancer of the cervix is becoming more controllable, endometrial cancer is moving into the predominant place, particularly as the life expectancy of women increases. Dr. Donald Austin, director of the California Tumor Registry, reported there was a 50 percent increase in the uterine cancer rate among women in the San Francisco Bay area between 1969 and 1973. The incidence of uterine cancer rose from 27.2 cases per 100,000 population to 41.4 in this five-year period. A similar trend was reported by researchers at the Los Angeles County–University of Southern California Medical Center. Dr. Austin said that the Connecticut Tumor Registry has reported a similar increase during the same period.

The rising incidence of uterine cancer coincides with the increases in sales of estrogen pills, which have more than quadrupled since 1962. As reported in the two articles in the *New England Journal of Medicine* in December 1975, the risk of endometrial cancer increased 5 to 14 times in women who took estrogen into the body from the outside, as in ERT. This information is important because of the large number of estrogen users in the country. "A recent survey in western Washington showed 51% of postmenopausal women had used estrogens."

It was pointed out by Dr. Austin that the increase of uterine cancer has been most notable among affluent white women over the age of 50; these are the women more likely to take estrogen. The point was underlined by Dr. Kenneth J. Ryan, who wrote in an editorial in the *New England Journal of Medicine*, "Racial and environmental factors . . . are also clearly associated with cancer occurrence. For example, cancers of the breast and endometrium have a higher incidence in the white than in the black" woman. The National Cancer Institute statistics show, however, that the rate for the black population has been rising since 1950, which is coincident with the steady migration to the northern cities. Dr. Smith reported that "patients with cervical cancer tend to be of a lower socioeconomic class than those with endometrial cancer and may therefore be less likely to be given estrogens." The disease is related to the habits of the affluent, for in the developing countries such as Asia, Africa, and South America, its occurrence is very low by comparison.

Other experts who acknowledge the use of estrogen as a crucial factor in the rise of uterine cancer think that other elements have also contributed to the rise in reported incidence. They include an increase in detection of the disease and dietary factors, particularly a trend toward more animal fats in the diet. It is interesting that "as the Japanese have adopted a Western-type, high protein, high animal-fat diet," their rate of endometrial cancer has increased. Also, in Israel, the Israelis of European origin have a Western pattern of cancer, which is high in uterine and breast cancer but low in cervical cancer, but the Israelis who are "of African origin have a so-called 'Oriental' mode" with the opposite distribution.

Evidence seems to point to animal fat and the Western diet as being a significant contributor to the developmental causes of endometrial cancer. It has been proven in other contexts that nutritional factors do impinge on the endocrine system.

Other factors, too, indicate a greater risk of endometrial cancer. The following ranges of risk have been specifically reported in the literature: hypertension (30-56 percent); obesity (28-63 percent); diabetes (9-32 percent); and nulliparity (never giving birth) (19-41 percent). Other high risk characteristics are tallness, infertility, failure of ovulation, and dysfunctional bleeding of the menopause. In addition, the incidence of endometrial cancer increases with age.

"Dr. Saul B. Gusberg has suspected this cancer association with the endometrium and breasts for 20 years." That is why his position has always been what was considered the conservative view in regard to estrogen replacement therapy. I have noticed, too, in the menopause literature, the language differs between those I call "the good guys" who are not patronizing toward women and the others, who are. They seem to go together: insulting language and estrogen pushers; respect for women and great caution with the prescribing of estrogen.

Cells must grow rapidly if cancer is produced, which makes it reasonable that the hormones (estrogens) responsible for the growth of endometrial cells should be involved in some way with the beginning of endometrial cancer. A substantial body of data exists indicating that the high levels of estrogens produced naturally in a woman's body, particularly estrone, which is one of the estrogenic hormones, predispose a woman to endometrial cancer. It now seems that a number of the risk factors for the disease can be explained on this basis, according to Dr. Gusberg.

Although comparisons are odious, they help one grasp the magnitude of the risk and put it into some sort of perspective. There is a 3- to 9-time increase in the risk of endometrial cancer in association with obesity alone, and a 17-time increase in the risk of death from lung cancer in those who smoke 20 cigarettes a day. In other words, the risks from taking estrogen can be compared to the risks that come from overeating or smoking.

If you are taking estrogen, it is a good idea to have an endometrial biopsy every six months. This test can be done in a doctor's office, although they are very new and not yet as common as the Pap test. Endometrial cancer can be detected in about two-thirds of the cases by the Pap smear. Another test, the Gravelee test, is considered more accurate because it directly washes out cells from inside the uterus. The most common symptom of the disease is vaginal bleeding after menopause. Early cases, the authorities say, are highly curable by surgery and radiotherapy.

Dr. Saul Gusberg, in discussing a strategy for the control of endometrial cancer before the Royal Society of Medicine in London, said, "Further consideration leads one to the speculation that dietary influence may play a role . . . for here nutritional status is significant and it impinges upon the endocrine system." For 25 years, Carlton Fredericks has been suggesting a dietary antidote for the cancer-producing potential of estrogen, both for birth control pill users and for menopausal and postmenopausal users. He recommends "copious intake of vitamin B complex, high in choline and inositol, and generous intake of high quality protein to aid the liver in changing the female hormone into a less active, and thereby less threatening form." His position is that this will help women in their resistance to the common diseases of endometrial and breast cancer.

In his presentation to the Royal Society of Medicine, Dr. Gusberg also reported on a new system of diagnosing endometrial cancer precursors that he is involved with at Mount Sinai Hospital in New York: "Our group has reported the accuracy of aspiration curettage and we believe that, since it does not require anesthesia it should be used as a histologic [tissue structure] screening measure for all high-risk women at the menopause, and perhaps when we gain more experience we shall apply it to all menopausal women."

Perhaps this test will eventually be used popularly to detect and control cancer of the lining of the uterus in the way the Pap test is used to detect cervical cancer. The aspiration method is similar in technique to the one used for early abortions by suction.

Women themselves are still their own best protection against a fatal breast cancer, since they can regularly check for suspicious lumps through self-examination of their breasts. Equally important is the next step: to report any new lumps to your doctor. Over 90 percent of diagnosed breast cancers are found by women, not doctors. So in addition to your regular monthly breast exam, it is important to feel your breasts when you are taking a shower or a bath or before going to bed, because to become intimate with your own individual conformation is the best and easiest way to become aware of any change.

New controversy has developed over the advisability of regular yearly mammography (x-raying of the breasts) exams, which has been referred to as "cancer's catch-22," because it could itself be a cause of cancer from radiation exposure. Dr. Irwin Bross, one of the world's leading authorities on radiation effects, noted that the unstructured use of this exam could produce "one of the worst iatrogenic [doctor-caused] disasters in medical history."

There is strong opinion against the use of mammography as a diagnostic tool. Dr. C. D. Haagensen, dean of American cancer surgeons, says, "I warn women to have mammograms only under special circumstances when clinical diagnosis is in doubt." He believes, basically, that cancer must be clinically diagnosed. "It depends on the doctor's observations," he says, "combined with the results of a biopsy [removal and microscopic examination of a small amount of breast tissue], which must be performed when certain symptoms, such as a dominant tumor, retraction of the nipple, etc., are present."

Most lumps are benign; indeed, close to 90 percent of those biopsied are. Before any treatment decision is made, biopsy should be performed and the result carefully explained. General anesthesia is not always necessary for a biopsy. Radical mastectomy (removal of the breast and overlying skin, the two big muscles of the chest wall, and all of the fatty tissue and lymph nodes in the armpit) is not the only treatment for breast cancer and has yet to be proven better than other treatments. Breast cancers are not all alike, and they call for individual treatments. Increasingly, combined treatments (surgery, radiation, and chemotherapy) are used. Whenever removal of a breast or uterus is recommended, it's vital to seek a second opinion from another specialist, preferably one affiliated with a different hospital than that of your first doctor.

If you can, and this is very important, have a good friend go along with you when you are being examined. Ask the doctor if your friend may come into the examining room with you, for when you discuss it later, she will be able to remember details that you may forget. It is also important, if you can work it out, to have the same friend go along for the second opinion, too. This is a time when we need support. Remember, you have a legal right to be told all the advantages and disadvantages of any treatment recommended. This is what you are paying for. You are not a cancer specialist, so don't worry about seeming dumb. Ask all the questions you can think of, as well as any that your friend can think of. In this way, you will not feel helpless, for you will have more information to help you with your decision. There are alternatives and you have a right to be told the known outcomes and what the risks may be, including the results, should you decide not to have any treatment at all. It is your right to refuse treatment or any part of the procedure at any time.

Doctors and nurses are used to their daily job but you are not used to being examined for cancer. Therefore, insist—with your friend at your side helping you—on learning the details. It is difficult, I know, for the situation is altogether full of stress, but keep uppermost in your mind that what is routine for the medical staff is extraordinary for you, and it's your body. You have a right to know.

FDA: BEST FRIEND TO THE ESTROGEN MANUFACTURERS?

The real danger of estrogen replacement therapy has been made clear by studies which have shown that the risk of cancer increases with use of ERT. The Food and Drug Administration (FDA) is the government agency to step in and take effective action. However, the FDA seems to be more sympathetic to the drug companies which manufacture estrogen than to the female citizens who take it. The fact is, the information was in the hands of the FDA before the studies were even published, but the agency didn't seem to want to move the red tape fast enough to put teeth into a constructive plan. However, many concerned citizens have begun to place pressure on the FDA. In January of 1976, Senator Edward M. Kennedy of Massachusetts, chairman of the Senate Subcommittee on Health, held hearings on the subject. When questioned, Commissioner Alexander M. Schmidt of the FDA told the committee that he believed there was "very strong" evidence linking the estrogen compounds prescribed for millions of postmenopausal women to cases of cancer of the lining of the uterus.

These hearings were held less than a month after an advisory committee recommended to the FDA that the use of estrogen compounds in the treatment of the symptoms and aftereffects of menopause be strictly limited. The recommendation was based on the findings published in December 1975 in the *New England Journal of Medicine.*

Dr. Schmidt, when questioned, acknowledged that the broad use of estrogen to ward off the effects of aging stems largely from "massive promotion and advertising" by Ayerst Laboratories. This is contrary to the ethical code of the Pharmaceutical Manufacturers Association. This association has known what Ayerst has been doing. Senator Kennedy requested that Dr. Schmidt evaluate the recent new studies. His reply: "We think the evidence is very strong that there are casualties. There must be more research, and there will be. But the evidence is strong enough now for us to be on guard against the over-use, misuse and casual use of these substances." A million and a half American women go through the menopause each year, estimated Dr. Schmidt, whereas the figures on the sale of estrogen indicate that at least five million women are receiving it. He considered this a "misuse" of the drug.

Now I ask you, if he considers the drug "misused" and the evidence "strong enough," why do we have to wait for more research before effective action is taken by the authorities? Despite the fact that many women and their doctors have been correctly frightened by the news and are not using estrogen anymore, plenty is still being prescribed, according to Jane Brody of the *New York Times.* I have heard women who are "hooked" on it say, "It hasn't hurt me yet," or "I don't have cancer."

When the executive vice president for scientific affairs for Ayerst Laboratories, C. J. Cavalitto, appeared at the hearings, he said, "We are not convinced that there is a cause-and-effect relationship" between Premarin and cancer of the lining of the uterus. Another company official defended the company's promotion of the drug as completely proper and said, when that question came up, that there "probably" may be some overprescribing of the drug.

The pressure against the FDA is mounting. When television conducts spontaneous and unrehearsed news interviews, they are truly using the medium to serve the public. In December 1975, "Face the Nation" had Dr. Schmidt as their guest, and the reporters did not mince words. Lesley Stahl of CBS News accused the FDA of being "charged with acting to please the drug industry instead of fulfilling its mandate to protect the nation's health." Morton Mintz of the *Washington Post* was pushing for "an informed consent law for dangerous drugs," which means the patient would sign a written statement that would read, "I am aware of the increased risk and lower reliability; I've been informed of this and agree to take the drug anyway." Specifically when it applies to estrogen taken in middle age, Morton Mintz would like the statement to read, "I am aware that the risk of endometrial cancer is increased sevenfold if I take this product for six months or more."

What the FDA said they are doing is requiring more explicit labeling of estrogen and the inclusion of "patient package inserts" so the patient is aware of the risks of taking estrogens.

We are justifiably angry at the slowness of government procedures in these matters, for we already have the case of diethylstilbestrol (DES), a synthetic nonsteroidal estrogen and proven carcinogen which is still being added to cattle feed to stimulate weight gain before slaughter. The use of DES gives the meat industry more pounds per animal and more dollars. It give us, the consumer, a known carcinogen. When Dr. Schmidt was questioned about this he said, "I do not believe that diethystilbestrol should be in the meat supply." But when it was banned in 1973 that ban was overturned in court on the ground of improper procedures. The FDA did not hold a further hearing on whether or not it was dangerous. The lobby for the meat packers has power. That DES is not permitted in animal feed in over 20 countries, and that many of those countries have a ban on the import of meat from the United States, says a lot.

Pregnant women were routinely given DES during the 1950s and 1960s to prevent spontaneous miscarriage. The tragic result is that in a number of these cases DES daughters were produced who in adolescence have developed rare cancers in the vagina and cervix. While these daughters were in the womb, the hormone was carried from the mother's bloodstream through the placenta into the fetus and had caused a change in a few cells in the developing baby. That little change developed into dangerous cancer. What had been thought only a female disease is emerging as one for males too. At the Chicago Lying-In Hospital, a new study is divulging that boys born 20 years ago whose mothers were given DES are showing genital abnormalities such as cysts, undersized testicles, and potential infertility. "The Food and Drug Administration has prohibited the use of such estrogens during pregnancy," but it is still being used in the feed of cattle.

I gave birth to three daughters in the early 1950s and wince every time I think of those millions of women whose doctors gave them DES. Barbara Seaman, author of *Free and Female,* says, "By 1953 it was established that DES didn't work . . . but that didn't stop doctors from using it." It was prescribed to pregnant women until 1971 and is still being used in the "morning-after" contraceptive pill. Why these dangerous drugs are used at all is too insane to fathom. For example, "about 40 million women have been given the suspect DES to help their breast milk dry up after childbirth" even though the process would normally occur without the use of a drug.

When the DES report was made public the big scare set in, for the frightening question had to be asked. If one estrogen preparation can cause cancer, what about all other estrogen preparations? It shed suspicion on birth control pills and estrogen replacement therapy as well as the numerous other uses of estrogen—a growth inhibitor for tall girls, for instance.

It is difficult to understand why the FDA cannot act swiftly on this matter. They did in February 1976, for example, when they asked for the market withdrawal of sequential oral contraceptives because new studies strongly suggested that these posed an increased risk of endometrial cancer compared with the combination-type oral contraceptives. The three companies, Mead-Johnson, Ortho Pharmaceuticals, and Syntex, all agreed to cease production at the agency's request.

The frustrating thing is that the FDA can act when they want to. One action they finally took which is greatly to their credit was to discredit Dr. Robert A. Wilson, who pushes estrogen replacement therapy in his book *Feminine Forever*. The Searle Company was informed that he is an "unacceptable investigator."

15
Estrogen Replacement Therapy

Estrogen replacement therapy is dangerous. It will raise your cancer risk. It may lead to vascular disease. It may even kill you. Synthetic hormones have been prescribed for women since their introduction 40 years ago, and some women have died from them. We are angry at the doctors who have prescribed them casually. And we are angry at the US Food and Drug Administration (FDA) for their lack of prudence and protection of our interest in preserving our health from this hazard. The lack of control over the onslaught of hormone propaganda from pharmaceutical houses who manufacture these hormones is also appalling. The fact that we are menopausal women and are looked upon as valueless by our culture is tragic in itself, but there is no excuse to allow violation of our bodies with harmful drugs.

If you're wondering why I'm so angry, it is because the evidence is frightening. The 1976 *Facts and Figures* of the American Cancer society tell us 168,000 women died from cancer in that year and 336,000 new cases appeared. Cancer has been clearly linked to menopausal and post-menopausal use of estrogen. "Eight million prescriptions annually are written to menopausal women for uses classified as 'probably effective' by the FDA." This agency is supposed to regulate and guarantee the safety and efficacy of these drugs; its function is consumer protection, yet it approves hormone drugs which have been "demonstrated" by the manufacturer to be safe only for short-term clinical use. Even this evaluation could be useless, for the latency period between taking the hormones and the development of cancer can be as long as 20 years.

I hope all women, in the interest of protecting and improving our health and life and that of our children and loved ones, will reject known carcinogens (cancer-producing agents) wherever they may appear—in drugs or food or in the air we breathe. If our refusal to tolerate carcinogens could become universal, we would shake the very fabric of this culture.

The greatest offender for popularizing hormone replacement therapy is Dr. Robert A. Wilson, whose book *Feminine Forever* promises the fountain of youth to all women who take hormones. He suggests starting in your thirties and continuing for the rest of your life. As menopausal women we have long stopped believing in fairy tales because we have all learned the hard way. There are no Prince Charmings and no happily ever afters. Life may be difficult, but we hope we can be reasonable about it. Unreasonable promises usually remain unreasonable. We knew even in fifth grade that Ponce de Leon was on the wrong track, that there is no such fountain of youth. Yet, when women are promised "the key" by doctors whom they admire and respect, whose credentials connect them with the biggest and "best" hospitals and universities, it has been irresistible. Who could refuse, when told this will keep them young, remove wrinkles, create beautiful skin, and make them sexy and desirable—even though it sounds impossible? When a visit costs between $25 and $50, the confusion between price and value is also involved. Magic is hard to oppose, especially when it comes packaged by authority and is easy to swallow in a pill.

Our value to the estrogen manufacturers was $80 million in 1975, almost five times the $17 million spent on them in 1962. A major proportion of those hormones were prescribed for healthy women, who were encouraged to take these pills routinely to help them through the problems of middle age. This escalating figure suggests both the number of possible victims as well as the reluctance of doctors and manufacturers to discontinue this heavy prescribing of estrogen, for the profit is huge. If you have been taking hormones, you must go back to your doctor and discuss the dosage; you must also have regular examinations.

Since the publication of various studies that expose estrogen replacement as more than suspect, some manufacturers have scrambled to claim that their estrogen is OK, not the "bad" one. The *Medical Letter,* a respected independent publication on drug therapy, says, "The consensus of informed opinion is that no convincing evidence has demonstrated that any one type of synthetic or natural estrogen is less likely to be carcinogenic than any other." They note that all estrogen originating outside the body, whether natural, synthetic, conjugated, or unconjugated, "should be considered potentially carcinogenic." True natural estrogens are those produced by the human body. Natural conjugated estrogens are laboratory produced but chemically similar to those produced by the body. The synthetic estrogens—stronger and cheaper to produce—are made chemically, and the formula is radically different from the natural.

THE NO. 1 MIDDLE AGE CON

The concept of estrogen replacement therapy is an affront to my sensibility. The implication is that if I must have something replaced it is because I have lost something, I am deficient in something. It is viewing me (or any menopausal woman) from an entirely wrong perspective. The term "replacement" implies in this context that I will be replaced to where I was when I was menstruating. Why? I don't want any more children, and I'm glad to be through with the nuisance of menstrual periods—I've had them for over 35 years and that's long enough. I've been looking forward to this freedom from conception and sanitary measures.

I accept that I'm a healthy woman whose body is changing. No matter how many articles and books I read that tell me I'm suffering from a "deficiency disease," I say I don't believe it. I have never felt more in control of my life than I do now and I feel neither deficient nor diseased. I think that the people who are promoting this idea—that something is wrong with me because I am 50—have something to gain or are irresponsible or stupid.

It is difficult for me to believe that trained medical people who are aware of the complexity and interplay of hormones can be so casual about prescribing estrogen and progesterone drugs when their need has never been proven, and they have never been proven to be safe. An estimated 25 million prescriptions a year are written in the United States alone for estrogen replacement drugs, and 5 or 6 million American women are believed to use the drugs for extended periods. It is creating problems for thousands of healthy women. There is even a medical word for that phenomenon: iatrogenic, induced by a physician. In a research project on menopause at New York University in 1975, it was found that almost 50 percent of the women seeing doctors took hormones. "Of these one quarter of them experienced negative side effects."

Let's go back a little and see how some of the false promises made for ERT really took hold. Where did they come from? It is interesting to go back to the beginning and see how this estrogen business developed. Two brothers, Drs. Edgar Allen Doisy and Edward A. Doisy, discovered in 1923 that the ovaries did far more than merely store and release eggs; the ovaries were a veritable chemical factory. This finding had enormous importance in understanding the function of the human female. (By the way, the human female is the only female species that has a menopause.) Further investigation proved that the ovaries produce two distinct hormones, estrogen and progesterone, which travel throughout the bloodstream to every part of the body. The messing around began upon this news. (The early research was carried out largely in agricultural colleges, with the hope that administering hormones to hens would encourage them to lay more eggs.)

The culture seems to have had an influence on creative minds, for it was in the late 1920s, when many people were going berserk, that a few doctors thought of using the hormones on the human female. Hens weren't interesting enough. Most of the medical profession who heard about it were aghast at the idea, but the few persisted and, in spite of the miserable side effects created in the women guinea pigs from the "crude extract made from dried sheep ovaries," the experimenters had their way. The hormones they prescribed caused women to suffer from nausea, headaches, skin rashes, cancer, and death.

It is only in the last ten years that this estrogen madness for menopausal women has boomed. How did it happen? There were three sources: the book by Dr. Robert A. Wilson, *Feminine Forever,* published in 1966, the women's magazines, and propaganda planted by Ayerst Laboratories.

The book sold thousands of copies both in hard and soft cover. The popular women's magazines picked up on the negative picture of the menopausal woman painted by Wilson, and they sold a lot of magazines by making flamboyant promises about how to avoid aging and how to remain feminine forever (the underlying implication in this absurd term is that we become neuters). To publish articles about menopause being a natural condition, about which we have nothing to fear, and giving helpful information, both physical and psychological, is, I assume, not interesting enough to them. It makes much more dramatic reading to give the "secret" of youth.

Many of those articles in the last ten years were written by men or edited by them. Not one of them reads as if they "know" what they're writing about. They don't have the ring of authenticity, and they certainly don't read as though any of them were written by a woman in her menopause. The articles talk about "them," meaning us, the ones with the menopause "disease."

Menopause is not like rape, a sudden violent act that can be reported on and discussed by everyone. Menopausal women, however, can talk about menopause if they're given the chance and not made to feel there is something wrong with them. Isn't that preferable to being told, by those who don't know, what we are feeling? Menopause is a slow, complex process involving the body and the mind, as well as their interaction upon each other. Its philosophic overtones include one's existential view of one's life. How dare those writers diminish us by treating us so flippantly and reducing us to our hormones? We objected when Freud did it and we object when anyone else does it, even if the modern version calls our destiny hormones instead of biology.

This travesty against us became enlarged because of action taken by Ayerst Laboratories, who manufacture the most popular drug used by the majority of women undergoing estrogen replacement therapy. The trade name of their pill is Premarin, and it is made from the urine of pregnant mares. This company placed ads in the medical journals and communicated—using the Wilson rhetoric—with the doctors who would prescribe estrogen. In addition, they maintained a public relations operation on Madison Avenue in New York City, the Information Center on the Mature Woman. How do I know this? When I was hunting for information on menopause I saw an offer for a free booklet. I sent away for it and received in the mail a patronizing slick booklet called *It's A Matter of Time*. This told me my doctor is my good friend who will see me through "the difficult time." It had the ring of those old-fashioned doctors who doped up women to have their babies with the don't-worry-honey, I'll-take-care-of-everything treatment. After telling me I'll be in trouble when my estrogen "supply is cut off," because "without estrogen we simply do not maintain all of our feminine characteristics," they warned me about "rather extreme changes" like sagging breasts and hair on my face. Then they tell me I've been a great giver to my family and they're grown so "now you have the opportunity to broaden your areas of giving" because "the world cries for love, for understanding." I know, it is hardly believable.

With the booklet came a Public Affairs pamphlet, *Your Menopause* by Ruth Carson. This was written in the patronizing style of the worst children's books, again very slick, and based on the assumption that the middle-aged woman is an idiot. Also enclosed was a list of "Recommended Reading on the Menopause." Naturally, everyone recommended ERT. The list was on the Information Center's stationery, which was beautifully designed. Above the logo was the note, "A Service For Media," and on the bottom of the stationery was the legend, "The Information Center on the Mature Woman is a service of Multidiscipline Research, Inc., through the support of Ayerst Laboratories." The message from the material is Wilson's style: when women enter menopause they are ready for the junk heap but the doctors, the saviors who can dispense estrogen, can save them from themselves.

The chief function of the Information Center's service for media was to write articles for any paper which would print them. They recommended ERT, of course. The Information Center also planted speakers on radio and television. I was telephoned by the Center in March 1975 because I had been the subject of an article in the New York *Sunday News,* in a regularly featured column written by Mary Reinholz. Among other things I was described as a 50-year-old woman who speaks on menopause. We set an appointment for 8 P.M. on March 25, 1975, at my house. Before I hung up, however, I said, "I want you to know, I'm against estrogen replacement therapy." Two days later I received a call telling me that the interviewer had been called out of town and would call me on her return. Well, you know that call never came.

Now, to get to the heart of *Feminine Forever,* the book that played the fundamental role in the estrogen drama. It did two things at once. It perpetrated the greatest number of insults (detailed in chapter 1) on the menopausal woman that has ever been documented, and it told women they could avoid those disasters by taking estrogen. The language used by Dr. Wilson is clearly biased against menopausal women, and its implications are oppressive. His frightening, degrading rhetoric reduces us to nonfunctioning human beings. It lays a perilously heavy load of dangerous expectation on the menopausal woman reader. This deceptive use of language has far-reaching and damaging effects, for it influences people who are in doubt.

The miracle he proposes, to avoid aging, the sine qua non, is, of course, estrogen. Is it any wonder women bought it? This is the promise of what estrogen will do for you; the quotes are from Wilson again. First, estrogen is defined as "the hormone of feminine attraction and well-being." It keeps "a woman sexually attractive and potent, it preserves the strength of her bones, the glow of her skin, the gloss of her hair. It prevents the development of high blood pressure, heart disease, and strokes. It tends to prevent diabetes and diseases of the urinary bladder."

That would certainly be enough reason to buy a pill, even though it sounds a little like the magic elixir that used to be hawked by traveling medicine men at carnivals, doesn't it? He erroneously again says that estrogen also "has a direct effect on a woman's emotional state" and provides "that mysterious life force that motivates work, study, ambition, and that marvelous urge toward excellence that inspires the best of human beings." As embarrassing as these statements are, he continues with more ways for you to be the perfect woman if you will only take the magic pill. "Estrogen acts as a natural energizer to both mind and body." It will give women "self-confidence, a sense of mastery over their destiny, the ability to think out problems effectively, resistance to mental and physical fatigue, and emotional self-control. . . . They never over-react hysterically, nor do they tend toward apathy. They are capable of facing the world with a healthful relaxed attitude and thereby able to enjoy their daily life. They are seldom depressed. Irrational crying spells are virtually unknown among them . . . estrogen makes women adaptable, even-tempered and generally easy to live with." And last but not least, "even frigidity . . . has been shown to be related to estrogen deficiency" (and we have been thinking that was due to careless lovers). Hear the ultimate: "the estrogen-rich woman is capable of far more generous and satisfying sexual responses."

These are all lies. They have been proven to be lies. Estrogen cannot fulfill these promises. "Only hot flashes (vasomotor symptoms) and genital atrophy are unique clinical features of the menopause and these are responsive to low dose estrogen therapy." This statement, published by the US Department of Health, Education, and Welfare in a publication *Menopause And Aging,* is a conclusion drawn from a report of the biggest conference ever held on the subject of menopause. In May 1971, in Hot

Springs, Arkansas, the experts gathered and 25 of the most illustrious names in the United States medical world presented papers about menopause—but not one of them was a woman.

Before we drop Dr. Wilson, let me tell you that he directs The Wilson Research Foundation, which has received funding from the manufacturers of estrogen: Ayerst, Searle, and the Upjohn Company. According to Morton Mintz of the *Washington Post,* Dr. Wilson has also been pushing the contraceptive pill as a "menopausal preventative," particularly Enovid, marketed by Searle. There is a 100 percent greater risk of heart attack for users of the contraceptive pill between the ages of 40 and 44 than for those 30-39 years old.

In spite of the evidence, the estrogen calamity has snowballed. As I noted, the popular women's magazines picked up the rhetoric of Dr. Wilson. The magazine article formula first uses scare techniques, then they supply the answer. This extract from a September 1974 *Ladies' Home Journal* article, entitled "Hormone Therapy," is a prime example: "symptoms of old age can descend upon her with astonishing speed." Of course, only two pages later we're given the panacea for avoiding old age, "the use of hormones to conquer aging." *Vogue,* January 1974, is slinkier and slicker because their article is titled: "Look Better—Feel Better—Can Hormones Help?" The menopausal woman is described first (scare technique) as having "an inability to feel, to act, or to love as one has usually done." That description is bad enough, but we are then discussed as though we are out of the human race: "The average menopausal patient is easily *controlled* [italics mine] with relatively low doses of estrogen, but some require large doses." Now, just in case you object to taking estrogen, which they catagorize as a "marked fear of hormones," they can still handle you. "Nonhormonal treatment consists of the use of sedatives, tranquilizers, and anti-depressants and/or education." Doping you up to quiet you down or giving you information, you have your choice. But I wonder why they don't quote information from a noted female authority on women's hormones, such as Dr. Katharina Dalton, who says:

It is only the faculty of childbearing which is lost at the change of life; the femininity, sexuality and attractiveness remain. To a woman in good health, physically and mentally, there is no reason any longer to fear what our grandmothers called 'the difficult age.' It is a time when there may be renewed vigor and when sex can be enjoyed without the ever-present fear of conception.

Instead we get opinions from terribly negative doctors, as in an editorial in *Good Housekeeping,* May 1973, titled "Should Hormone Therapy Be Used In Menopause?" The chief authority cited for estrogen is Dr. Maxwell Roland, professor of obstetrics and gynecology at the French Polyclinic Medical School in New York: "Dr. Roland and other gynecologists believe that hormones should be given to *all* women as soon as their estrogen level begins to decrease, sometime after age 40. Replacing estrogen at this time in a woman's life, they say, would prevent the menopause altogether. . . . These gynecologists view the menopause as a deficiency disease."

And there are doctors who are not only for ERT but for a lot of it. Dr. Robert Greenblatt of the Medical College of Georgia says, "I'm not such a great believer in minimal dosage. If minimal amounts are good, a little more may be even better."

The outrageous claims made for hormone therapy by some doctors are not shared by others, who have advised against the routine use of estrogen for all women. One of those is Dr. Saul B. Gusberg, at Mount Sinai School of Medicine of The City University of New York. He notes that there is no objective evidence that correlates general physical deterioration (or aging) with lack of estrogen. "It is more likely that an emotional reaction during the menopause is a response to basic changes in the woman's life, such as children growing up and leaving home, and not to lack of estrogen."

The irresponsible doctors claim that ERT protects women from heart disease and osteoporosis (bone loss), but the more reasonable and responsible doctors feel that little convincing evidence now exists that estrogen is an effective preventative of either of these conditions. Dr. Howard W. Jones, Jr., professor of obstetrics and gynecology at Johns Hopkins School of Medicine in Baltimore, says, "For example, we know that exercise can retard bone loss, and that diet and exercise play vital roles in whether heart disease develops, but we do not know the precise relationship of estrogen to these diseases."

In spite of the negative way the media has described menopause, the 1975 New York University survey on menopause found that "the total number of women reporting menopause as a (net) positive experience (68%) is noteworthy in view of the traditional characterization of menopause in our culture."

ERT: PROS AND CONS

As we have already seen, there is much disagreement among doctors over the benefits of ERT in treating menopausal symptoms. Those against it think the risks far outweigh the benefits. *Newsweek* reported that many doctors have "criticized it as a fad exploiting the American woman's vain quest for enduring youthfulness."

Differing views were expressed when the California figures on the increase in cancer were published. Dr. Paul Morrow of the Los Angeles County University of Southern California Medical Center said, "The benefits are to improve the comfort and well-being of the patient, but estrogen may not be a benefit to her health." Dr. Jessie Marmorston, another USC physician, firmly believes the opposite. "Not to give estrogen to a post-menopausal woman is close to criminal."

Another school of thought, called a moderate position by some, is taken by Dr. Robert Kistner of Harvard Medical School. If ERT is properly managed, he claims the risk of cancer can be minimized. Dr. Kistner claims that the problem is that some gynecologists prescribe too much of the hormone. It is well known, he adds, that estrogen can cause uterine hyperplasia (an overgrowth of the endometrial glands lining the uterus) which can evolve into cancer. Physicians should periodically conduct a biopsy of women on ERT, says Kistner, so that when hyperplasia is detected, the patient can be taken off the hormone until the conditon disappears. By occasionally replacing the estrogen with progesterone, an antiestrogenic hormone that causes the uterine lining to slough off as in a menstrual period, hyperplasia—and cancer—can also be prevented, he says. (A number of doctors do prescribe the two hormones, estrogen and the synthetic progestin, regularly and cycle them, which does create a regular menstruation.)

For over 50 years, controversy has surrounded the hypothesis "that estrogen [whether produced by the body or taken in] is causally related to the development of endometrial carcinoma." That is why hormones have generally not been given to women who have a history of thrombophlebitis (blood clots in veins) or kidney, liver, or cardiac disease, or a family history of breast or endometrial cancer, or if a woman suffers from irregular bleeding or benign tumors of the breast or uterus. There are possible additional risks for sufferers from migraine headaches and excessive smokers, who are also contraindicated for ERT.

Speaking of endometrial cancer, Dr. Carmel J. Cohan, director of gynecological oncology at Mount Sinai Medical Center in New York, says, "It is a disease of affluence, obesity and high-fat diets, as well as estrogens." He goes further to make his point and notes that endometrial cancer is rare in women from low socioeconomic groups but increases in incidence as these groups become more affluent. The disease, which hardly exists in native Asian women, approaches American statistics among Oriental women who come to the United States.

Estrogenic hormones have "profound widespread metabolic effects," say two researchers who have made this area their specialty, Drs. Chull S. Song and Paul Beck. They add that the "evidence is strong that estrogens can contribute to the risk of thromboembolic disease, cerebral accidents and coronary disease and the effect appears to be dose-related with an increased risk in the older age groups."

Among the selling points that have convinced some women to take estrogen was that, because estrogen decreases in the body after menopause, we are more likely victims of heart attacks. The estrogen was supposed to be a protection against this. It is not so. Coronary heart disease and the menopause has been the subject of research by Dr. Robert H. Furman of the University of Indiana School of Medicine. He notes, "The acceleration of coronary artery disease mortality with age in women is similar in pre- and postmenopausal periods." He further substantiates his conclusions: "Retrospective survey of medical and autopsy records do not establish a protective effect of estrogen or ovarian function against coronary artery disease." In addition, there is an increased vulnerability to blood clot accident with estrogen administration, says Dr. Furman. The facts are exactly opposite those given us by the estrogen pushers.

As for osteoporosis (bone loss), Dr. Robert P. Heaney, chairman of the Department of Medicine at Creighton University of Medicine in Omaha, Nebraska, says, "If by 'success' we mean increase in bone mass and decrease in bone fragility, then plainly estrogens have not proved successful in treatment of osteoporosis."

Atherosclerosis (damaged tissue surrounded by fatty deposits) is a slow-developing process, and it naturally increases with advancing years. Postmenopausal women who have taken hormones such as those in oral contraceptives during their childbearing years are more likely to have an increased risk of developing thrombosis (blood clots). If estrogen is continued after menopause, as in ERT, "she may be subjected to additional hazards both of spontaneous thrombosis and of further acceleration of atherosclerosis," says William H. Inman, senior medical officer of the Committee on Safety of Medicines, in London.

The booklet on menopause published by the National Institute on Aging tells us "scientific studies to date have not established a clear-cut relationship between ailments such as depression or insomnia and estrogen deficiency, or the relief of such ailments by estrogen therapy."

Dr. Harry K. Ziel, who directed one of the major studies linking ERT with cancer, said about hormones, "This is not an innocuous drug that can be used like salt and pepper. Doctors should restrict its use to women with incapacitating symptoms since it has a life-threatening risk."

The theory of estrogen replacement therapy is not useful to us because it does not bring order to the confusion and chaos of menopausal facts; too many of the claims made do not relate to each other. A useful theory should provide a logical explanation, without contradiction. The group of doctors who believed ERT could "cure" the symptoms of menopause have been proven wrong.

That small doses of estrogen for short periods do bring relief from hot flashes and vaginal problems has been established. Why not determine the reasons for these problems? Some good guesses have been made, such as relating the hypothalamus (the body's thermostat) to hot flashes, but they have not been validated. It seems that the combination of cultural, emotional, and physical circumstances of a menopausal woman's life are all related to the cause of the symptoms.

There do seem to be alternatives to the general use of estrogen, for I have talked to about 1,000 women, 95 percent of whom have not taken estrogen and were more than "getting by." Without question, the women do not represent a cross section of the population, and I do not claim they represent the women in the country. They were mostly from New York, New Jersey, and Connecticut, and practically all of them worked outside the home. The common denominators for the large majority may indicate some sort of trend. These women were interested in nutrition and most receptive to the idea of the relationship of food and good health. And of greatest importance, they did not feel isolated, for they were women who gathered in groups to talk.

What these women are doing—getting together and talking—is exactly the prescription recommended by Drs. Pauline B. Bart and Marlyn Grossman, feminist behavioral scientists. Their chapter on menopause in the forthcoming book *The Woman As Patient* claims that women have been treated with ERT too often for conditions which are cultural rather than hormonal.

I'm going to tell you a story about ERT that may strike you as unbelievable. I was surprised by it, but after giving it some thought, I remembered that when I was studying mushrooms I had read a similar story about the Uzbecks in Siberia. I was visiting a friend in the country, and she told me I must meet Josephine and Helen, two sisters, 89 and 94, because they were unusually vigorous and most interesting. We called on them and were graciously served delicious carrot cake and mint tea. I told these bright, talkative women that I was writing a book and was interested in what they attributed their good health and high energy to. Their diet was superb; they baked their own whole grain bread and hardly used any canned food. They also drank eight ounces of their first urine of the day and had been doing it for 20 years. "Why?" I asked. "To return the estrogen," they replied. And they suggested I do it, too, by starting with a teaspoon of urine in an eight-ounce glass of orange juice every morning, then adding another teaspoon until all of the orange juice was replaced. They were convinced that returning the estrogen was keeping them in such good shape.

Shocking as this story is, I then remembered the Uzbecks who got a second high from their *amanita muscaria* mushrooms by drinking their urine. I do not recommend drinking one's urine to replace estrogen because the amount of estrogen is minute and the urine contains toxins, and I seriously question if that is "the secret" of the sisters' good health. However, when one realizes that pregnant mares' urine is used in the preparation of hormones, the sisters' story becomes less farfetched. But, as you know, I don't care for the concept of replacement.

MY OWN EXPERIMENT

Although I am well aware of the complexity of our hormones, I couldn't resist trying out an idea of my own. If the medical thinking is that our estrogen level falls dramatically at menopause (which I have always questioned), I began to wonder if perhaps there may not be a way to stimulate greater production from within.

This is how I reasoned. If one is sexually celibate for a period of time and then chooses to change that condition, intercourse, which is not quite so easy and comfortable at first, in short order becomes easy and pleasurable. The body adapts, secretions become activated from use. Maybe, then, we could raise the level of our sex hormone production by introducing some natural element that would stimulate them. After all, if our bodies manufacture the hormones in the first place, that production must be stimulated as a result of something we take into our bodies. We know that junk foods with preservatives and additives do not benefit us, because the body resists foreign chemical substances. We also know that the body accepts that which comes from nature. Therefore natural foods must be the answer to producing those elements known as precursors, the raw material our glands transform into hormones. The question was then which natural foods to use.

Betty Lee Morales is a woman worth listening to because she is certainly doing something right—at 70 she looks 50. When talking about older women at the University of California, Los Angeles, she told about research in Germany which suggested that bee pollen and royal jelly could act to stimulate hormone production. I then remembered reading about Russian scientists who discovered that pollen is the active substance in honey responsible for honey's rejuvenating property. "The rationalization for using these two supplements is that pollen represents the male and royal jelly the female hormone precursor." OK, we have male and female hormones in our bodies. What besides hormone production (if that is what it is) is involved here? Bee pollen contains vitamins, proteins, and minerals. I figured those can't hurt. I take vitamins anyhow, so it didn't seem too risky an idea. I knew honey, seeds, and nuts are also supposed to be excellent, and since they are a natural part of my diet, pollen and royal jelly seemed to fall in easily.

The bee gathers the fine powder produced by flowers and manufactures it into pollen by impregnating it with nectar. It's altogether poetic. The pollen, a mass of male germ cells, contains a plant hormone similar to the pituitary hormone gonadotrophin, which stimulates the sex glands. Royal jelly, which is very rich in pantothenic acid as well as other B complex vitamins, is the food of the queen bee, who lives ten times longer than the worker bees. A highly nutritious secretion of the honey bee, it is supposed to have a regenerative effect on the human body. Surely this must be better to take than medicine or a drug or the estrogen made from pregnant mare's urine?

I gave bee pollen and royal jelly a try early in October 1976. I had used them singly, but never together before. As the kids say, "I got off on it."

The idea charmed me. I added a 500-milligram tablet of bee pollen (it comes loose or pressed together) and a 50-milligram capsule of royal jelly to my daily supplements. After about three weeks, my breasts were too heavy for comfort. They had become enlarged, a familiar premenstrual feeling (I had not had a period since the middle of March). In the middle of October I had a day and a half of staining, not what one would call a "real" period. I stopped taking the bee food and tried again at the end of November to test it further. After a couple of weeks, my body again felt exaggeratedly premenstrual with bloat and extremely tender breasts. I was certain the level of estrogen was very high in my body, but was there enough progesterone to create a period? How I wished for it just to get relief. You can be sure I stopped taking the stuff. In December, when I was 52¼, I did get a "real" period: three days of flow, and two and a half more days of staining.

This was not a scientific experiment. I do not know if the bee pollen and royal jelly brought on the period or if it was just coincidence. It was a hunch I felt like trying. It didn't seem irresponsible, but too much estrogen in the body can be dangerous, even if it's natural. I do *not* recommend it as a way to build estrogen. But it is interesting and pollen and royal jelly are nutritious supplements. However, if you're in your menopause and your hormones are hopping around, perhaps it's a better idea to leave these foods alone, until your hormones settle down. One never knows when the periods are entirely over until a year, some say two years, later. Not enough is known about our hormones, but luckily some of the "good guys" are studying them further.

16
The Menopausal Woman as Hero

The search to learn what was happening to my body at menopause almost made me feel like Jason in quest of the Golden Fleece. It took me into highways and byways I hadn't expected to journey through, and to new and unfamiliar places such as New York's 103rd Street and Fifth Avenue. Jason's travel was by water, which is the symbol for intuition. I too was symbolically journeying far from my home base, being led by my intuition, which told me there must be better explanations of menopause than the ones I was getting from the books written about it.

The Golden Fleece was guarded by a dragon who never slept. We too have our dragons to slay to try to learn what is happening to our bodies at this time.

One is generally suspicious of people who claim to have *the* answers, who seem to oversimplify the complicated business of menopause. Our biggest dragon is Dr. Robert A. Wilson, but there are so many all over the place, and they are dressed up so prettily with their credentials that even spotting them is a struggle. Becoming a dragon-spotter became a challenge.

If you are smiling at my imagery, and perhaps think of heroes only in the shape of men, particularly tall, young, handsome men, let me tell you that they come in all sizes, shapes, and ages. Even in the shape of a 50-year-old menopausal woman who is searching for the truth about herself. I do not really mean to imply that I am a hero simply because I wanted to know, for example, if I was at great risk of getting endometrial cancer because my body felt like it was producing a lot of estrogen. This is not an uncommon feeling among women who are in the last year of their menstruation, when they are skipping some periods. You see, some women produce quite a bit of estrogen during that year, but some months they do not produce enough progesterone to create a menstrual flow. Both those hormones are necessary in order for the endometrium, the lining of the uterus, to slough off—the action that creates bleeding. When your body makes a lot of natural estrogen but not very much progesterone, one has the feeling of being premenstrual for quite a long time. So my motive was frankly selfish—which, by the way, Dr. Hans Selye, the stress specialist, says is a healthy way to be if you want to live longer. My quest felt heroic, nevertheless, because in a sense I was challenging many doctors, thousands of whom had written $80 million worth of estrogen prescriptions in 1975 alone, and a large part of these were for healthy women.

Let me expand this hero idea, because I want you to be included. I want you to view the menopausal woman in a perspective different from that which most people use. She cannot, indeed must not, be stereotyped. I have been saying throughout this book that we are, each one of us, individual, unique. We all have distinct and separate rhythms and are each in our own particular space that no one dare judge. We learn from each other and get courage and support from each other to move forward and to grow without fear or hesitation, but each woman grows at her own pace, in the way that is comfortable for her. It is harder to grow when we are made to feel that something is wrong with us, that we are worthless. That makes our struggle even more difficult. The problem is compounded when people who don't really know us or care for us tell us what we should do. Remember, at the beginning of the book we threw out the word *should*. When a menopausal woman says *no* to the traditional role this culture places on her, she is behaving in a heroic manner. She is not accepting the role of being inferior.

Why, you may ask, do I pursue the task of learning about my body with such relentless passion? It is because I must understand this multidimensional self that I am. As menopausal women we are essentially viewed with a myopic vision that is blurred to our humanness. It is customary to be ashamed of being in your menopause, but I do not see that as something to be ashamed of, or to hide, even though menopause makes us, in terms of this youth-oriented society, nonbeings, women of no value.

Let me give you a concrete example of what I mean. CBS television news was going to do a story on menopause in November 1976. Great. I loved the idea of their saying the word loud and clear, not as a joke, but for all to hear, not covering it up with euphemisms. They hunted to find women to speak about their menopause but couldn't get women to say, "I'm in my menopause." The women were ashamed. CBS called me because in June 1975 I had been a panelist on a program, presented by The New York Society of Clinical Psychologists, celebrating Women's International Year. At that event, I had spoken about menopausal women from the point of view of being one. CBS knew this. Yet, because menopause has such a rotten reputation I was offered these options if I would participate: I would not have to give my name, I could be photographed from the back or I could be photographed in shadow so I wouldn't be recognized. "Are you kidding?" I asked. "I'm not ashamed to be identified as a menopausal woman. I want to be photographed face forward and tell my name and age. I'm not hiding it under the rug." That's revolutionary because it is contrary to what is being done. OK, OK. It was more than CBS had hoped for.

Back to heroism. When we are in our menopause, we are also trying, because of our age and the conflicts and complexities inherent in a woman's life at that time, to confront and acknowledge without illusion the fundamental facts of life—facts that are sometimes as incomprehensible as they are ugly. We are trying to view our basic realities, with all the existential ambiguities, in such a light that they are made life-affirming in spite of the absurd nature of existence. This is heroism.

In order to do this, we must try to understand ourselves, try to know our bodies and our minds, not as separate, unrelated entities but as related parts of an integrated harmonious whole human being. We cannot be reduced to our anatomy, or our hormones. But we also can't dismiss them as being unimportant either and blame only the culture for what we are feeling. Trying to learn what is happening in our bodies will enable us to get closer to understanding how and why we are responding and behaving the way we are to everything around us. It is of immediate and fundamental interest to us, for armed with this knowledge we can alleviate many fears. Most often it is fear that keeps us from growing.

By learning about our bodies, we're not trying to take over the medical profession. We are dependent on medical technology and need it. However, we are trying to do many things with that information. First and foremost, by understanding ourselves better we are also schooling ourselves to be more intelligent medical consumers. This is part of what taking control of one's life means, to know the things that are happening both to your body and mind. With the menopause, for example, by knowing the possibilities, a woman who finds herself for the first time having night sweats, will know that having to change her nightgown because it is soaked is nothing to panic about. That can happen to a woman in her menopause and she is not sick. But if we don't know that, we can be very scared. The point is that, by knowing the possibilities, because they have happened to millions of other healthy women, we are relieved and don't have to run to a doctor for every little ache and pain.

Then when we do go to a doctor, we can ask questions without fear and guilt for taking their time. We're not expecting gentle, concerned Marcus Welby. We know he doesn't exist and is only a figment of fantasy. What we want is to be treated with dignity and humanity. We do not want that separation of big, smart, medical doctor and little, dumb, pest, me. We also don't want our uteruses cut out when a D and C would do just as well. We want to be active participants in our health care and be informed about what is taking place. Some women who have had hysterectomies, for example, don't know if their ovaries were also removed.

So far in this book, I have reported what I have learned. For instance, although many doctors tell us we stop making estrogen, they are wrong, for others whom I trust say we make it from an extraglandular source at and after menopause. The rate of cancer of the uterus is rising, and that risk is increased by too much estrogen if taken as estrogen replacement therapy or if produced by one's own body. How much is too much? Why haven't we been told in the popular articles that our bodies make it? If our bodies produce extraglandular estrogen, why do some women have pain during intercourse because the walls of their vaginas are thin? Doesn't the extraglandular estrogen help that? If the extraglandular estrogen is in the body, including the fat of the body, then will a fat woman have plenty of estrogen to prevent pain in the vagina but have too much for her uterus? Can the extraglandular estrogen be measured? Does it affect fibroids? These are only some of the questions that concerned me.

I hunted for more information but couldn't find as much as I wanted in the medical journals. There was only one thing left to do. Ask. Go to a source and ask the person whose articles had already told me quite a bit about extraglandular estrogen. Go to the person whose research is the relation of extraglandular estrogen to endometrial cancer in post-menopausal women. Go to the one who has contributed significantly to the knowledge recently published in the *New England Journal of Medicine.* I did. I sent some questions to Dr. Saul B. Gusberg, professor and chairman of the Department of Obstetrics and Gynecology at Mount Sinai School of Medicine of The City University of New York. His answers follow.

AN INTERVIEW WITH DR. SAUL B. GUSBERG

Reitz: If the main source of estrogen at and after menopause is extraglandular, would you say the reason women get relief from hot flashes with estrogen replacement is because the extraglandular production is not yet high enough?

Gusberg: I have your questions in front of me. To each of these questions the answer cannot be a very direct one because they're rather subtle questions.

R.R.: Oh, I didn't mean them to be, that was not my intention.

S.G.: No, no, it's not because of the way you have structured them, it's the way they *are* scientifically. They're very complicated questions, that are not entirely understood.

R.R.: That's why I'm asking you, because you're the authority and I'm trying to find out.

S.G.: There are many things we don't know about the menopause and need more research. In some people the amount of so-called extraglandular estrogen is more than in other individuals, but it's not a matter of working itself up. Some women are more sensitive.

You see, nobody quite knows why people have hot flushes except the absence of estrogen. Some people believe that it's because the pituitary overworks, which it does. You understand—I'm sure you've read all this—when the menopause happens the ovarian function ceases and the pituitary overworks in an attempt to whip it into action. If you give estrogen, the hot flushes go away and the gonadotrophin, the pituitary, stop working so hard, so people have assumed in the past that they are related, that the overwork of the pituitary causes the hot flushes. This may not be so. It's possible that they are just concomitant, that they are related temporally but not casually, OK?

R.R.: Fine.

S.G.: Why do a minority of women have severe hot flushes? The majority either have none or they are minor. We don't know the answer to that, but it is true that in some the extraglandular production of estrogen is apparently enough so that their equilibrium, their glandular readjustment so to speak, is gradual enough so that it doesn't bother them. The same holds true for vaginal atrophy. After all, a great many women have vaginal thinning without complaint, and the majority have no complaint. Do you have children?

R.R.: Yes, I have three daughters.

S.G.: The average woman who has had children, even when she has vaginal thinning, has no complaints, the complaint usually being discomfort during sex relations. Whereas a woman who hasn't had a child would be much more prone to have discomfort from vaginal atrophy than the woman who has had children.

R.R.: If the extraglandular estrogen is produced in body fat, does that mean that thin women have less?

S.G.: Correct.

R.R.: Then in some ways, fat would be a positive, at least in relation to vaginal atrophy, wouldn't it?

S.G.: Do you mean a thin woman would be more prone?

R.R.: If a thin woman produces less extraglandular estrogen, would she then not be more likely, perhaps, to have a problem with the thinning vaginal walls?

S.G.: Possible. This is a logical deduction but unproven.

R.R.: You speak of estrogen overstimulation, where estrogen is elevated for a prolonged period. How long is a prolonged period?

S.G.: Continuous estrogen over a period of three to ten years, continuous meaning without progesterone modifying it. You see, progesterone is the hormonal antagonist, and in the normal cycle of a fertile woman. . . .

R.R.: But we're past the cycle.

S.G.: But I'm going back for a moment for background. In a fertile cycle, a woman has a good deal of estrogen but she has it modified constantly by this progesterone. On the other hand, when she gets menopausal, even the relatively low border of estrogen that is converted from extraglandular spaces, wherever they may be, fat or whatever, constantly bombards the uterus without progesterone. That makes a difference.

R.R.: There's a point I'd like to clarify, if you'll bear with me. Too much estrogen, even if it's made by one's own body, is dangerous because it may cause cancer of the endometrium, right?

S.G.: We believe now that it does place people at higher risk. Too much for a short period probably wouldn't make any difference.

R.R.: Because many women who are just in that one year. . . .

S.G.: That wouldn't bother me.

R.R.: I know for myself that my body produces an enormous amount of estrogen.

S.G.: How do you know that?

R.R.: Because of my breasts.

S.G.: How old are you? You don't need to tell.

R.R.: I'm 52 and delighted to tell, that's absurd. I'm beyond that. Because the way my breasts feel at different times, I can guess when I have more or less estrogen in my body. Do you pooh-pooh that?

S.G.: No, not at all.

R.R.: I like that you speak about diet, but you are never specific.

S.G.: One cannot be specific as yet. Nutrition is one of the most difficult things to investigate, even among cultivated people. I'll bet if I asked you what you ate last Thursday you wouldn't know.

R.R.: I probably would, since I bake my own whole grain bread. I'm one of those. If you see the list of menopause foods in the nutrition chapter you can guess my menu. It will not contain meat, white bread, or sugar.

S.G.: Unless one interviews people personally day after day, diet is a very difficult thing to investigate. Oriental women, Japanese, for example, get thinner as they get older whereas Western women get a little plumper when they get older. The Japanese diet is very low in animal fat and low in calories in addition. In Japan, endometrial cancer is almost unknown, it's a rarity. In Western countries it's common and getting more common. When Japanese immigrate to this country and, in a second generation, begin to take on a Western diet, they begin to take on Western style cancers. This is true of cancer of the breast as well, which is rare in Japan.

R.R.: Dr. Gusberg, after hormones, nutrition is the biggest chapter in my book so I was pleased to see that you spoke about that.

S.G.: It's very important, and the amount known about it is very meager.

R.R.: Among the women I was involved with in the menopause workshops, I noticed that the women who ate less sugar had less hot flashes.

S.G.: Menopause Anonymous?

R.R.: No [laughter] because it wasn't anything we were trying to get rid of, but something we were trying to find out about. The books all said to take estrogen and I didn't want to. I didn't think I had a "deficiency disease."

S.G.: That's nonsense.

R.R.: Of course it's nonsense, but you don't know how it's affected this whole culture. But you do know.

S.G.: I do know. But there's a whole new cycle now. People are beginning to be more sensible about this and realize that not a great trauma has happened to the average woman going through menopause.

R.R.: It seems that the ones who have been pushing estrogen have also been the ones who have been insulting to menopausal women.

S.G.: They haven't listened to their patients enough.

R.R.: That's exactly what I say. That's the reason you're the only one I'm interested in speaking to.

S.G.: Have I answered your questions?

R.R.: Yes, thank you, but may I ask you another?

S.G.: Yes.

R.R.: This has concerned me very much. If women do produce this extraglandular estrogen, it would make itself apparent in the urine, right?

S.G.: Yes and no. Some would appear, but the amount would be so small. It's just that even during the cycle it is small. The quantities that are observable even in a cycling woman are terribly small to be measured. They are measurable by very careful scientific methods.

R.R.: I see. Because if they were easily measurable and were very clearly apparent then it would make the people who say we stop making estrogen look altogether silly.

S.G.: The whole story about this is not fully in yet—the whole story of the aromatization and the production of estrogen.

R.R.: Women are told not to have fibroids removed at around the age of 35 or 40, because after the menopause the fibroids will get smaller because they will not be producing so much estrogen.

S.G.: Right. To some extent. Some need removal in any case.

R.R.: What about the extraglandular estrogen?

S.G.: It's much lower in amount than the cycling woman's estrogen. The amount necessary, for example, to prevent thinning of the vagina is much less than is necessary for producing bleeding from the uterus, so that a woman can be quite comfortable without vaginal thinning and yet she doesn't have a period.

R.R.: That's the crucial point. This aspiration curettage you're doing at Mount Sinai, could that do for endometrial cancer what the Pap test has done for cervical cancer?

S.G.: We hope it will. It's going in that direction.

R.R.: How does a person like me have such an experience?

S.G.: More and more doctors are using that technique, though it's not universal as yet. We think it's terribly simple to do and can be done by any physician but it's not as simple as doing a Pap smear. But the Pap smear is highly inaccurate for endometrial cancer, whereas it is highly accurate and efficient for cervix cancer.

Let food be your medicine.

Hippocrates

17
Nutrition and Middle Age

"Tell me what you eat and I will tell you what you are" said Brillat-Savarin in 1790, and although it sounds frivolous, the concept is true. By looking at the food people eat we can learn a lot about them. I, too, asked the women I interviewed what they ate. Without question, the ones who felt and looked better, had clear complexions and healthy hair, were the women who were eating a nutritious diet and taking dietary supplements.

Think, for example, of a person who boasts, "I'm a steak-and-potatoes man myself." Doesn't he usually look like one—puffy? He probably is not a flexible person who will try other foods, he sticks to what he knows, is probably not an experimental lover (aren't the senses all related?), and probably has a high cholesterol count.

There is a difference in appearance in middle age between a hamburger-and-french-fries eater and a salad-and-yogurt eater. Look for yourself and you will see it, especially in skin tone. Look at the people in the supermarket and you can learn a lot about them from the food in their carts.

Does diet make a difference in menopause? Everyone agrees it does. Even the doctors who automatically give tranquilizers and estrogen to every woman patient 40 or over wouldn't disagree. They may, but often do not, mumble something about the necessity for a well-balanced diet as they hand you the prescriptions.

It has been well said that a person digs her grave with her teeth. I want to live to be 100 and feel well. I don't want to settle for today's national average age of 74.5 for women because there is too much I want to do. One of the ways I plan to do it is to build up my body's resistance and defenses against disease. Good nutrition will do it, for if the tissues, cells, and organs are strong and healthy, it is much easier to resist and fight diseases.

Of course, factors other than nutrition also determine how we feel as we age—the ways we handle stress, our capacity for and enjoyment of pleasure, our way of dealing with anger, the ways we feel validated on a daily basis, and the amount of exercise we do. This chapter, however, is about nutrition.

As we age, our bodies require less food. Our chances for living longer increase when we carry less weight, because it relieves stress on our vital organs. Thus, being overweight is of great concern to us.

Diet books for weight loss are all over the place, and I have known many people who have used them religiously. I do not like standard diets because we are all so different. I am not addressing myself to people with specific diseases such as diabetes who are under doctor's care but to women in their menopause who are generally healthy. The food we eat is related to many things, and eating carries such a huge emotional load that for anyone but yourself to decide what you should eat is ludicrous. Prescribed diets always seem temporary. My aim is for a rest-of-your-life way of eating.

First of all, if you're old enough to read this book, you know a lot about yourself and diets. You know that two slices of toast is more fattening than one slice. You know that a wedge of apple pie is more fattening than a raw apple. Only you can come to terms with how and what goes into your mouth.

For anyone to tell you a cup of yogurt is better for you than a cup of ice cream is unnecessary; you know that. You, yourself, must come to the decision that eating yogurt is a plus for your body, while eating ice cream with its sugar is a minus. This is very complicated, for we want to function from choice rather than from deprivation. And unless we do, the diets don't work; that's why most of them are failures. The essential point is that we are grown-up-women-in-control who need to make our own choices from reasoned good sense; that is where we want to be.

Furthermore, by the time we come to middle age we should not do drastic things to our bodies. We must make changes gradually and not switch dramatically, overnight. For example, I used to be a big coffee drinker and was fussy about every detail. Then I decided I did not want all that caffeine and saccharin. By the end of the month, I was using only decaffeinated coffee, with honey. During the next month, instead of reaching for coffee, I reached for fruit. I could not break a 30-year habit easily. We become addicted to the rituals surrounding an act as well as to the act itself. We cannot disregard a way of functioning that we have grown accustomed to, even if we wish to change it. Now I drink Postum or Pero, cereal beverages with no caffeine, but I also began trying different herb teas.

Weight Watchers seems to have taken hold the way none of the other popular diets have. Their success is based partly on some fine nutritional principles (and partly on advertising), but their heavy use of nonnutritive sweetening agents makes me uncomfortable because the body's tolerance of them is suspect. I do not like their use of chemically treated and processed foods, particularly diet sodas. Have you ever read the label on a diet soda?

The whole concept of this low-cal, no-cal industry that has become a part of our lives is based on keeping our bodies trim, but for the wrong reasons—not for health, but for looks, so that we can compete sexually. If health were the goal, we would see attractive individual containers of honey in restaurants instead of packets of sweeteners. Our culture has evolved a curious distortion of what comprises beauty. True beauty lies in a healthy, well-functioning body.

Foods that have been processed with heat and chemical additives are less nutritious than those not prepared in this way. If we are trying to love ourselves, respect for our bodies is a part of the process. We therefore don't want to put junk into our bodies. We all can *see* that women who are nutrition-conscious have fewer wrinkles and age more attractively. I've noticed, too, that women who are self-accepting seem to age more easily and have fewer health complaints and look different from those who are continually finding fault with themselves and still trying to compete with the models in the ads.

You may say, "I accept your propaganda. I, too, want to be healthy and look good as I age. What do your recommend?" There is no pat formula and no set of rules. You are the one who will make decisions about what, when, how, and why you eat the food you do. Think about it, talk to your friends, and read—especially the labels on the foods you buy.

When you start respecting your body and loving it you will find you will stop polluting it. Instead of pain-killers, some women have found vitamin C with calcium helps, or perhaps for you a cup of herb tea will do it. Or maybe you'll just live with the pain and not fight it, or maybe you will try a combination of the three ideas. You will certainly not eat cottony white bread or candy bars, for they are empty calories. Whole wheat breads without additives and preservatives are now available in most supermarkets. You won't eat processed cheese because you now can easily buy natural ones. As part of loving yourself, you'll read the printing on the yogurt cups and will buy only the natural ones rather than the brands that contain a lot of sugar and gelatin, food starch, citric acid, artificial color, and flavorings. Add your own fresh fruit and honey if you want extra sweetness.

By examining labels seriously you will find differences in many common products, even cottage cheese. For example, some of them are natural while others contain vegetable gum, or carrageenan, stabilizers for longer shelf life; some even have artificial flavor added. Who needs those additives? The manufacturer—not the individual who cares about her body. Since we are weight conscious, it's a good idea to avoid cheeses that are made with cream and whole milk because the butterfat is too high in calories and cholesterol. Instead, select cheeses made with part skim milk, such as cottage and farmer cheese, Jarlsburg, Tilsit, Iceland, Port Salud, Danish Havarti, Finland Lappi, skim Ricotta and Mozzarella (but check labels to be sure).

We are aiming for a nutritious diet to create and maintain a healthy body with all of its parts absorbing and utilizing the food we eat. Since we want to live to be 100—and we want those years to be useful and pleasurable, not painful—we do not want to tax our complex machinery with toxic foods that the digestive process has to work overtime to try to excrete through the kidneys.

Our healthy bodies are constantly building and replacing body tissues, antibodies, hormones, enzymes, and blood cells. For this we require proteins which break down into amino acids that pass into the blood and are carried through our entire bodies. As we age, our physical problems emerge because blood proteins, hormones, enzymes, and antibodies are not being manufactured in the amounts our bodies need. This is among the reasons why we start seeing wrinkles and begin to lose muscle tone. Attractiveness, vigor, and energy start by our eating proteins. When your energy is low and you are tired too often and look it, examine the amount of protein in your diet. Remember, steak is not a synonym for protein, a mistake popularly made by people who are not nutritionally oriented. Protein comes in many shapes and sizes. Dr. Louis V. Avioli, a nutrition specialist at Washington University School of Medicine, notes that in women over 35, protein is required but not entirely in animal form, and "maybe we should all be vegetarians."

GOOD FAT

Our bodies need less food as we age, so we must be more discriminating about what we select. Also, our body's ability to handle fats decreases, and it takes longer to metabolize the fat that entered our blood from dinner. It would seem reasonable then, especially since we have a tendency to put on weight, to eliminate fat. However, this is not exactly true, for there is animal fat—Bad Fat because it is saturated—and there is Good Fat (which is polyunsaturated). In-between is hydrogenated fat. All do different things for us. Animal fat is high in cholesterol and comes largely from meat, butter, and cream. It can accumulate in our arteries and attach itself to the walls, thus reducing space for the flow of blood. This fat is also more difficult for the body to utilize.

Fat-free diets are a mistake. Our bodies need fat, but only specific kinds. Good fats, the polyunsaturated ones, are the natural vegetable oils: corn, soybean, sunflower, safflower, peanut, and cottonseed—*not* olive or coconut oil. They supply more than ten times the amount of the valuable essential fatty acids than margarine or even hydrogenated fats (solidified cooking fats). Good fats work for us. Other fats work against us. Good fats are broken down by our digestive processes and supply our bodies with the essential fatty acids that combine with other nutrients to help transport the nutrients where they are needed for building new cells. We also need fat for multiplying the positive bacteria in our intestinal tracts and for the absorption of vitamins. Our hormones of the adrenal cortex and our sex glands are made of particular kinds of fats.

Strange as it may sound, we are sometimes overweight because we eat too little fat. To eliminate salad dressing in order to save 100 calories or so of oil is a huge error, for no reducing can be nutritionally successful without polyunsaturated oils. Some of us are waterlogged, and a daily salad with dressing made of vegetable oil can actually help us lose weight.

Can you think of times when you feel terribly hungry, starved in fact? This may be because, when the supply of essential fatty acids is too low, our bodies try to make up the shortage by changing blood sugar to fat. This makes our blood sugar level plunge, causing urgent hunger. Fats satisfy because they remain in the stomach longer than most other foods; therefore to eat salad without dressing will probably trigger more eating of starch and sugar.

We also need some fat to stimulate production of bile and the fat-digesting enzymes. Eliminating fats completely may cause serious gall bladder difficulties. Some stored fat, believe it or not, is necessary. For example, a small amount around the kidneys supports them. A fat layer under the skin protects the muscles and nerves and helps maintain body temperature.

Another thing about oil is that if taken internally it makes our hair and skin look better. Your hair is more likely to be shiny and glossy if you use oil on salad than if you buy expensive shampoos. Skin looks less patchy and altogether softer and smoother. Use the same oil for your skin as for your salad—it is cheaper and better for you than cosmetics. My favorite oil is apricot kernel oil. I use it inside and outside, carefully, because it is expensive. I put it on my salad and on my face and also use it as a body oil rub. It is fragrantly delicate, cold-pressed with no preservatives, and rich in polyunsaturates. Much of what we put on the skin will be absorbed and eventually will find its way into the bloodstream.

Sex, too, comes into the fat story. Adelle Davis, the late nutritionist, said, "Persons on seemingly adequate diets except for oil have reported increased sex interest after dietary improvement." Did you know that a little daily oil could do all that for you? I have no authority to cite for this idea, but it is my guess that the condition medically described as "atrophic vaginitis" (meaning that the cells lining the walls of the vagina are dry) would also be helped by using oil. It makes sense that if oil improves outside skin, it should have the same effect on the inside.

Much as I sound as if I love good fat, this is by no means a case of "if a little is good, a lot is better." While a daily tablespoon or two is superb, any more than that will be stored—most of it just where you've always been a little plump.

Since I have turned 50, I have become a more selective person. I don't want my body to work trying to metabolize junk food that does not feed me properly. I want food to nurture me. I respect my body too much to waste all that activity, all the energy necessary for the process of digestion, for my heart to pump all that blood, for the filtering process through my liver, gall bladder, and kidneys. Think about that—you'll never eat a potato chip again for the rest of your life.

VITAMINS, MINERALS, AND SUPPLEMENTS

Vitamins, like love, is one of those subjects no one can be against. Just as some people need and want more loving than others, some need extra vitamins. Many doctors will tell us we get all the vitamins we need in a well-balanced diet. They are not against vitamins; they feel we get enough of them. I'm not sure how many people eat this well-balanced diet or even exactly what it is. It always reminds me of those panty hose and bras labelled "One size fits all." You can guess how my 38C is accommodated.

We are, each one of us, specifically individual with wide variations in body frame, life-style, dietary habits, exposure to and ways of dealing with stress. My body's responses and their effect on my biochemistry were different when I was working at a 9 to 5 pressure job with overtime than they are now when I am working in a self-regulating way at home. We cannot be lumped together as a group of "middle-aged women who need such and such." The daily requirement for each one of us is different. We have our own unique biological make-up with distinct needs. What may be fine for one may be inadequate for another.

Many people feel that our food is impoverished because the soil in which it grows is impoverished. In addition, many people are not happy about the chemical fertilizers and pesticides added to that impoverished soil. Either way, they feel, the final products lose nutritive value before they reach our table. Also, the "fresh" foods we do consume are usually a long way from the field. Therefore we need supplements to protect us against deficiency. And since the number of intelligent people taking them is growing by leaps and bounds, and they seem to be thriving, I think the subject is worth serious consideration.

What is a vitamin? Unlike minerals, which are simple inorganic substances, a vitamin is a complex substance. It is organic; that is, it is found in living things. Vitamins are necessary for health, and they cannot be made by the body but are supplied by the food we eat. If specific vitamins are absent from our diets, specific diseases result. Around the turn of the century, a biochemist, Dr. Casimir Funk, investigated widespread and destructive diseases: beriberi, pellagra, rickets, and scurvy. He found that in each case, a specific substance was missing from the food eaten by the people who had the disease. In 1912 he named these substances vitamins (from the Latin word *vita,* life) and pointed out the relationship betwen vitamins, health, and disease.

A hormone is made by the body while almost all vitamins must be taken into the body. Our body's cell machinery depends upon vitamins; therefore, if a vitamin is lacking, the machinery breaks down and a vitamin-deficiency disease appears. Our interest is to keep our bodies in super good health. We must be certain we have the vitamins and minerals that our cells need to do the constant job of tissue repair and growth our bodies demand. We are not so much worried about deficiency diseases as we are about mild deficiencies, those that can cause increased susceptibility to infection and injury, lack of alertness, and depression.

There is a huge amount of literature on treatment of disease by nutrition. It is even full of dramatic stories about people eating particular foods that were missing from their diets and achieving miraculous cures. To cite those here would be digressing, but I can't resist mentioning the last one I learned about because it is so startling. It is the discovery of vitamin B_{17}, laetrile, which has been successfully used in the treatment of terminal cancer. The active substance seems to be cyanogenic glucoside, found primarily in apricot kernels and, some say, in almonds. Apricot kernels are hard to find, but many people now are eating three almonds every day as a preventive measure against cancer. Almonds are a super food, rich in protein, high in vitamins A and B, and in the minerals calcium, phosphorus, magnesium, and potassium. And they are delicious. But remember, they have calories, too, so don't get carried away.

If you have not taken supplements before and if you should decide to do so, please, as with anything we do in our middle age, *take it easy.* Start slowly. Whether one is jogging or taking vitamins, start gradually and build up to it. When you buy vitamins, read the labels. You may be surprised to discover that a vitamin-mineral tablet can contain 20 or more different substances. However, you will also discover that no one tablet can contain all the things you will want.

If you decide to take brewers' yeast (a food, not a vitamin), it may take you a while to integrate it into your daily eating plan. Some people cannot tolerate the taste of the flakes or the powder, even if mixed with a liquid. Others have difficulty swallowing the large number of tablets necessary if you take it in that form. Feel your own way. Once you decide you want the benefits of this single food that contains more concentrated nutrients than any other known food—it is especially rich in B vitamins and full of protein—you'll figure out how to take it.

Minerals should always be taken with vitamins, for there is a strong interrelationship between them, and they work in harmony with each other. Try to buy vitamin-mineral supplements labeled "natural" or "organic" rather than synthetic ones. Supplements are not food; they are taken in addition to food. (If you're taking vitamins, you do not have an excuse to eat junk!) Supplements are best taken in conjunction with food, and after meals is best for optimum absorption.

Vitamins

Vitamin A is a fat-soluble vitamin. It is helpful for digestion and bone formation, and is needed by skin and hair to prevent dryness. It helps the body resist infection, and also helps eyes adjust to light changes. Vitamin A is found in fish, liver, eggs, dairy foods, vegetables, and fruits as carotene, the provitamin that the body converts to a double amount of vitamin A.

Vitamin B₁, or thiamin, is a factor in helping carbohydrate metabolism. It increases energy, mental alertness, and aids in digestive disturbances and constipation. Some people have had partial or total relief from headaches with thiamin supplements. Crankiness or being forgetful may be due to lack of thiamin or the body's inability to use it effectively, for some older people do not utilize it well and should take more. It is water soluble and found in many foods, especially whole grains.

Vitamin B₂, or riboflavin, works in conjunction with vitamin A. It is needed for the eyes, skin, and nerves and builds resistance to attacks by fungus which can cause vaginal itching or athlete's foot. It seems also to help ease tension and anxiety. It is found in dairy products and whole grains.

Vitamin B₃, also called niacin or niacinamide, is one of the B complex group. It affects the functioning of the brain and nervous system and is profoundly involved with the health of the soft tissues of the mouth and vagina. It is especially important for smokers, for this vitamin is related to the build-up of tartar. It is a help for depression, headaches, indigestion, and diarrhea. It is found in whole grains, peas, beans, and peanuts.

Vitamin B₆, pyridoxine, is important in the metabolism of fat and protein, and is necessary for the healthy function of the brain, nervous system, muscles, and skin. It also combats stress, tension, and anxiety, gives relief from swelling and bloat due to edema and helps leg cramps. It is found in whole grains, milk, yeast, egg yolk, rice, and bran. One slice of whole-wheat bread has six times the amount of B₆ in a slice of typical American white bread.

Vitamin B₁₂, or cobalamin or cyanocobalamin, is involved with the condition that leads to pernicious anemia. It is used in postoperative and convalescent patients to speed recovery and is part of the B complex group related to keeping one's "prime-of-life" feelings longer. It is found in brewers' yeast and eggs.

Vitamin B₁₅, known as pangamic acid or calcium pangamate, was discovered in this country by Dr. Ernest T. Krebs, Jr., in 1952. It "increases oxygen efficiency of the entire body and aids in the detoxification of waste products." It is also supposed to greatly increase physical strength and stamina. Soviet scientists have found it effective in retarding the aging process. The US government has not officially recognized that B_{15} is of value, although it is used in Russia, Japan, Yugoslavia, France, Spain, and Germany. It is found in small amounts in seeds, especially sunflower seeds, and usually in the company of other members of the vitamin B complex group.

Vitamin B_{17}, or laetrile, found in natural foods containing nitriloside, is also known as amygdalin. Reports about its use as a treatment for cancer can be found in *Laetrile: Control for Cancer* by Glenn D. Kittler and *World Without Cancer: The Story of Vitamin B_{17}* by G. Edward Griffin. It is found in apricots, peaches, cherries, plums, prunes, berries, buckwheat, millet, alfalfa, chick peas, broad beans, barley, flax seed, and lentils.

Biotin, a B-complex vitamin, although sometimes it is called vitamin H, helps relieve eczema and hair loss. It is also needed for the utilization of fat and carbohydrates in the body. It is available in many foods, especially yeast.

Choline, a B-complex vitamin helpful in lowering cholesterol levels in the blood, is important for smokers and overweight people. It is found particularly in soy products and whole grains.

Folic acid, a B-complex vitamin important for cell growth, interacts with female hormones and is thought to be a precursor to the formation of estrogen. Dr. Harold Rosenberg, author of *The Book of Vitamin Therapy* and past president of the International Academy of Preventive Medicine, notes: "Irregular or excessive menses, more folic acid." Foods that contain it are milk, whole grains, and green vegetables, especially spinach.

Inositol, a B-complex vitamin, is an essential factor in growth of new cells and a lipotropic factor involved with fat. The skin, appetite, and cholesterol level are affected by it. It is found in whole grains and peanuts.

PABA, another B-complex vitamin, is the common abbreviation for para-aminobenzoic acid. It is sometimes called the "anti-gray hair" vitamin, but a large dose is required for that and should be supervised by a nutritionist or a physician. It is claimed to be important in metabolism of adrenal and pituitary hormones and estrogen. Some say it is a factor in slowing down aging because it interacts with many hormones. It may help arthritis. It is found in brewers' yeast and whole grains.

Pantothenic acid is a B-complex vitamin. Varieties of this vitamin are called pantothenate, calcium pantothenate, or pantheonol. It is helpful in reducing uric acid in the blood and thus may help prevent gout and possibly arthritis and heart attacks. Nutritionists think it may preserve the functions of the adrenal glands and act to keep hair from graying. This vitamin is known as an antistress one; it is also essential for cell growth. It is found in soybeans, wheat germ, peanuts, yeast, egg yolks, whole grains, broccoli, salmon, and royal jelly.

Vitamin C has many uses in the body beside decreasing the incidence of infection and ameliorating the severity of the common cold. It checks many kinds of viruses and infections, especially in the gums, as well as helping wounds heal and checking skin problems. It is important for smokers and people under stress. Insufficient vitamin C can cause a deficiency in connective tissue. Connective tissue is largely responsible for the strength of bones, teeth, skin, tendons, blood-vessel walls, and other parts of the body. Linus Pauling, twice winner of the Nobel Prize, recommends 1,000 to 2,000 mg per day. It is found in citrus fruits, tomatoes, rose hips, acerola berries, red and green peppers, black currants, broccoli, parsley, Brussels sprouts, cabbage, cauliflower, and green leafy vegetables.

Vitamin D is also known as calciferol or ergocalciferol. The body actually manufactures this vitamin in the skin upon exposure to ultraviolet rays of the sun. It is important in aging, for it regulates calcium and phosphorus in bone and tooth formation and helps in absorption of calcium from the blood. It is found in fish-liver oil, some fish, eggs, and milk.

Vitamin E comes in four forms, which together are called tocopherols. They occur together in food and when bought in capsules may be labeled "vitamin E complex" or "mixed tocopherols." They contain the alpha form—the one most active in our bodies—and beta, gamma, and delta forms, which protect the alpha form from destruction. Vitamin E is also sold in the alpha form alone, which is cheaper but is not recommended. Vitamin E helps keep up the adrenal and sex hormones and oxygenates the blood. It eases leg cramps and asthma, and helps heal deep wounds and burns. It helps dissolve blood clots, especially those of varicose veins and phlebitis. The work of the Drs. Shute in Canada in the treatment of heart problems is well known. If there is a single vitamin I would claim as "the menopausal vitamin" it is vitamin E because it revitalizes the entire system. I have seen dramatic effects in women after only one week of taking vitamin E for almost continuous hot flashes and night sweats. Dr. Henry A. Gozan reported that 59 of 66 menopausal women to whom he gave vitamin E for flashes, headaches, and nervousness were completely relieved of these symptoms. Dr. Evan Shute says, "One of the most generally recognized uses of alphatocopherol is for hot flashes and headaches at the change of life (menopause)." It is best taken with vitamin C, since the two enhance each other. It comes from wheat germ oil, and is found in wheat germ and whole grains (especially oatmeal), in corn, soybean, and cottonseed oils, peanuts, navy beans, and salmon.

Vitamin K, needed for normal blood clotting, is found in many foods. Antibiotics taken by mouth kill intestinal bacteria and can cause a loss of vitamin K as well as loss of some Bs. Yogurt will help replace beneficial bacteria.

Vitamin T, though not often listed, is supposed to help memory. It comes from sesame seeds and their oil.

Bioflavonoids, rutin and hesperidin, are sometimes called vitamin P, but there is controversy about this name. The utilization of vitamin C is aided by these substances because they protect it in the body and encourage its antihistaminic and antiallergic effects. They also strengthen the capillaries and blood vessels in the hands and feet. It is in most citrus fruits. Eat some of the white pulp of orange, which is a good source. Rutin is also in buckwheat groats.

Minerals

Vitamins and minerals work in harmony with each other. There is an interrelationship between them. Minerals help the body absorb vitamins and boost their effectiveness after they are absorbed. Minerals are necessary to healthy blood, bones, teeth, nerves, hair, and heart. One does not feel in top shape if there are mineral deficiencies.

Calcium is very important to us as menopausal women because we are susceptible to osteoporosis, a thinning of the bones. Calcium helps maintain strong bones and teeth. Adelle Davis says overnight relief from "hot flashes, night sweats, leg cramps, irritability, nervousness and mental depression" can be achieved from a combination of vitamin C and calcium. She also says it helps insomnia, soothes nerves, and is a pain killer. Others say it helps alleviate premature aging, promotes the healing process, especially bone fractures, and improves hair and nails. It is in milk, yogurt, buttermilk, and cheese as well as mustard, dandelion, and turnip greens, watercress, and kale. It can also be taken as bonemeal or dolomite.

Iron carries oxygen in the blood, forms red corpuscles, and is necessary for tissue respiration. A lack of it causes anemia. It is in blackstrap molasses, wheat germ, whole grains, spinach, eggs, and apricots.

Magnesium is related to the proper functioning of many enzymes in our bodies. Many new claims are being made for it, such as that it quiets the nerves, but it surely improves the utilization of calcium. As a component of chlorophyll, it is easy to see why the best source is green leafy vegetables. It is in soy products, nuts, whole grains, sea salt, milk, egg yolk, and citrus fruits.

Phosphorus is necessary for growing tissue and for calcium absorption and retention. Phosphorus is also important for nerves and kidneys and hormone production. It is found in most natural foods, especially raisins and nuts.

Trace minerals. Many trace minerals are needed in smaller quantities than the other minerals, but they play a role in the total healthy functioning process because they interact with vitamins and other minerals. "They are the basic spark-plugs in the chemistry of life, on which the exchange of energy in the combustion of foods and the building of living tissue depends." Sea salt and kelp provide many trace minerals, as do green leafy vegetables, seafood, fruit, nuts, and grains.

MENOPAUSE FOODS

Some people may look at the title of this section and wonder how far can I carry this. I cannot carry it far enough to outweigh the damage that our culture has done to the image of the menopausal woman. Psychologically, the negative image alone would be a serious enough violation, but it has gone far beyond that. Our bodies have been seriously violated and damaged by the medications and operations that have been prescribed for our "health."

Among the women I interviewed I found that those who were concerned with the food they ate were experiencing their menopause with more ease. Good nutrition is unquestionably an important factor in the degree of severity of menopausal symptoms.

I hope these reminders or suggestions will be useful, for we tend to forget some of the things we like and mean to do. We fall into food patterns out of habit. By periodically scanning this chapter, you might remember to buy some of the healthier foods when you go to the store. If you have them, you'll eat them. For example, buttermilk is a food people seem to forget. If it's in the refrigerator you'll use it. There is hardly anything better for us because of its calcium and protein content and because it helps digestion and absorption of nutrients.

We are our own best healers. The dictionary gives us an important message, when we look under *health*. Among its various listings: "to make sound or whole, to restore to original purity or integrity; the condition of being sound in body, mind or soul; freedom from physical disease or pain; flourishing condition; well-being; vigor of body and mind; hale; robust; vigorous." Who doesn't want to be healthy? If we feel physically healthy we are not fragmented, thus we are more capable of dealing with the problems of life as they present themselves.

Prevention may appear to some of us, at first, as self-indulgence. For example, when I first bought my juice extractor I went through a guilt trip about shopping for and consuming all those vegetables, just for me. Not only did no one care, no one was even interested. I still went through my guilt number.

Caring about your own healthy body is investing in yourself. No health insurance can pay the dividends that your sense of well-being can give you.

Foods to Limit

Before I list the positive foods, I want first to mention the negatives. The list is short, but it is important because these can do a great deal of harm. Watch these foods carefully, and limit your intake of them severely:

salt	alcohol	tea	red meat
sugar	coffee	(herb teas are fine)	butter
white flour		chocolate	cream

Salt, or sodium, is one of the minerals we need to keep our body fluids in proper chemical balance. Most health authorities feel we consume too much salt in our diets. Studies have shown that a high intake is related to hypertension, or high blood pressure. The body dilutes salt deposits by water-logging the tissues, which makes for swelling and bloat.

Sugar is an undesirable form of carbohydrate. Not only are its nutrients stripped in the refining process, but the utilization of man-refined sugar requires vitamins (especially the B-complex ones) which come from other foods. The doubledecker demand can cause vitamin deficiency despite a theoretically sufficient diet. Man-refined sugar contributes to tooth decay, indigestion, and diabetes. After menopause, sugar raises the level of cholesterol in the blood. Many nutritionists believe eliminating sugar helps alleviate pain, including menstrual cramps.

Sugar is called "The Quiet Killer" by Dr. John Yudkin, author of *Sweet and Dangerous* (sounds like a murder story and is). He believes that man-refined sugar plays an important role in many diseases, especially coronary thrombosis. From his research into low-carbohydrate diets, which contain little sugar, he concluded that "sugar irritates the lining of the upper alimentary canal—the esophagus, stomach, and duodenum." He also claims that "sugar can induce sizeable alterations in the levels of potent hormones" and by avoiding it you will "increase your life span." Connections between sugar consumption and cancer are also being made. Dr. Otto Meyerhoff of the University of Pennsylvania Medical School, a Nobel Prize winner, refers to "the appetite of tumors for sugar."

If you eat sugar, have it *after,* not between, meals (after you have eaten, a gentle rise in blood sugar will already be taking place).

White flour is a waste of calories, because many nutrients are missing from it. These nutrients are easily obtainable from whole-wheat flour. Carlton Fredericks tells us that "at least twenty-three factors are depleted in the processing of white flour, and at best, some six are restored."

Alcohol, like coffee and sugar, can be called a deceiver. All three pick us up, but then they drop us. We become addicted to the lift, but not the let-down, so we have some more. They stimulate the production of adrenal hormones, which cause blood sugar levels to increase, giving us that temporary boost. The nervous system is negatively affected and the normal functioning of our glands is disturbed.

Our B vitamins, which we need significantly, are ravaged by alcohol, as is the mineral magnesium. Cirrhosis of the liver and brain damage are common diseases caused by excessive alcohol intake. The Sloan-Kettering Institute in New York confirmed the Carter report that six ounces or more of hard liquor drunk daily makes one 700 percent more prone to cancer of the larynx. Dr. Joseph G. Molmar emphasizes the caloric count in alcohol; alcohol not only adds fat but also irritability and impotence.

All this refers to heavy daily drinkers, not to people who are in good physical condition and enjoy a nutritious diet. For us, a glass or two of wine once in a while can be absorbed without detrimental effects. This, by the way, is one of my ideals—to extract the good from any situation.

Caffeine is a poison. A white crystalline alkaloid hidden in our dark cup of coffee, it is the fourth biggest commodity in world commerce, according to the *Wall Street Journal.* Every day, 8 out of 10 adult Americans drink coffee. After drinking a cup of coffee, the stomach temperature rises 10° to 15°F., your hydrochloric acid output increases 400 percent, the salivary glands produce twice as much saliva, your heart beats faster, while the blood vessels narrow in your brain but widen in and around your heart. Your metabolic rate and the uric acid level in your blood increase, and your kidneys manufacture and discharge up to twice as much urine.

The usual cup of coffee contains 80 to 120 milligrams of the poisonous drug caffeine. A cup of tea has about half that amount. A five-ounce cola drink has about 20 milligrams, and four average chocolate bars contain the caffeine equivalent to a cup of coffee. Coffee, tea, cocoa, and chocolate are thus prime sources for this drug.

No one denies coffee has an invigorating effect that temporarily stimulates the brain and wards off fatigue. However, if you drink too many cups you'll also overstimulate your pancreas and wash away B vitamins. More seriously, studies by Dr. Philip Cole of Harvard's School of Public Health relating coffee-drinking to bladder cancer found that for women who drank a cup a day the risk was two-and-a-half times greater than that of nondrinkers of coffee.

Remember, we are against doing damage to ourselves. However, as rotten as coffee is for you, if your body is used to drinking it, it is also used to the hydrochloric acid coffee stimulates. If you stop all at once, you may have gas, bloat, constipation, and even cramps. True, you're working for the greater good by cutting coffee out, but do it gradually, easily. Give yourself a transition period. Wean yourself perhaps by using half coffee, half Postum for a few days and then gradually lessening the amount of coffee. Try prune juice and eat yogurt if constipation is bothersome during your transition period.

Tea is composed of caffein, tannic acid, and oils. We have already rejected caffeine for our health. If that weren't enough, tannic acid is used to convert raw hides into leather. Who knows what conversions it can create in our insides? Besides, we know the herb teas are beneficial soothers rather than activators. The original healers, the witches, were always concocting herbal brews to make someone feel better. I put my trust in their instincts.

Chocolate always comes with sugar and saturated fat, and we don't want any of that. Without the sugar it is cocoa, which is a concentrated food containing about 40 percent carbohydrates, 22 percent fat, 18 percent protein, and 6 percent ash. The stimulant comes from theoromine and a small amount of caffeine, and "it provides approximately 2,214 cal. per pound."

Red meat, a cholesterol-producing food, contains many calories. Some researchers now question whether a high intake of cholesterol-producing foods and a high level of cholesterol in the blood are related, but others are sure it is. Until someone disproves the idea that red meat is associated with cholesterol buildup and heart attacks, it would seem sensible to eliminate red meat, or at least go easy on it. All red meat contains a high percentage of fat, even the lean cuts.

Diethylstilbestrol (DES) is a hormone used to fatten cattle. It is an extremely dangerous drug, yet the FDA still allows it to be used for cattle even though it has clearly been established as carcinogenic. It is also being used in contraceptive pills. Until it is banned from the United States altogether, as it is in many countries, the meat-packing industry will continue to use it. Another reason I do not eat red meat is it makes me feel heavy and loggy and seems to tax my whole metabolic process too much.

Butter and *Cream* are high in both calories and animal fat. As we age these are not utilized as easily by the body as are vegetable fats. They will also raise your cholesterol count.

Super Foods

The resource list below is intended to help expand your ideas about foods that will nurture you. It is not all-inclusive, but I hope it will remind you to eat more parsley and use more garlic and try to incorporate other "high-potency" foods into your regular eating system. Each item was chosen because of its particular value to us in our menopause, and the reasons follow. I made these particular choices based on our special needs, and the items mentioned are the ones that would be underlined, for emphasis, on a much longer list. Bon Appétit!

apricots	garlic
brewers' yeast	gelatin
brown rice	herbs
buttermilk	kelp
cabbage	lecithin
celery	milk (nonfat)
cheese	molasses (blackstrap)
cucumber	nuts
dried fruit	oil (polyunsaturated)
eggs	oatmeal
fish	parsley
fowl	peppers (red and green)
fresh fruit	sea salt
fresh vegetables	seeds

sprouts
Swiss chard
tahini (sesame paste)
vinegar (natural apple cider)
watercress

wheat germ
whole grains
whole wheat bread
yogurt

Apricots are good fresh or dried and are rich in vitamins and minerals, especially B₁₇. They are a staple food of the Hunzas of the Himalayas who live to be 100.

Brewers' yeast is one of the best sources of all the B complex vitamins, and it supplies protein, too. It is probably the least expensive food you can buy that supplies the greatest number of nutrients.

Brown rice is not polished and is rich in protein, thiamine, riboflavin, niacin, and minerals and is very easy to digest. Brown rice is to white rice what whole-wheat bread is to white bread.

Buttermilk, like yogurt, is one of the very best foods for us, since it contains calcium, protein, and B vitamins. As we digest the milk sugar we create lactic acid, which stimulates calcium utilization.

Cabbage is a most underrated vegetable. We like it because it is high in calcium and contains vitamins C and A. It is also a natural diuretic. Forget the cole slaw cliché and just cut some thin slices into your salad. If you have a juicer, add cabbage to your carrots, a delicious combination.

Celery has a poor reputation because it's always been one of those low-calorie things we are "supposed" to eat when we're really starved for something else. It will give us calcium for our bones, as well as sodium, magnesium, and iron. Even half a stalk cut into your salad is worth the trouble.

Cheese, the low-fat kind, is a good source of protein and calcium.

Cucumber is important to us for it is a natural diuretic and prolongs agility. It is high in potassium and full of many other minerals.

Dried fruit satisfies that "something sweet" craving. Prunes are especially good when you feel your digestion is sluggish. Be careful to read the labels, because many supermarket dried fruits contain sulfur dioxide, which destroys B vitamins and has been suspected as being carcinogenic.

Eggs have many good things in them: protein, vitamin A, thiamine, riboflavin, iron, calcium, biotin, and choline. They also contain cholesterol, but better eliminate meat and keep the eggs. Look for fish with eggs, called roe; they, too, are superb.

Fish is full of nutrients that are good for us, in addition to protein. Most fish are comparatively low in calories. Shellfish are high in cholesterol and are to be avoided.

Fowl is excellent for protein.

Fresh fruit is one of our best purifiers. Eat at least two pieces a day. They all contain vitamin C, and the natural sugar in fruit is totally positive and easily digested.

Fresh vegetables are the best things you can eat. Like fresh fruits, they supply us with vitamins, minerals, and enzymes in their best forms. Enzymes are very important to us because they act as catalysts in the digestion of the food we eat and produce energy. They are very delicate and can easily be destroyed by cooking or processing. Because they are so perishable we must eat plenty of natural, uncooked food to get the benefit of these marvelous enzymes.

Garlic is a potent herb, literally and figuratively. It can do an enormous amount of good, for it works on the secretions of your gastric juices and promotes diuretic action. It is an old folk remedy, especially for viruses, and is called the natural antibiotic. Some believe it helps get rid of toxins in the body, even through the pores of your skin. I once had a dear friend who couldn't stand the smell of garlic, so I stopped using it. But I was young then.

Gelatin is a source of extra protein. It contains glycine, one of the amino acids that seems to give a lift to the metabolism. Some people find it helps blood circulation. Many take the unflavored powder mixed in some fruit juice. Do not buy prepared gelatin—it is worthless, or worse, since it contains 85 percent sugar along with chemical additives and artificial color and flavor.

Herbs are our best friends. They can do so much for us—quiet us down, pep us up, make pedestrian food exotic, heal us. They are truly Mother Nature's gift to us. Get acquainted with them, use them, learn the ones you like best.

Kelp is dried seaweed and a good source of minerals, especially iodine, potassium, and phosphorus. Dr. Curtis Wood, Jr. "has reported relief from pain in arthritic patients by the use of kelp. . . ." I put the powdered form in my salt shaker and use less salt that way.

Lecithin comes from soybeans, and it helps utilize fat and fatty substances. It is also believed to lower cholesterol in the blood and keep it from being deposited on the walls of the arteries. It, too, has been suggested to relieve pain from arthritis.

Milk (nonfat) is high in calcium and protein. Try to use extra powdered milk to enrich such foods as cooked cereal, but add it after you take the pot off the heat. It is best to buy the noninstant types, where the heat used in preparation is not so high and more vitamins are preserved.

Molasses (blackstrap) is very rich in iron and B vitamins. It is one of those marvelous foods I have had difficulty integrating into my life because I don't like the taste. I finally succeeded by using a small amount with honey in my morning Postum. It's OK there.

Nuts are high in protein and unsaturated fats and full of vitamins (especially Bs) and minerals (particularly the trace elements). Do not buy them roasted or salted. Almonds, cashews, peanuts, pecans, and pistachios have the highest protein value for their calories. Brazil nuts and walnuts have higher calorie counts, so avoid them.

Oil (polyunsaturated) is needed by the body because it contains the essential fatty acids. A tablespoon or two a day will help absorb vitamins, give us clear skin and healthy hair, and help keep up our vitality.

Oatmeal is one of those rare food items that is good and cheap. It contains protein, calcium, iron, vitamin E, and the Bs. Buy it only as a whole grain, not processed and certainly not instant. "Rolled oats have been found to lower cholesterol."

Parsley is especially good for us. It should go on everything you can put it on, and I don't mean only as a garnish—I mean a lot. Chop a hefty handful into your raw salad. It stimulates gastric activity and it is loaded with potassium, vitamin A (even more than carrots), and contains three times as much vitamin C as does lemon juice and four times as much iron as spinach. Garnish, indeed. It's better than almost anything it usually decorates.

Peppers, green or red, are very high in vitamin C. They also contain minerals that are especially important for our nails and hair. Red peppers, though they taste sweeter, have almost the same value as green peppers.

Sea salt, the iodized kind, should be used instead of processed salt because it is dried salt from the sea and so contains many more minerals.

Seeds contain the germ of life for they have the ability to sprout. Eat them whenever you find them in such fruits as apples and lemons. Sunflower seeds are sweeter than nuts and are a superb snack.

Sprouts are one of the healthiest foods you can eat because the vitamins growing from a seed are enormously concentrated. Marvelous in salads, they are good on protein foods too. Heat destroys their valuable nutrients; therefore, place them directly on the plate with other food, never cook them.

Alfalfa sprouts are easy to grow at home. Place a tablespoon of dry seeds in a glass jar, add 2" of water, cover with cheesecloth held by a rubber band, and place in the dark under your sink. The next day, pour off as much water as you can through the cheesecloth and rinse with fresh water. Rinse three times every day, and leave the jar on its side on a counter top. Three days later you'll have a jar full of sprouts, and in two more days they'll be growing little green leaves. And their taste is something else— savory and delicate.

Swiss chard is on this list because it is a very rich dark green vegetable that is sweeter than many others and so much more palatable. Although it is absolutely loaded with good nutrition, it is not used nearly enough. Besides being delicious just steamed with garlic for three minutes (no more), uncooked, cut in thin strips, it is a fine addition to a raw salad.

Tahini (sesame butter), crushed sesame seeds, is richer in calcium than milk. It contains the esoteric vitamin T, which helps memory, and is a perfect source of unsaturated fat. Get to know this food and use it mixed with some salad dressing.

Vinegar has an extraordinarily high potassium count and creates hydrochloric acid in the digestive system. It contributes to healthy blood vessels (veins and arteries) and to building red blood. It must be natural apple cider vinegar *only*.

Watercress is for us because it is loaded with vitamins and minerals, especially calcium, and is tasty and spicy. Use it up within a few days before the leaves turn yellow.

Wheat germ is one food we really must incorporate into our daily lives for it is a rich natural source of vitamin E and the Bs. Raw is better than toasted but not as easy to find.

Whole grains contain three principal parts of the cereal: the inner germ, the endosperm, and the outer layers of bran. When cereals are put through the milling process they lose nutrients and no replacing, restoring, or enriching ever puts them all back. That is why we are against eating white rice or foods made with white flour. Whole grains contain protein, vitamin E, the Bs and more.

Whole wheat bread is much better for you than white bread because it has more nutrients. "Enriched" white bread is not as rich as whole wheat because only about a quarter of the nutrients removed are restored.

Yogurt, alphabetically last on this list, is really very high on my list (see "Yogurt Therapy" following).

CHOLESTEROL

Cholesterol, although it is necessary for life (it has many uses in our bodies and is produced all through it), can be dangerous. I know of no doctor or nutritionist, nor have I read a single text, that relates cholesterol to hot flashes, but I firmly believe there is a relationship. Everyone mentions vitamin E and calcium to ease hot flashes—and I am in complete agreement with that. They also talk about keeping the cholesterol level down to avoid heart disease. However, no one has spelled out the meaning of cholesterol in the arteries during a hot flash. This is the way I see it: when there is an excess of cholesterol in the bloodstream, it starts to build up on the interior walls of the arteries, making the walls of the blood vessel thicker and the passage narrower. Since a hot flash occurs when blood vessels abruptly dilate, does it not seem reasonable that if the thickened blood vessels cannot dilate fully and the blood has to squeeze by a mushy substance, that that flash will have to be more uncomfortable than a flash that doesn't have to work so hard?

Can it be that doctors have not figured this out? If they have, why don't they recommend watching the cholesterol level for hot flashes? Not one woman ever told me that when she went to a doctor for help with hot flashes she was asked about her diet. It makes me angry. That's why I'm writing this book. We menopausal women suffer from lack of concern.

We're important to ourselves and want to watch the buildup of cholesterol which is indirectly responsible for heart disease and stroke. The arteriosclerotic process can be reversed if fat and cholesterol are reduced. One way to do this is by taking in less cholesterol in the food we eat and another is using vitamin E. Since a high amount of cholesterol comes from animal products, it appears obvious that they should be cut down. The level of cholesterol is not the same in all animal foods. For example, red meat is much higher than veal. There is no cholesterol in foods that come from plants.

As we age, we put on fat unless we are careful. Each new pound increases the cholesterol count. If it concerns you, get your cholesterol count the next time you go for a check-up. The American average is around 220; if you have 150 or less, your cholesterol level is in very good shape and your chances of having a heart attack are ten times less than the average adult's.

The Department of Internal Medicine at the University of Iowa has prepared a *Low Cholesterol Diet Manual*. The following are their "no no's," foods high in cholesterol according to their tables: kidney, liver, brains, sweetbreads, whole milk, butter, cream, certain cheeses (Limburger, Roquefort, cream, American, cheddar, bleu, mozzarella, Swiss, Gouda, Parmesan), and most shellfish (shrimp, crab, lobster, oysters, scallops, and clams).

Since our goal is to get the most from the food we consume, we want to be careful about its preparation. High temperatures when cooking cause greater loss of vitamins and minerals. Steaming food, using little water, and cooking food for shorter periods altogether helps preserve nutrients. Keep the pot covered, to contain vapors, for they contain nutrients which are important to the integrity of your tissues, gums, joints, and muscles. Drinking anything scalding hot or ice cold shocks your internal organs. Wash your fresh fruit and vegetables unless you are sure they are organically grown. Who wants to ingest the chemical fertilizers and pesticides?

Some people, when they first get "into" natural foods, have a tendency to overeat. They eat the good things, like nuts, in *addition* to meals instead of as part of them. Also, there sometimes is a tendency to eat too much of things you feel are "good for you." Without doubt, raisins and almonds are a much better snack than a Danish pastry, but they are highly concentrated foods and can put weight on you. Just because it's healthy and natural does not mean it doesn't have calories. Watch this.

Don't get carried away by honey. Just because it's a natural food and good for you does not mean unlimited amounts are OK. A little goes a long way, for it is sweeter than sugar. It contains fruit sugars and their valuable vitamins, and it is easier on the pancreas. But it is still sugar. Too much sugar in any form can cause strain in the body's regulation of carbohydrates. The last thing we want to do is add strain on our bodies particularly when we are having hot flashes. Therefore, hot flashes mean cut out sugar altogether, except in fruit. You'll be more comfortable.

Frequent small meals make weight control and weight loss easier, for they tend to reduce levels of blood cholesterol and improve sugar tolerance.

YOGURT THERAPY

Sounds crazy, doesn't it? What does yogurt have to do with therapy or menopause and aging? A lot. Yogurt is probably the most important food you can eat for a healthy aging. It is superb nutrition and can be used as "medicine" and as cosmetic. However, use *only* pure yogurt, never the type with additions such as sugar, fruit, or stabilizers—sugar creates a breeding ground for disease. Add your own fruit, honey, nuts, or raisins.

Some people think yogurt is a dieting aid. That is not true, but it is healthy and good for you and not a high calorie food. An eight-ounce cup of plain part-skim yogurt is some 130 calories. Add 20 for a teaspoon of honey, 25 for a teaspoon of wheat germ, and 25 more for a tablespoon of bran and those 200 calories are super nutritious. The soft-frozen yogurt which is presumptuously competing with the quintessential American dessert, ice cream, is less caloric—but don't forget, it contains plenty of sugar.

Allow yogurt to remain at room temperature, uncovered, for 15 minutes before eating. I learned this from the late Joseph Metzger, who was the owner of Dannon Yogurt and the father of the current chairman of the board. He graciously consented to talk to my class at the New School for Social Research when I was giving a course in 1961 on the folklore and mythology of food—cultured milk was a perfect illustration of many of my points.

Practically all the books that have been written about menopause recommend estrogen replacement therapy with deadly seriousness. ERT can be deadly but that isn't looked upon as crazy. Many doctors are still prescribing estrogen today to healthy women after the proof has been clearly established and documented in the *New England Journal of Medicine,* December 1975, that it can raise the risk of uterine cancer. Yogurt, the single most beneficial food and a home remedy for numerous ailments, inside as well as outside the body, is looked upon by some as a joke. Joke indeed. It can neither harm nor incapacitate you, unlike ERT, let alone cause your death, and it has helped many—from checking flatulence to relieving vaginal infections.

Yogurt has been called the "miracle rejuvenator" by some because it works hard for us by helping to keep the intestinal tract free from destructive bacteria. When Gaylord Hauser suggested eating it in the late 1940s before it became popular, he was dismissed by most people as a "health food nut." Carlson Wade, a current health food writer, says yogurt "sets the foundation for helping to improve the digestive system, enrich the bloodsteam, clear the skin, send a wave of vitamins, minerals and protein throughout the endocrine system and rejuvenate the hormones, key to youthful health."

If you question yogurt therapy, consider some of the ideas presented here. I have tried most of them, as have the women I have interviewed and the women who attended the menopause workshops.

Scientists are exploring the mysteries of the yogurt culture and their discoveries are extraordinary, but the exact reason that makes yogurt so unusual remains elusive. The Jewish Memorial Hospital in New York has had success with their studies on the use of yogurt for curing infant diarrhea and old-age constipation. At New York's Mt. Sinai Hospital, liver specialists are said to be performing geriatric experiments with yogurt enemas (also used during World War I for the treatment of intestinal ailments). Dr. George V. Mann, associate professor of biochemistry and medicine at Vanderbilt University, has conducted experiments which have resulted in lowering the blood cholesterol level by inhibiting the amount produced by his subjects. The patients are eating between 1 and 4½ quarts of yogurt a day. "Their serum cholesterol was reduced by 20 to 50 percent. Dr. Mann is presently trying to isolate and characterize the material in yogurt that will explain his findings." An unexpected result of a geriatric experiment for constipation with chronically ill people was the clearing up of diabetic ulcer sores. When the patients stopped eating yogurt the sores and the constipation returned.

What is this strange food that is taking more shelf space in supermarkets and appearing in cafeterias, movie lobbies, sports stadiums, planes and trains, airports and stations? The American public spent $300 million on yogurt in 1975. Yogurt, an ancient food, is fermented milk with a custard consistency. It supplies lactic acid to the body. It aids digestion, reduces the acid content of the blood, and is beneficial in restoring and maintaining a normal intestinal flora. It probably originated in the Middle East. Yogurt is probably the oldest prepared food in existence, for wherever there is milk, there is some form of fermented milk.

Every kind of milk—cow, buffalo, sheep, goat, mare, camel, reindeer— can become fermented. Other names for the lactic fermentation of milk, from Iceland to South Africa, follow:

busa	koumiss	mazun	skyr
chass	kuban	mazzoradu	taetioc
dahi	laban	nejah	taette
gioddu	lassi	pauira	tarho
huslanka	leben	plimae	tyre
kaelder-milk	madzoon	saya	urda
kefir	mattha	skuta	whey champagne

As soon as humans discovered they had more milk than they could consume before it soured, they learned to turn it into curdled, fermented milk which could be kept much longer than fresh milk. Remember Little Miss Muffet, eating her curds and whey? She was eating a form of yogurt. If sometimes your yogurt separates, the thick white part is the curd, the basis for cheese, and the watery part is the whey. Do not pour that liquid out—it contains valuable nutrients.

Yogurt is richer in protein than milk and contains more riboflavin. It can be eaten when milk cannot be digested due to lactose intolerance. The "friendly" bacteria in yogurt culture fight off the "destructive" bacteria in the intestines and create a positive flora. Scientists have not been able to explain fully what the constructive bacteria in yogurt does or exactly how it works, but they do know, for example, that it is the acidity of yogurt that is the important element in the body's utilization of calcium. Assimilation of calcium is of prime importance to us in avoiding osteoporosis, to which we are more prone after menopause. The American Medical Association, never a group that goes overboard for a new old idea, views the benign bacteria benignly, for animals anyhow. An editorial in their journal noted it has some value when commenting on the work of DuBos at Rockefeller University, "who had found that administration of the friendly bacteria (of yogurt) to animals had increased their resistance to infection and prolonged their life spans."

Yogurt was "rediscovered" around the turn of this century by Russian scientist Ilya Metchnikoff, director of the Pasteur Institute in Paris, who strongly believed the secret of aging was directly related to the food one put in one's mouth. He was awarded the Nobel Prize in 1908 for his contributions to physiology and medicine. Metchnikoff, fascinated by the longevity of the Bulgarians, discovered that they ate large quantities of yogurt. He analyzed Bulgarian yogurt and discovered the specific that killed the putrid bacteria in the intestine, *Lactobacillus bulgaricus*. (In the three known cultures today, where people commonly live to be 100, their diets are rich in cultured milk.)

Doctors commonly prescribe yogurt when they prescribe antibiotics because such drugs overwhelm all bacteria, good and bad, and yogurt restores a beneficial balance of microflora in the intestines. Antibiotics do the same thing in the vagina creating a new vulnerability in both areas. It is a good idea to eat yogurt three times a day if you are taking antibiotics.

Vaginal infections are also being treated with yogurt, and it is popular among women who are involved in the self-help health movement. I have heard the complaint, "Yogurt in the vagina? Ugh! It's so sticky!" Creams and jellies are sticky and yogurt doesn't contain any harmful chemicals like those in many douches, vaginal spray deodorants, and the fruit-flavored preparations designed for camouflaging a woman's natural taste and smell. It is applied in various ways. You can add a few tablespoons of yogurt to warm douche water, or remove a tampon from its tube and replace it with yogurt. The woman lies on her shoulders and upper back with her legs up and inserts the yogurt, then remains in that position for a few minutes. Another method is to place the yogurt on a long spoon and insert it through the opening of a plastic speculum. Judith Hennessee, writing about yogurt in *New Times,* tells us "the normal acidity of the vagina, which prevents infections, also sustains a population of lactobacilli. When the acidity and the lactobacilli are disturbed—by antibiotics, for example—monilia fungi seize the opportunity to grow. Theoretically, yogurt should restore the vaginal flora." It does for most women, not all. Many doctors pooh-pooh the idea but some have used it when nothing else worked. Women are also using yogurt for cystitis, inflammation of the urinary bladder, which sometimes occurs as a result of vigorous intercourse and creates a burning sensation when urinating. Amazingly, yogurt has brought immediate results for some women after only one application.

I know of women in New York City who were using estrogen cream for their mature vaginal condition of thin walls, called absurdly by the medical profession, "atrophic vaginitis." When the news was published that the use of hormones can cause uterine cancer, they looked around for an alternative. This was their reasoning: anything you put in or on your skin eventually finds its way into your bloodstream; therefore they didn't want to use the cream because they didn't want the estrogen in their bodies, even in minute amounts. Also, they weren't entirely sure how much help they were getting from the estrogen or the cream. These are women who are familiar with the self-help movement and had already heard of yogurt's use in the vagina. They were also familiar with the use of polyunsaturated oil for body massage and on the genitals, both male and female, during sex. It was, therefore, an easy step to trying this new idea.

The women are using one tablespoon of yogurt and one teaspoon of oil, stirred together in a glass custard cup, and are applying it with their cream inserters once a week. One can purchase a plunger applicator at the drug store that is made for contraceptive jelly or cream. It's messy because cream or jelly has a more cohesive consistency, but with practice one develops dexterity. The yogurt-oil mixture is inserted while lying on one's back before retiring. (One learns to lift the hips in such a way so that more of the mixture is on the inside than the outside—place a towel on the bed before you begin.) The oil is pure vegetable, cold-pressed, without preservatives.

When you are going to visit another country, eat plenty of yogurt before and after, especially if the country does not have it easily available, Mexico for instance. Yogurt is the perfect antidote for Montezuma's revenge. If prone to poor digestion when you travel, take yogurt with you in tablet form. Vitamin stores carry them. People in the Middle East and Africa eat some form of yogurt because dysentery and diarrhea are common, due to a lack of health regulations for food. Those who eat yogurt generally do not suffer these illnesses—if they do, yogurt is almost the only food they can stomach. Yogurt helps constipation, too, which seems incongruous. The reason for this is that it acts as a corrective and the positive bacteria create a healthy intestinal flora—which is also the reason it is effective for hangovers.

The best known outside use for yogurt is as a facial (see chapter 5). Yogurt protects the skin from the ultra-violet rays of the sun at the beach. It doesn't show so much when it is mixed with oil but in the case of sunburn, apply it heavily to help remove the heat and then dab it off with cotton dipped in cold water. People have found relief from itching skin, especially from eczema, and the general condition improves from applying yogurt. It is also used as a shampoo and is an ingredient in a "hot oil." Mix it with oil and rub it into the scalp and allow it to "cook" by wrapping a hot towel around the head or wearing a plastic bag for half an hour.

Don't forget how versatile yogurt is. Use it in salad dressings, in soups, sauces, desserts and in health drinks, and on rice and vegetables. It is a good low-calorie replacement for sour cream. Yogurt achieves another dimension when salt is added to it.

Let me warn you not to expect to become rejuvenated from eating one or many cups of yogurt. It works best when integrated into your daily diet. Yogurt a few times a day, even if only in small amounts, is more beneficial than the same amount consumed at once. One can make pure yogurt easily and economically. Consult any good cookbook. If you don't feel like making it, buy quart containers, which are cheaper.

Who doesn't want to live longer? Yogurt will help you.

FOOD FOR SEX

We don't believe in aphrodisiacs, but there seem to be foods that work to give us a kind of vigor. I've listed a small number below for emphasis and strongly suggest incorporating them into your daily diet. Fresh fruit and vegetables are of prime importance, of course. The function of this list is to remind you of the goodies this group can supply that will keep you feeling zippy.

When we talk about foods for sex, there are those who snicker and say, "That's because you think so." That's right. A lot is to be said for that point, for no doubt there is probably an element of belief involved. The people who use these foods do so because they think the foods will work for them in a positive way.

almonds	honey
peanuts	kelp
protein	whole grains
brewers' yeast	sprouted seeds and grains
sesame seeds	yogurt
sunflower seeds	wheat germ

Seeds, nuts, and whole grains are good sources of zinc. Several studies have indicated that a deficiency of the trace mineral zinc may be associated with genital disorders. All raw seeds and nuts are rich in protein and enzymes, but almonds and peanuts are lower in calories than others.

Legend has it that many centuries ago women in Babylon ate candies made of sesame seeds and honey to improve their sexual responsiveness. Honey, when raw, unstrained, and unpasteurized, contains minerals and amino acids, especially aspartic acid, which is believed to act as a sexual tonic. Sesame seeds are rich in magnesium and potassium. Simmered together they produce an excellent supply of valuable trace minerals.

The hypophyseal hormone, which stimulates sexual activity and is produced by the pituitary gland, is made from protein, according to Dr. James Leathem of the Bureau of Biological Research at Rutgers University. Therefore the body requires protein in the diet for this hormone's production. Protein also repairs and builds cells.

Brewers' yeast, one of the most concentrated and least expensive forms of protein available, is also the cheapest source of B vitamins. More nutrients are concentrated in yeast than in any other known food, and yeast cells are "living food" for enzymes.

Kelp is a rich natural source of iodine and other minerals. An iodine deficiency can disrupt the normal thyroid functions which are necessary for hormone production. Thyroid hormones are linked to sexual drive and stimulus; an underactive thyroid can diminish sexual vigor.

Sprouts are supercharged enzyme food and contain a root auxin, a plant hormone, that helps enzymes and amino acids in producing young cells and in renewing old ones.

Yogurt, made from milk but easier to digest, is a source of protein, minerals, and vitamins with emphasis on casein, the protein of milk that is needed for healthy functioning and production of sex hormones. It also contains vitamin B_{12}, which is found in the uterus and in seminal fluid and is essential for sexual activity.

Wheat germ is a good source of vitamin E and also contains the precursor for the formation of estrogen in the body. Hops are also supposed to be good in the same way, and although used mostly for beer, one can use hops to brew a refreshing drink. The germ contains life-generating substances and has been proven to increase endurance. There's so much fun to be had, who doesn't want to endure?

18
Male Menopause

The term *male menopause* has come into recent usage, in spite of the laughs it gets, because people *do* use it when they talk and write about middle-aged men. Language develops from usage. The word *menopause* is no more applicable to men than it is to women. As was pointed out earlier in the book, when used about women the word more correctly should be "menocease," for it is not a pause in the monthly cycles but an end to them. However, *menopause* has come to mean a combination of the elements a woman experiences at the same time her menstrual flow stops. We can apply the term to men, too, even if they don't menstruate, for it is more the combination of life's circumstances that occur around the age of 50, sometimes beginning as early as 40 for some, that creates the condition labeled menopause. We women want to learn about it to understand our male friends and relatives better—and we hope that they will want to try to understand us.

There are many things women and men of middle age have in common, and to know about the other is to learn more about oneself. A sympathetic viewing of female menopause would teach men a lot about their own. As Plato says in the myth of the Androgynes, "The organism of the male supposes that of the female. Man discovers woman in discovering himself and inversely it is in so far as she incarnates sexuality that woman is redoubtable. We can never separate the immanent and the transcendent aspects of living experience: what I fear or desire is always an embodiment of my own existence, but nothing happens to me except it comes through what is not me." The physical phenomenon we obviously share is a diminishing production of sex hormones in the body. In women it's the ovaries, in men it's the testes, which are similiar in size and shape to the ovaries. It is curious that as the cultural sex roles are becoming less rigid there is a more open move toward comparison—but of the similarities of the sexes rather than of the differences. There was no talk of male menopause at the turn of the century when "a man was a man" and a woman knew her place.

More than six years ago, letters started coming in to Dr. Theodore Isaac Rubin, the house psychiatrist at *Ladies' Home Journal*, inquiring if men go through menopause. His answer: "Even without a comparable physiological syndrome, men between the ages of 35 and 55 do go through an emotional menopause." However, psychiatrist Helen Kaplan, director of the Paine-Whitney Sex Therapy Clinic, Cornell Medical School, when speaking about male menopause, said, "A well-integrated man adjusts to the decline in control and sexual power; he has no climacteric."

Some members of the medical profession prefer the terms *male climacteric* or *male crisis* or *midlife crisis* or *middle age crisis*. In Europe, *climacterium verile* is popular. The phrase *menopausal syndrome* is the most foolish of all for it implies the menopause causes the syndrome, when in fact the hormonal part of the picture is far less important than are the problems of being middle-aged in a culture that worships youth and looks down upon age. There are sticklers who feel "male climacteric syndrome" is closer to the biology of the matter and prefer it. I like Gertrude Stein's way of describing the period as "middle living." Peter Chew says that "male menopause is more than faintly silly" in his book *The Inner World of the Middle-Aged Man.* "Change of life" is a phrase used for women, but I've not heard it used for men.

I remember when I first heard the term *male menopause.* My immediate response was, of course, that it was like *couvade* in some pre-literate cultures when men go through a simulated birth process while their mate is delivering, which is supposed to safeguard the infant's welfare. They wanted the experience and felt it, too, and their male companions were genuinely sympathetic and supported their "birthing" friend in a couvade hut. So, it must be the same with menopause, I thought—taking over another female function. However, after I delved into the concept of male menopause I changed my mind about its being similar to couvade, for I think there is truly something to it. The term is unfortunate, but it is unfortunate for women, too, and that seems to be what we've got. The word *climacteric* is related to *climax,* and I don't see why middle age should be looked upon either as a crisis or a climax. The original Greek from which the word *climacteric* is derived has to do with a rung on a ladder, but why should middle age rather than any other phase be described that way? Such words don't make any more sense than the word *menopause.*

Much that is attributed to menopause is not caused by the condition but is rather a result of having lived a particular number of years, so being menopausal applies equally to men as to women. Gail Sheehy says in

Passages, "At 50, there is a new warmth and mellowing. Friends become more important than ever, but so does privacy. Since it is so often proclaimed by people past midlife, the motto of this stage might be, 'No more bullshit.' "

By whatever name, what is *it*? And what are *its* symptoms? Male menopause is an exceedingly complex scheme of physical, social, cultural, psychological, and philosophical realities coming together to make some men around the ages between 45 and 55 feel, at best, occasionally uneasy and at worst, very uncomfortable with pain. The male menopause resembles female menopause because it is often triggered by hormonal changes as well as social pressure.

What are the symptoms? Martha Weinman Lear, a brilliant writer who understands male menopause, lists them in the *New York Times Magazine* in "Is There a Male Menopause?" There are

> nervousness, decrease or loss of sexual potential, depressions, decreased memory and concentration, decreased or absent libido, fatigue, sleep disturbances, irritability, loss of interest and self-confidence, indecisiveness, numbness and tingling, fear of impending danger, excitability; less often, headaches, vertigo, tachycardia, constipation, crying, hot flashes, chilly sensations, itching, sweating, cold hands and feet.

Sound familiar? Other lists I've seen include the 50 symptoms mentioned in chapter 2 in defining women's menopausal symptoms, plus others such as hypochondria and heartburn. Most doctors emphasize male depression because that seems to accompany the other symptoms. Every male, however, doesn't get depressed during the middle years just as every female doesn't, but many do. I have not come upon anyone yet who doesn't sometimes feel blue. Menopausal? No one really knows.

Do men have monthly cycles like women? According to the endocrinologist Dr. Estelle Ramey, professor at Georgetown University Medical School, "Men *do* have monthly cycles. The evidence of them may be less dramatic, but the monthly changes are no less real." She describes a 16-year study conducted in Denmark in which male urine was tested for the fluctuating amounts of male sex hormones it contained. The result: a pronounced 30-day rhythm was revealed through the ebb and flow of hormones. Her opinion is that men respond to their cycles in a way that is a function of their "culturally acquired self-image. They deny it." This is a fact to be lamented, for it is no doubt the reason the largely male scientific community has not drawn on the information about biological rhythms for the treatment of disease or for protection against disease. Dr. Ramey says, "Menopause in men has been studied somewhat more than the effects of their monthly cycles, but not enough."

The Australian scientist Margaret Henderson, who teaches at Melbourne

University, became interested in male monthly temperature cycles while she was examining disorders such as migraine headaches, depression, asthma, and alcoholic bouts. She found that such attacks in women often occur when the body temperature rises slightly, and she discovered that men, too, have a periodic temperature cycle of from 17 to 35 days, depending on the individual.

All living things—humans, plants and animals—have time cycles. In humans they are biologically represented in a metabolic process that is our rhythmic nature, which is cyclic. But "cyclic change is so unexpected even among medical doctors and scientists that it is often mistaken for abnormality." So says Gay Gaer Luce in her extraordinary book *Body Time, Physiological Rhythms and Social Stress,* which focuses upon human time structure and elaborates on our daily, weekly, monthly, yearly, and life cycles. At menopause, both women and men are entering a new life cycle, and it brings bodily changes. Is that then what male menopause is?

Ms. Lear puts it succinctly and with wit:

The hormone-production levels are dropping, the sexual vigor is diminishing . . . the children are leaving, the parents are dying, the job horizons are narrowing, the friends are having the first heart attacks; the past floods by in a fog of hopes unrealized, opportunities not grasped, women not bedded, potential not fulfilled, and the future is a confrontation with one's own mortality.

Psychological or not, these problems are enough to make anyone feel depressed, and menopause blues is not only the prerogative of women.

However, the endocrinologists and the sex therapists who see the male truth laid bare are the best guessers available to us about what male menopause is—and they disagree with each other on the treatment in the same way that the gynecologists disagree about the treatment of women's menopause. For instance, there are those who are for hormone replacement therapy and others who are against it.

DO MALE HORMONES RAGE?

Dr. Herbert S. Kupperman, associate professor of medicine at New York University Medical Center and chief of endocrinology at three hospitals, emphasizes that "primary testicular insufficiency" is the only "pure" male climacteric. He does not use the term when referring to secondary testicular insufficiency, which is the common variety of impotence of psychological origin. His view is that if a man is sexually dysfunctional with his wife but can perform with another woman, or gets an erection at a movie, he is not in the male climacteric. Kupperman notes that "The true climacteric is a physiological cessation of testicular function accompanied by vasomotor symptoms [hot flashes], neurological symptoms, and psychosomatic symptoms. If the symptoms occur without physiologic expression of diminished testosterone production, and increased gonadtropins, then it is not the male climacteric.'' He is saying, in other words, that if a man has hot flashes, is depressed and impotent but does have ''enough'' testosterone in his blood stream, he is *not* menopausal.

The way the lines are drawn amazes me. It has the ring of semantic quibbling. If a man is depressed and impotent, whether the trouble is ''pure'' or not hardly seems to matter. He's in trouble. Kupperman, when dealing with male patients, prescribes testosterone hormone replacement therapy. When prescribing for females the hormone used is estrogen. He claims that within six weeks most men start to improve and function again sexually. He also claims to be able to separate the physiologically induced cases of impotence from the psychologically induced ones by the use of placebos. It sounds extraordinarily oversimplified, doesn't it? Dr. Norman Zinberg, professor of psychiatry at Harvard Medical School, in discussing testosterone-level variations, tells us the variability is enormous ''from month to month, from day to day, and even from hour to hour, with no known cause and no visible effect.''

Dr. Harold Lear believes sexual problems are overloaded with anxiety and may cause depression which can become so intense ''that raising his testosterone level will not affect his depression.'' Lear is head of the Human Sexuality Program at Manhattan's Mount Sinai Hospital. He left the field of urology at the age of 50 to become a sex therapist, better to understand the problems of impotence. He elaborates by describing a patient: ''He'll say, 'I'm over the hill, Doc.' Now that becomes a self-fulfilling prophecy. So that even if you rectify the physiological disability but don't treat the psychological overlay, you're not doing him any good. So you give him the testosterone he needs and he walks out, and he still stays impotent.''

Dr. Ivan Popov, medical director of the Renaissance Revitalization Center in Nassau, the Bahamas, is involved with the problems of aging. He uses the cell therapy originated by the famous Swiss doctor Paul Niehmans, who was his teacher, instead of hormone therapy, which he feels is destructive to the total person. His position is that

they create a dependency and they also create lazy endocrine glands. Glandular secretions work on the feedback system. Shortage of a hormone in the blood is registered by the anterior part of the pituitary gland and the hypothalamus, which in turn secrete other hormones in minute quantities. When these hormones, circulating in the blood, reach the gland to which they bear the message, this gland follows the orders and starts secreting the missing hormone. When the hormonal level in the blood rises, the anterior pituitary and the hypothalamus send a message to stop production. Artificial introduction of a hormone overtakes this cycle, and the gland that is supposed to do the work no longer needs to. There are sufficient hormones in the body and no need for the pituitary to give any order at all.

It does seem reasonable to theorize that if hormones are injected, the body doesn't have to trouble to produce them itself.

The job, the wife or partner, the home, the children, one's existential search for meaning in life, one's relation to the universe, the realization of one's mortality all pale in the light of the two major problems that are the most common in male menopause. Both of them stem from the prostate, the producer of male sex hormones. They are called prostate disorders and impotence. They can occur separately or together.

What is impotence? I dislike the word as much as I dislike "frigidity" when it is applied to women's sexuality. We are dealing with one of man's most delicate biologic mechanisms, and measuring the level of testosterone in his blood does not strike me as being the way to begin to solve the problem, because by removing stress that level can increase and the measure will change. I do not mean to simplify the complexity of the combination of elements operating, but impotence is not, after all, castration. The equipment is there. Except in the smallest percentage of cases, labeled "prime," the number of men with an organic problem is very small. How to nurture it back to health in a nonthreatening way would seem the place to start.

The known specialists discussing impotence argue about hormones and sex therapy but they do not discuss the endocrine system as though it were part of a man's total physical health. Endocrinologists and psychiatrists do not pay much attention to nutrition, but I cannot help feel that if a man concerned with impotence were to limit his intake of sugar, alcohol, animal fats, coffee, and cigarettes, his total health picture would improve, including his endocrine functioning. A man doing business over a rich lunch, drinking martinis and coffee and dining heavily again in the same day, with perhaps time out to get his testosterone shot is hardly acting in a reasonably healthy way. There is mounting evidence that biochemical principles underlie the "food-to-mood" phenomenon and that a person's diet has a profound influence on the way he feels and perceives the world around him.

Drastic changes are demanded and must be instituted in the life-style of the person when sexual problems appear, because depression causes loss of energy and it becomes a self-perpetuating cycle: impotence, depression, exhaustion. Then what finally can we say impotence is? I have seen it defined as the inability of a man to achieve and maintain an erection. The question is then, an erection for how long? Impotence, a condition that may be temporary or longer lasting, relates to a man's sex drive. It manifests itself as his being interested in sex and not being capable of fulfilling that interest in the way he has preconceived it. Or it may show itself as a man's having little or no interest in sex. What one man may consider impotent another might consider successful sexual fulfillment. For example, five minutes of vigorous sexual intercourse could be viewed by one as a very good experience and by another as fifteen minutes short of what he had hoped for. The degree of sexual disturbance is relative. Having no sex drive whatsoever, or the inability to get an erection at all is, of course, a more clearly defined situation.

Prostate disorder, also called "male trouble," is the commonest affliction of the modern middle-aged man. Well over half of the American male population over 60 have some enlargement of the prostate, and the proportion rises to almost every male by age 80. By itself, it is nothing to be alarmed about; it is part of the normal condition of aging in the human male. No symptoms may show themselves when it is simple enlargement, but if inflammation of the gland occurs (prostatitis) it is "almost certain to do so in painful and embarrassing ways." If an active infection can be found, it can be controlled and probably cured with drugs, but when there is distress without locating an infection, that is more difficult to cure. Any "disorder of the prostate is likely to cause painful, difficult and too frequent or incomplete urination." Doctors advise men over 50 to have semiannual or annual prostate examinations in which the prostate is palpated for early detection and diagnosis in case there are growths.

Cancer is the most feared of prostatic diseases because "cancer originating in this gland is the third commonest malignancy among North American males, and the third ranking cause of cancer deaths among men." As many as 60,000 men in the country will have prostate cancer diagnosed this year and 20,000 will die from the spread of the disease. Although the prostate gland in the male is associated with sexual function, testosterone is produced chiefly in the testes. We relate the ovaries in woman to the testes in man because they are both called *gonads* from the Greek word for "seed." The prostate gland is remarkably similiar to the female breast under the microscope. When it becomes cancerous, the disease is related to and sometimes controlled by the sex hormones. The prostate surgeons have the same problem as the breast cancer surgeons, namely how radical an operation to perform or whether to perform one at all. Unlike the breast, the prostate gland is not visible because it is inside the body, against the wall of the rectum.

Gilbert Cant, the former medicine editor of *Time* magazine, says in an article in the *New York Times Magazine* that this last quarter of the twentieth century is the age of prostatism for the male half of the population. The reason more attention is paid to menopausal and post-menopausal problems in women is that we are living longer. So are men, and this is when prostate problems develop. And as mastectomies are "going public," it is inevitable that prostatitis will too. The age of quiet suffering in the dark is happily disappearing because early detection is more readily possible when there is light on these matters through consciousness-raising about their existence.

The tricky thing about prostatitis is that it is difficult initially to distinguish between the more serious variety and the benign enlargement, for the symptoms are essentially the same. In the words of Cant, "The most common, and usually the earliest to appear, is the need to get up in the middle of the night to micturate. Despite its urgency, urination then may start slowly, there will be increasing need for frequent urination throughout the day, and in still more severe cases, pain in the lower back and perineal region will be experienced."

Some doctors believe cancer cells flourish in the presence of testosterone when it is injected, and since the estimates are that about a quarter of American men over 40 have a dormant possibility of prostate cancer, hormone therapy could be dangerous. Dr. Jay Rosenblum, neurologist at the New York School of Medicine, says that if hormones are taken when there is cancer of the prostate, it "is like pouring gasoline into the fire. It will accelerate its growth. So, hormones are potentially very dangerous, unless administered under good, medical supervision." Moderate enlargement, according to Cant, can cause some slight discomfort with erection and a lot more with ejaculation. Yet he claims this is psychological rather than physical.

This brings up the same question asked about female menopause. How much is it the hormones and how much is it the culture (which creates the psychological)? Dr. Lear says

> When the hormonal loss is gradual and normal, as in the climacteric years, the realities of his diminishing energy and changing sexual response are undramatic, but they are still realities. How a man handles them depends not only on how he sees himself but also, very much, on how the culture sees him. In a culture where old age brings dignity, honor, status, would we find the same syndrome? I doubt it.

In the land of the Hunzas in the Himalayas where we have learned the aged are revered for their wisdom, they do not have prostatitis or cancer.

We are not living in that Shangri-la, however; therefore we must look at our own specifics. The production of male reproductive hormones starts declining before he reaches 20 and continues to decline very gradually until old age. In the female, her peak of estrogen production is around 23, and the decline is very gradual. Some women and some men have greater hormonal fluctuations at menopause, but I do not agree with those who claim women's estrogen supply is "cut off" then, nor do I agree men's testosterone supply "drops sharply." There is too much evidence to the contrary. So, what have we here? The majority of women and men move into their menopause gradually as far as their biology is concerned. Then why is it common in middle living for men to become alcoholic, depressed, promiscuous, hypochondriacal, and even suicidally inclined?

DEPRESSION

Dan Levinson, psychologist at Yale University, recently completed a five-year study, funded by the National Institute of Mental Health, of these problems in men aged 35 to 45. He claims that a reason for the kind of shock that hits men at this time is that they have been busy working in their twenties and thirties focusing on career. Then sides of their nature which have lain dormant emerge. Depression can be triggered by the resurgence of childhood dreams, conflicts in need of resolution, new erotic longings and fantasies, the sadness over opportunities not taken, or a new questioning of values. All of this, probably coupled with a search for meaning in life, can cause most of the depression at this time.

Middle age depression is attributed to the realization that "the individual has stopped growing up and has begun to grow old," says Elliot Jaques, a British psychoanalyst. Depression is a mild word, for some men go into panic over aging. The cosmetic industry is booming, in spite of the new natural look for women, because they're exploiting this male aging fear. They call the merchandise "grooming products" to remove the female curse of make-up, but pancake is pancake. John Revson of Revlon says the biggest buyers are middle-aged men "because they're looking for that fountain of youth. Everybody is looking to maintain a youthful image today."

It's more than that—it's also taking inventory or, as some put it, stocktaking time. The realization that more than half of one's life has been lived is frightening, and time becomes more precious. There is worry over all the things undone, and there doesn't seem to be enough time for everything—which gives the feeling of missing out on a chunk of life. Is there ever enough quiet time to reason out one's existence, to try to bring the chaos of one's experience into some kind of order for internal peace? How does one become a "whole" person without feeling inadequate in so many areas of life? These are questions menopausal men ask. Psychiatrists have a term for the condition when middle-aged men's questions go along with a yearning to chuck their current lives and escape to another world. It is called the "Gauguin Syndrome," but the seemingly voluptuous worlds of Tahiti or San Francisco or Greenwich Village also have their problems, which are never considered.

The developmental view of adulthood which Dan Levinson holds will, he hopes, help menopausal men understand themselves better. When the demons strike, Levinson hopes that they will know they are not alone, but rather that the midlife transition or crisis "is a natural developmental process, and that while the losses are all too obvious at this time of life— and while the losses are going to increase—men should be equally aware of the not-inconsiderable gains, and be prepared to take advantage of them." The first sizable celebration of middle age in this country was the publication of *Life Begins At Forty* by Walter B. Pitkin in 1932. It was a very popular book during the Great Depression, maybe because everyone was depressed and this was one thing to feel good about that didn't cost money.

Some are convinced that underlying the menopausal man's depression is the fear of death. Ernest Becker, whose book *The Denial of Death* won him a Pulitzer prize, argues brilliantly that man's horror of death and the "overwhelmingness" of an incomprehensible world is the trigger pursuing success. "The idea of death, the fear of it, haunts the human animal like nothing else; it is a mainspring of human activity—activity designed largely to avoid the fatality of death, to overcome it by denying in some way that it is the final destiny of man."

Almost everyone acknowledges that the American drive for success can be a killer. Men who are engaged in activities other than the daily job for a living, who have avocations that give them pleasure unrelated to money, who have their "play" which is highly sustaining, are less likely candidates for depression. It is unbalanced to be so busy with getting ahead that the pleasures of life are missed. The Talmud warns against that: "Man will be called to account for all the permitted pleasures which he failed to enjoy."

STRESS

The way middle-aged men have been coping with stress in their lives before will, as with women, largely determine the way in which they cope with it at menopause. Everyone admires people who are busy with their creative pleasure projects, be it building shelves, gardening, or serious reading. These are people who find retirement less of a shock, too. A man I admire especially in this way is former prime minister of England, Edward Heath, who played in a professional jazz band.

As addicted as we are to the work ethic in America—it has been called the "national neurosis"—and even though that commitment deprives many men of leisure, that isn't the worst of the problem. The immediate fallout of stress coming from work pressure is more destructive.

Stress affects the amount of testosterone in a man's bloodstream. Men's hormones, as we know, fluctuate just like women's; they are not a static phenomenon. The more stress, the less testosterone. It's almost as simple as that. If the testosterone level falls too low, we know what that means—sexual problems—and that brings depression. Dr. Hans Selye, director of the Institute of Experimental Medicine and Surgery at the University of Montreal, is the granddaddy of the stress experiments which started in the 1930s. He has proved through his studies of the body's hormonal secretions during stress that stress is a cause of disease and aging. Stress sets a whole series of actions going in the body; this in turn affects not only the hormones but creates changes in the blood, breathing, and muscles as a defense. It taxes the pituitary gland by increasing its secretions, which in turn stimulates the adrenal cortex to produce corticoid hormones.

Medical research and popular perception implicate heavy stress as a prime cause of heart attacks. It is the number one killer in America. In 1975, of the estimated one to three million Americans who had heart disease, close to 675,000 will die of it, 175,000 before they reach 65.

Recent research suggests that the biological mechanism is responsible for this link. The immediate cause of a stress-induced heart attack, says one view, is the buildup of cholesterol deposits on the walls of the arteries. Stress lowers the level of testosterone and increases the level of cholesterol in the bloodstream. These deposits form plaques, which narrow the vessels. If these plaques decay and tear away from the artery walls, they form clots that close off the channels of one or more of the coronary arteries, already narrowed by plaques. The result is heart attack.

We are born with a specific amount of adaptive energy, which gradually becomes used up by stress. This means that our aging process is directly related to the total amount of drain on the supply of our adaptability. If the stress response is activated too often or lasts too long, it takes a heavy toll. For example, the muscles of the head and neck can stay contracted, which is how headaches are born. Dr. Jerome E. Singer, consultant for the book *Stress*, published by Time-Life Books, tells us five good ways to cope with stress: 1) take it easy; 2) consider the bright side; 3) try to avoid surprises; 4) give yourself some choices; 5) think long-term.

Now, how to remove oneself from stressful situations is not easy, but one step in that direction is awareness. Some people think it's heroic to keep stress undercover. They don't even admit to themselves when they're in the pressure cooker. That kind of bravado can cost a man his life. He must decide not to accept stress on a day-to-day basis as inevitable. It is less stressful when he responds to problems differently, at a slower pace. For instance, when people come to learn their own time structure and know what hours of the day they can handle stress more easily, that can be a revolution in self-insight because it will create a change in their image. They will learn to use themselves better by giving in to body demands and avoiding stress. People do change, they change in their jobs and in their lives. In fact, many men in their menopause change.

However, "a great deal more research into the male menopause needs to be done if men are to be relieved medically from some of its symptoms, and to suffer less from the personal implications of trying to deny biological facts," concludes Dr. Estelle Ramey.

Male menopause is news these days and has been found to be worthy of national attention. There have been prime-time programs on television and large articles in national news magazines. The New York public educational channel called their program "The Pause that Perplexes" when they staged a roundtable discussion in the late 1970s. I would like to see discussions take place for both female and male menopause.

Appendix

The following extract is from an article in *Majority Report,* vol. 6, no. 20 (February 5, 1977). *Majority Report,* a women's liberation newspaper founded in May 1971, is published biweekly in New York City. In its February 5, 1977 issue it printed a 1,500-word letter dated December 17, 1976, from an executive vice-president at Hill and Knowlton, Inc., a public relations firm, to the president of Ayerst Laboratories. The purpose of *Majority Report* in publishing the letter was to expose the cynicism of drug company public relations tactics.

The heart of the letter was a list of eight suggestions for "continuing activities" to counteract "adverse publicity . . . [and] negative damaging commentary in the medical, scientific, and lay media" against estrogen replacement therapy. The writer was referring to the studies which have shown that women who have taken estrogens for more than a year have an increased risk of developing cancer of the endometrium and that use of estrogen during pregnancy is linked to birth defects. The eight suggestions were vital in the opinion of the writer because "menopause remains a fashionable topic, cancer is always current. . . ." His suggestions:

1. Placement of a comprehensive article on the menopause in a major women's magazine. The prime targets here would be *McCall's, Ladies' Home Journal, Family Circle,* and *Redbook.* A possible theme is the stages of life that women pass through—the triumphs, tragedies, challenges of each.

2. Placement with syndicated columnists on newspapers' women's page. These sections are the second most widely read (after sports) and have substantial impact. Writers such as King Features' Phyllis Batelle should be contacted with a variety of approaches for column material.

3. General magazines. The interest of such writers as Walter Ross at the *Reader's Digest* should be fueled with the latest favorable reports, research statistics, and other information.

4. Science editors. Writers such as Alton Blakeslee should be provided help in assembling data on menopause.

5. Editorial service. Features and shorter fillers should be distributed to suburban and small town daily and weekly newspapers through Hill and Knowlton's service that provides, free of charge, material in ready-to-use form. These news items are sent to more than 4500 "grass roots" publications across the U.S., either on a one-time basis or as a regular series. The newspapers are carefully selected for their use of this type of material, and the clippings that return are numbered in the hundreds and often reach four figures.

6. A film on the menopause. Production of a high-quality film could provide a highly persuasive message to a variety of important audiences including television, women's clubs, and medical conventions. It is important again to stress that the benefits of estrogen replacement therapy should not be explicitly stated, but rather should flow from a general exposition on the menopause.

7. Television spokeswoman. We suggest a resumption of the program of securing television interviews in U.S. cities. If the spokeswoman is properly prepared and rehearsed, these appearances could avoid violating in any way the letter or spirit of regulations. In fact, they should be portrayed as public service ventures.

8. TV film clip. A section of the film could be edited for use in the television presentations. This technique would not only add visual impact to the interview, but also have the added advantage of interjecting a segment of two minutes or so that would proceed without interruption from the host or other participants on the program.

In conclusion, the writer stressed that at least two Ayerst spokesmen be groomed (by a training course the writer's company had designed) to "deliver a prepared or spontaneous comment confidently and convincingly."

Notes

For complete publishing information consult the Bibliography

P.v   "Bless̀ed sister, holy mother. . . . ": T. S. Eliot, "Ash Wednesday," in *Collected Poems and Plays, 1909-1950* (1952), p. 67.

1. Why This Book?

P.1   "Good talk seems to pass. . . . ": Edith Wharton, *A Backward Glance* (1934), p. 171.

P.3   two books have come out. . . . : *Menstruation & Menopause* by Paula Weideger (1976) and *The Menopause Myth* by Sheldon H. Cherry (1976).

P.3   "Menopause—The Loss of Womanhood . . . ": Robert A. Wilson, *Feminine Forever* (1966), p. 92.

P.3   ". . . the ovaries shrivel up and die . . .": ibid., p. 40.

P.3   ". . . the woman becomes . . . a eunuch.": ibid.

P.3   "I have known cases . . . committed suicide.": ibid., p. 43.

P.3   "no woman can be sure . . . living decay.": ibid.

P.3   ". . . most women . . . menopause cripples them.": ibid.

P.3   "I have seen untreated women . . . caricatures. . . .": ibid., p. 44.

P.3   "Though the physical suffering from. . . .": ibid.

P.3   "Outright murder. . . .": ibid., p. 94.

P.3   ". . . this common aberration.": ibid., p. 95.

P.3   "To be suddenly desexed. . . .": ibid., p. 96.

P.4   ". . . she is incapable of rationally perceiving. . . .": ibid., p. 97.

P.4   "The transformation . . . of a formerly pleasant. . . .": ibid.

P.4   "In a maze of longing and delusion. . . .": ibid., p. 102.

P.4   "Enlightened physicians . . . curable deficiency disease. . . .": ibid., p. 105.

P.5   "A considerate woman usually makes a valiant effort. . . .": Miriam Lincoln, *You'll Live Through It* (1950), p. 188.

P.5   "Talk . . . mountains out of molehills.": ibid., p. 189.

P.5   Helene Deutsch, whose "presumptive mistakes. . . .": Rosetta Reitz (using the name Rachael Goldman), "The Liberation of the Yiddisha Mama," *Village Voice* (February 11, 1971), p. 53.

P.5   "servant of the species": A common phrase for Deutsch, used frequently to differentiate a child-bearing woman and to separate women from each other. Helene Deutsch, *The Psychology of Women* (1945), vol. 2, p. 459.

P.5   Benedek modernized the Freudian view: Therese Benedek, "Climacterium, a Developmental Phase," *Psychoanalytic Quarterly* vol. 19 (1950), pp. 1-27.

2. Menopause—What Is It?

P.11   "I do not want to simplify. . . .": Adrienne Rich, "From an Old House in America," in *Poems: Selected and New 1950-1974* (1975), p. 240.

P.11   "It is a condition . . . frustrating to women. . . .": Isaac Asimov, *Human Body* (1964).

P.11   "Ovarian Dysfunction": *The Merck Manual of Diagnosis and Therapy,* 11th ed. (1966), p. 474.

P.12   "The transitional phase. . . .": ibid., p. 477.

P.12   "and often attended by a complex imbalance. . . .": *The Merck Manual,* 10th ed. (1961), p. 462.

P.12   "large doses of estradiol benzoate.": ibid., p. 463.

P.12   "critical point in human life. . . .": *Dorland's Illustrated Medical Dictionary,* 25th ed. (1974), p. 329. The concept of male menopause is fairly new, and the 25th edition is the first to include men under the word *menopause.* The 24th edition, published in 1965, does not.

P.12   ". . . the end or cessation of menstrual periods. . . .": Sheldon H. Cherry, *The Menopause Myth* (1976), p. 2.

P.12   "The problem is really a social problem. . . .": statement by Dr. Marcia L. Storch, gynecological endocrinologist at Roosevelt Hospital, New York City, panel discussion hosted by Frank Field, "What You Should Know About Estrogen," NBC-TV, May 23, 1976.

P.14   "Strangely enough, it is usually just those women. . . .": Katharina Dalton, *The Menstrual Cycle* (1969), p. 88.

P.14   "is no ovulation . . . during the last couple of years. . . .": ibid.

P.16   less estrogen . . . extraglandular sources also exist.: Pentti K. Siiteri and Paul C. MacDonald, "Role of Extraglandular Estrogen in Human Endocrinology," in *Handbook of Physiology,* edited by R. O. Greep and E. B. Eastwood (1973), vol. 2, pp. 615-629.

P.17   *Endgame:* A play by Samuel Beckett. Beckett interestingly gives the name Nagg to the male of the couple in garbage cans, and the woman is called Nell. I have always loved Beckett for not falling into using a stereotypic view of women, especially older women, by calling *her* Nagg instead of Nell.

P.17   "Forecasting studies by the Rand Corporation. . . .": Josef P. Hrachovec, *Keeping Young & Living Longer* (1972).

P.17   "a move away from sexual polarization. . . .": Carolyn G. Heilbrun, *Toward a Recognition of Androgyny* (1974), p. ix.

P.17   "And gives to every power. . . .": William Shakespeare, *Love's Labour's Lost,* act 4, scene 3, lines 331-332.

P.17   "Dionysus appears to be neither. . . .": As quoted in Heilbrun, p. xi.

P.17   "The truth is, a great mind must be androgynous." Samuel Taylor Coleridge, as quoted in Heilbrun, p. xx.

P.20   fibroid tumors. . . . "They are so common. . . .": Sherwin A. Kaufman, *The Ageless Woman* (1967), p. 109.

P.20   "Clots are simply the result. . . .": ibid., p. 106.

P.21   separate the fear of aging: Lena Levine and Beka Doherty, *The Menopause* (1952), p. 50.

P.21   most talked about symptom of menopause,: Bernice L. Neugarten and Ruth J.

Kraines, "Menopausal Symptoms in Women of Various Ages," *Psychosomatic Medicine* vol. 27 (1965), pp. 266-273.

P.22 bizarre because of their names: *The Merck Manual,* 11th ed. (1966), p. 477.

3. Hot Flashes

P.25 "By facing her own emotion. . . .": M. Esther Harding, *Woman's Mysteries* (1973), p. 242.

P.25 "hot f. a vasomotor. . . .": *Stedman's Medical Dictionary,* 22nd ed. (1972).

P.26 ". . . temporary error of the thermostatic control. . . .": Katharina Dalton, *The Menstrual Cycle* (1969), p. 93.

P.28 the risk of cancer . . . linked to estrogen replacement: Harry K. Ziel and William D. Finkle, "Increased Risk of Endometrial Carcinoma Among Users of Conjugated Estrogens," *New England Journal of Medicine* vol. 293 (1975), pp. 1167-1170.

P.29 "About sixty percent of women get distinct hot flashes. . . .": Sheldon H. Cherry, *The Menopause Myth* (1976), p. 19.

4. Weight Gain Is Not a Crime, Only Dangerous

P.32 "You not only are what you eat. . . .": From "Live Longer and Like It," a feature science article by the American Medical Association's Department of Science News (1968), as quoted in Ruth Winter, *Ageless Aging* (1973), p. 76.

P.32 We receive too little respect for our experience: Simone de Beauvoir, *Second Sex* (1961 [French edition, 1949]), pp. 541-561. In chapter 20, "From Maturity to Old Age," the author discusses this topic from a philosophical view, better than anyone has yet or since. In spite of its being written over twenty-five years ago, most of it more than holds up. It's worth rereading.

P.32 Our bodies need less food: Louise Page and Lillian J. Fincher, *Food and Your Weight,* (1960), p. 3.

P.33 The behaviorists tell us: Kathryn Mahoney and Michael J. Mahoney, "Fight Fat with Behavior Control," *Psychology Today* (May 1976), p. 39.

P.33 "Reach for your mate instead of your plate.": Abraham I. Friedman, *Fat Can Be Beautiful* (1974), p. 188.

P.33 For every pound of fat: Ruth Winter, *Ageless Aging,* p. 76.

P.33 "If you can control your diet. . . .": As quoted in Winter, p. 76.

P.34 Endometrial cancer . . . is linked with obesity . . .:Saul B. Gusberg, et al., "Carcinogenesis and Estrogens," in *Menopause and Aging* (1971), p. 5.

P.34 the case of Betty Rose Hall: Peter Chew, *The Inner World of the Middle-Aged Man* (1976), pp. 188-189.

P.34 she "was on the plump side. . . .": As quoted in Chew, pp. 188-189.

P.34 Eminent authorities . . . agree: Friedman, p. 86.

P.35 Dr. Judith S. Stern . . . relapse rate . . . 95 percent: Zonia P. Krassner, "Review of the Symposium on Nutritional Disorders of American Women," *Women & Health* vol. 1, no. 2 (March/April 1976), p. 27.

P.35 "the craving for sweets disappears. . . .": Adelle Davis, *Let's Eat Right to Keep Fit* (1954), p. 17.

P.35 "We can allow ourselves to be plump. . . .": Dr. Scholten quoted in Friedman, p. 86.

P.36 "In the hypothalamus . . . specialized 'hunger'. . . .": Solomon H. Snyder, *Madness and the Brain* (1975), p. 219.

P.37 calorie requirements diminish: Friedman, p. 186.

P.37 Our fat problem grows as we age: Krassner, p. 26.

P.37 Dr. Sami Hashim . . . fixed satiety level . . .: ibid., p. 27.

P.37 "Factors such as smell. . . .": ibid.

P.37 Carol Munter: Personal interview, February 16, 1975.

5. Other "Symptoms"

P.42   "Beauty—be not caused. . . .": *Final Harvest: Emily Dickinson's Poems,* edited by Thomas H. Johnson (1961), p. 128.

P.42   skin as active . . . interrelated body organs: "How Strong Is the Skin?" *Medical World News* (October 2, 1970).

P.43   self cleansing mechanism: J. Bedford Shelmire, Jr., *The Art Of Looking Younger* (1975), p. 29.

P.43   It represents about one sixth: Ivan Popov, *Stay Young* (1975), p. 180.

P.43   dries . . . furniture . . . and our skin.: Marvin Chernovsky, "Dry Skin and Its Consequences," *Journal of the American Medical Women's Association* vol. 27, no. 4 (March 1972), pp. 133-145.

P.44   "the glands of the skin . . . decrease. . . .": Ruth Winter, *Ageless Aging* (1973), p. 63.

P.44   "natural foul smell": As quoted in "Government Response to Contraceptive and Cosmetic Health Risks" by Jerry L. Weaver, *Women & Health* vol. 1, no. 2 (March/April 1976), p. 8.

P.44   profits from vaginal deodorants: Ellen Frankfort, *Vaginal Politics* (1973), p. 97.

P.45   Beauty aids were the number two cause: *New York Times* (April 14, 1971), p. 56.

P.45   a 1973 report of 1,031 eye cosmetic products: Weaver, p. 7.

P.45   A 1975 survey showed 40.5 injuries: *Los Angeles Times* (June 29, 1975), pt. 1, p. 14.

P.45   The Food, Drug and Cosmetic Act of 1938: Weaver, p. 7.

P.45   As for estrogen cream . . . experiments: Winter, p. 64.

P.45   melanin "builds up in our skin. . . .": Winter, p. 60.

P.46   stretch marks . . . sesame oil: Mildred Jackson and Terri Teague, *The Handbook of Alternatives to Chemical Medicine* (1975), p. 115.

P.46   a pot of pine needles: Virginia Castleton-Thomas, *My Secrets of Natural Beauty* (1971), p. 95.

P.50   apple cider vinegar . . . rinse: Joan T. Keim-Laughran, "Condition Your Condition," *Well-Being, A Healing Magazine* no. 1 (February 1977), p. 11.

P.50   The primary nourishment for hair: Abraham I. Friedman, *Fat Can Be Beautiful* (1974), p. 209.

P.50   Hair is constantly being renewed: Winter, p. 71.

P.51   hirsutism. . . . Hair increase: Robert H. Glass and Nathan G. Kase, *Woman's Choice* (1970), pp. 86-90.

P.51   "Deficiencies of at least four B vitamins. . . .": Adelle Davis, *Let's Eat Right to Keep Fit* (1954), p. 73.

P.52   tells about . . . hair color changes: Linda Clark, *Get Well Naturally* (1972), p. 131.

P.52   Nails contain calcium: Popov, p. 186.

P.56   *osteoporosis* . . . bone tissue becomes porous: *Menopause: The Experts Speak* (1975), p. 10.

P.56   "Osteoporosis is the commonest chronic. . . .": Robert P. Heaney, "Menopausal Effects on Calcium Homeostasis and Skeletal Metabolism," in *Menopause and Aging* (1971), p. 59.

P.56   around one quarter of all white women. . . .: Heaney, pp. 59-66.

P.56   Almost 20 percent . . . die from hip fractures. . . .: Robert P. Heaney, Eugene Eisenberg, and C. Conrad Johnson, Jr., "Postmenopausal Osteoporosis," in *Menopause and Aging* (1971), pp. 7-8.

P.56   "plainly estrogens have not proved. . . .": Heaney, p. 66.

P.56   "is no definite evidence that osteoporosis. . . .": Chull S. Song and Paul Beck, "Metabolic Effects of Steroid Hormones," in *Menopause and Aging* (1971), p. 11.

P.56   Dr. Avioli believes day-to-day muscle pull. . . .: Zonia P. Krassner, "Review of the

Symposium on Nutritional Disorders of American Women," *Women & Health* vol. 1, no. 2 (March/April 1976), p. 26.

P.57 "maybe we should all be vegetarians.": Louis Avioli, as quoted in "Nutritional Problems of Women Discussed by Medical Experts" by Enid Nemy, *New York Times* (November 22, 1975).

P.57 "Women who have passed through menopause. . . .": Leon Root, *Oh, My Aching Back* (1973), p. 79.

P.57 not a natural part of aging: "Does Low Calcium Intake Cause Osteoporosis?" *Journal of American Medical Association* vol. 218, no. 2 (October 1971), p. 263.

P.57 "In many osteoporotic individuals. . . .": As quoted in *The Book of Vitamin Therapy* by Harold Rosenberg and A. N. Feldzamen (1975), p. 114.

P.57 calcium has many "other bodily functions. . . .": ibid.

P.58 back pain occurs most often for two reasons. . . .: Hans Kraus, *Backache Stress and Tension* (1972), p. 22.

P.58 organic disease causes only a small. . . .: ibid., pp. 70-74.

P.58 "may afflict . . . 100,000,000 Americans.": Arnold P. Friedman, Shervert H. Frazier, Jr., and Dodi Schulz, *The Headache Book* (1973), pp. 1-2.

P.58 comes from nerves in the walls: Daniel Goleman, "Why Your Temples Pound." *Psychology Today* (August 1976), p. 41.

P.58 "monthly changes in water retention. . . .": Gay Gaer Luce, *Body Time* (1971), p. 233.

P.59 "blood coursing through swollen vessels. . . .": Goleman, p. 41.

P.59 symptoms . . . reduced to two: hot flashes and dryness: *Menopause: The Experts Speak* (1975), p. 7.

P.59 breasts get fuller: George Crile, Jr., *What Women Should Know about the Breast Cancer Controversy* (1974), p. 134.

P.59 stress specialist: Hans Selye, *The Stress of Life* (1956).

P.60 "This means . . . that excess aldosterone. . . .": Katharina Dalton, *The Menstrual Cycle* (1969), p. 13.

P.60 "when diuretics are used. . . .": ibid., p. 68.

P.60 Potassium depletion can be corrected: William D. Snively, Jr., and Jan Thuerback, *The Sea of Life* (1969), p. 79.

P.60 not to use . . . if we "tend to swell . . . during menopause." ibid., p. 71.

P.60 pyridoxine (vitamin B₆) to remove fluids: John M. Ellis, *The Doctor Who Looked at Hands* (1971). This is a 300-page book entirely devoted to this vitamin.

P.61 "Home remedies always will have. . . .": Dr. E. Vincent Askey, as quoted in *Get Well Naturally* by Linda Clark (1972), p. 26.

P.61 New Medicine . . . "holistic health": George Leonard, "The Search for Health," *New West* (January 3, 1977), pp. 14-15.

P.61 not just the absence of overt disease: Jonathan Kirsch, "Can Your Mind Cure Cancer? *New West* (January 3, 1977), pp. 40-45.

P.61 "cancer personality": ibid.

P.61 "If all abuse of tobacco. . . .": Dr. Phillip R. Lee, as quoted in "The New Medicine & Holistic Healing," *New West* (May 10, 1976).

P.62 "Doctors haven't been trained for health. . . .": Dr. Leonard Duhl, as quoted in "The New Medicine & Holistic Healing," *New West* (May 10, 1976).

6. Blues Ain't Necessarily So

P.64 "middle-aged women concerned about wrinkles. . . .": Carol Nowak, as quoted in Arthur J. Snider, "The Magnetism of Middle-Aged Men," *New York Post* (May 7, 1976), p. 30.

P.65 "Women become 'depressed' long before. . . .": Phyllis Chesler, *Women and Madness* (1972), p. 41.

P.66   "Bleeding, violent purges. . . .": Barbara Ehrenreich and Deirdre English, *Complaints and Disorders* (1973), p. 32.

P.66   "In some cases leeches. . . .": ibid., p. 33

P.66   "Everyone is depressed. . . .": Solomon H. Snyder, *Madness and the Brain* (1974), p. 2.

P.68   "It is suggested . . . the ovary produces insufficient. . . .": Katharina Dalton, *The Menstrual Cycle* (1969), p. 63.

P.69   "The amount of calcium in a woman's blood. . . .": Adelle Davis, *Let's Eat Right to Keep Fit* (1954), pp. 177.

P.70   may want a younger . . . woman: I. P. Bell, "The Double Standard," *Trans-Action*, vol. 8, no. 1–2 (1970), pp. 69–74.

P.70   When children grow up and leave: See Pauline Bart, "Depression in Middle-Aged Women," the classic work on the subject, in *Women in Sexist Society*, edited by Vivian Gornick and Barbara K. Moran (1972), pp. 177–183.

P.70   "Woman has ended her existence. . . .": Helene Deutsch, *The Psychology of Women* (1945), vol. 2, pp. 459–461.

P.71   "women are in a continual state of mourning. . . .": Chesler, p. 41.

P.71   "Society labels as crazy. . . .": Thomas Szasz, as quoted in Snyder, p. 5.

P.72   "Madness need not be all breakdown. . . .": R. D. Laing, *The Politics of Experience* (1967), p. 136.

P.72   "We have been had.": Lolly Hirsch, personal interview, April 18, 1975.

P.72   "The climacteric is the time. . . .": Isabel Hutton, *Woman's Prime of Life* (1937), p. 128 ff.

P.72   "Above all, we can learn to love ourselves. . . .": Madeline Gray, *Changing Years* (1951), p. 195.

P.72   "Anything which tends to limit. . . .": Clara Thompson, "Middle Age," in *Woman: Body and Culture*, edited by Signe Hammer (1975), pp. 224–227.

P.73   "a time for finding *one's own*. . . .": Eda LeShan, *The Wonderful Crisis of Middle Age* (1974), p. 18–19.

P.74   Tranquilizers are the most commercially: Deborah Larned, "The Selling of Valium," *Ms. Magazine* (November 1975), p. 32.

P.74   "Of the 23 major active ingredients. . . .": *Newsweek* (December 15, 1975), p. 97.

P.75   "been associated with a battery of unwanted side effects. . . .": Deborah Larned, "Do You Take Valium?" *Ms. Magazine* (November 1975), pp. 26–30.

P.75   De-Fear Yourself: My ideas for this section became crystalized after I read David Cooper, *The Grammar of Living* (1974). His precise articulation helped me to formulate mine. I am in his debt.

P.77   "cumulative menstrual losses. . . .": Davis, p. 191.

P.77   "Like sodium and potassium. . . .": Gay Gaer Luce, *Body Time* (1971), p. 256.

P.77   "It is as though the emotional brain. . . .": Carlton Fredericks, *Look Younger, Feel Healthier* (1975), pp. 52–53.

7. Let Loose Anger—Learn to Love Yourself

P.79   "I am hoarding anger. . . .": Ethel Seldin-Schwartz, "Diary of a Middle-Aged Divorce," *Ms. Magazine* (April 1976), p. 86.

P.79   We have not been taught to express anger: For this idea and the ones following on this page I leaned heavily on David Cooper, *The Grammar of Living* (1974), pp. 81–103.

P.80   man's property: Susan Brownmiller, *Against Our Will* (1975), p. 17.

P.84   "And once I saw her menstrual blood. . . .": Philip Roth, *Portnoy's Complaint* (1970), p. 46.

P.84   "As the estrogen is shut off. . . .": David Reuben, *Everything You Always Wanted to Know About Sex* (1970), pp. 292–293.

P.84   the people in Turkey; as cited in "The Menopause: Reward or Punishment?" by Marcha Flint, *Psychosomatics* vol. 16 (4th quarter 1975), p. 163.

P.84   Ashanti in Africa: From Dr. Ruby Leawitt, anthropologist emphasizing cross-cultural view of women, personal interview May 17, 1975.

P.84   the Tiwi of Australia: C. W. M. Hart and Arnold R. Pilling, *The Tiwi of North Australia* (1969).

P.84   the Magars of Nepal: John T. Hitchcock, *The Magars of Banyan Hill* (1969).

P.85   "the need of a reorientation. . . .": Kenneth Burke, *Permanence and Change, An Anatomy of Purpose* (1965), p. 169.

8. Move to Save Your Life

P.90   ". . . a soul in which knowledge passes. . . .": George Eliot, *Middlemarch* (1964), p. 220.

P.91   "It is necessary to walk. . . .": Dr. Ida M. Golomb, personal interview, August 15, 1976.

P.92   the rope is the right length: Lenore R. Zohman, *Beyond Diet*. A 36-page booklet on exercise for fitness and heart health, available for the asking from Best Foods Exercise Booklet, Dept. ZFC, Box 307, Coventry, Conn., 06238.

P.94   Muscle makes up 40 percent of our total body weight: Ruth Winter, *Ageless Aging* (1973), p. 92.

P.94   creatine, a chemical contained in muscle. . . .: Paul Dudley White, "The Role of Exercise in the Aging," in *Health Aspects of Aging*, American Medical Association booklet (1965).

P.94   "level of physical activity. . . .": Lawrence E. Lamb, *Stay Youthful and Fit, A Doctor's Guide* (1974), p. 192.

P.94   clears away the buildup of adrenalin: ibid., p. 193.

P.95   retarding effect . . . of arteriosclerosis: Winter, p. 100.

9. Me and My Speculum

P.96   "Most people, don't you see? . . .": Henry James, *The Sacred Fount* (1953), p. 133.

P.97 $80 million worth of estrogen: See note for p. 180 in chapter 15.

P.97   In the spring of 1971 Carol Downer inserted: From personal interview with Lolly Hirsch, a member of the collective which publishes *The Monthly Extract, An Irregular Periodical* and from the specific issue vol. 3, no. 1 (March/April 1974).

P.97   "If any woman in that room had sniggered. . . .": *The Monthly Extract* vol. 3, no. 1 (March/April 1974), p. 2.

P.98   "Men began taking over obstetrics. . . .": Margaret Mead, as reprinted in *The Monthly Extract* vol. 3, no. 1 (March/April 1974).

P.98   "Now we must ask ourselves: WHAT MAN WOULD BE. . . .": Jeanne Hirsch, as reprinted in *The Monthly Extract* vol. 3, no. 1 (March/April 1974).

P.99   unconscious collusion: The idea comes from David Cooper, *The Grammar of Living* (1974), p. 56.

P.99   33,000 women died from breast cancer, that 89,000 new cases. . . .: Jane E. Brody, "Estrogen after Menopause Held No Bar to Cancer," *New York Times* (August 17, 1976).

P.99   lung cancer . . . on the increase: Jane E. Brody, "Coast Study Finds Sharp Rise in Uterine Cancer," *New York Times* (November 1, 1975).

P.99   over 30 percent . . . have hysterectomies: J. B. Bunker and D. W. Brown, Jr., "The Physician-Patient as an Informal Consumer of Surgical Services," *New England Journal of Medicine* vol. 290 (1974), pp. 1051-1055.

P.100 Vaginal Ecology: I am indebted to the Vaginal Infections Research Group, Portland Women's Liberation School for this phrase. This is also the name of a four-part piece printed in *Portland Scribe* (August 5 to September 2, 1976).

P.101   "gynecological disturbances are often an expression. . . .": Laura Hanks, Joanne Demers, and Margaret Alic, "Vaginal Ecology, Part 2, Prevention," *Portland Scribe* (August 12, 1976).

P.102   Diabetics must be careful. . . . : Joyce Prensky, ed., *Healing Yourself,* 6th rev. ed. (1976), p. 36. Available from Healing Yourself Collective, P.O. Box 3203, Eugene, Oregon 97403, at a cost of $1.50 plus 25¢ postage.

P.102   Stay away from . . . vaginal deodorants: Jerry L. Weaver, "Government Response to Contraceptive and Cosmetic Health Risks," *Women & Health* vol. 1, no. 2 (March/April 1976), p. 8.

10. The Language of Menopause

P.103   "We do not realize . . . language . . . enslaves us. . . .": Alfred Korzybski, *Science and Sanity,* 4th ed. (1958), p. 90. My interest in language stems from the late '40s when I first read this book, the basic primer of semantics. I am also indebted to I. A. Richard's and Charles Ogden's *The Meaning of Meaning* and William Empson's *Seven Types of Ambiguity,* both of which stimulated a fundamental questioning about the way ideas are articulated. These influences are part of the bedrock underlying the creation of this book.

P.103   "middle living": a phrase used throughout *The Making of Americans* by Gertrude Stein, published in Paris in 1925. This phrase designates active maturity from around 40 to 60 years of age and is much preferred to the commonly used *middle-aged.*

P.103   semantic environment, polluted environment: These ideas come from Eve Merriam, *Sex and Semantics: Some Notes on BOMFOG.* I read the full article printed by *KNOW, Inc.,* feminist publishers, P.O. Box 86031, Pittsburgh, Pa. 15221. *KNOW, Inc.* also reprinted the original, which was half as long and showed the deleted sections that were too radical for *New York University Education Quarterly* vol. 5, no. 4 (Summer 1974).

P.103   how anti-woman [language] is: Haig A. Bosmajian, *Language of Oppression* (1974), p. 7.

P.104   creating harmful effects: Benjamin Lee Whorf, *Language, Thought and Reality: Selected Writings of Benjamin Lee Whorf,* edited by John B. Carroll (1956), p. 134.

P.104   Twinge List: George Orwell said, "Silly words and expressions have often disappeared . . . [from] the conscious action of a minority." George Orwell, "Politics and the English Language" in *The Borzoi Reader,* edited by C. Muscatine and M. Griffith (1971), p. 88.

P.106   In communicating meaning. . . .: Jessica Murray, "Male Perspective in Language," *Women: A Journal of Liberation,* vol. 3, no. 2 [no date], p. 50.

P.106   "definite morbid process. . . .": *Dorland's Illustrated Medical Dictionary,* 24th ed. (1966), p. 428.

P.107   "preservation of a serviceable vagina.": *The Merck Manual of Diagnosis and Therapy,* 12th ed. (1972), p. 1184.

P.107   "cultural sexism . . . female degradation. . . .": Susan Brownmiller, *Against Our Will* (1975), p. 389.

P.107   a thinning of the cells. . . .: This clinical description of atrophic vaginitis is from *Menopause: The Experts Speak* (1975), p. 7. This booklet, USDHEW Publ. No. (NIH) 75-756, is available for the asking from National Institute on Aging, Bethesda, Md., 20014.

P.108   "senile woman": William H. Masters and Virginia E. Johnson, *Human Sexual Response* (1966), p. 238.

P.108   "As the human female experiences endocrine starvation. . . .": ibid., p. 237.

P.108   *involution: Webster's Seventh New Collegiate Dictionary* (1963).

P.109   "Conduct and character are largely determined. . . .": Aldous Huxley, *Words and Their Meaning* (1940), p. 9.

P.109   "We have not been free to . . . name ourselves.": Mary Daly, *Beyond God the Father* (1973).

P.109   "male supremist language": Haig A. Bosmajian, "The Language of Sexism," *ETC.* vol. 29 (1972), pp. 305-313.

P.110   "the deleterious effect. . . .": Ethel Strainchamps, "Our Sexist Language" in *Woman in Sexist Society,* edited by Vivian Gornick and Barbara K. Moran (1972), p. 348.

P.110   "any language that expresses stereotyped attitudes. . . .": Casey Miller and Kate Swift, "One Small Step for Genkind," *New York Times Magazine* (April 16, 1972), p. 36. This idea is reinforced in "De-Sexing the English Language" by the same authors in *Ms. Magazine* (Spring 1972), p. 7.

P.110   "Manglish": Varda One, *Manglish,* KNOW, Inc. (address in n.p. 103 semantic environment . . .), four-page pamphlet.

P.110   "cooped up" with her "brood": Alleen Pace Nilsen, "Sexism in English: A Feminist View," in *Female Studies 6,* edited by Nancy Hoffman, Cynthia Secor, and Adrian Tinsley (1972), p. 102-109.

P.111   "cocks" do not age: Pointed out in a personal interview with Dr. H. Lee Gershuny, Professor of Communications and Linguistics, The City University of New York, June 3, 1976.

P.111   Males roar, bellow, and growl: Peter Farb, *Word Play* (1973), p. 141-144.

P.111   "woman's language": Robin Lakoff, "Language and Woman's Place," *Language in Society* (1973), vol. 2, pp. 45-79.

P.112   differences in intonation patterns: Mary Ritchie Key, "Linguistic Behavior of Male and Female," *Linguistics* (August 15, 1972), pp. 15-31.

P.112   "women's speech reflects the stereotyped roles. . . .": Cheris Kramer, "Women's Speech: Separate But Unequal?" *Quarterly Journal of Speech* vol. 60 (February 1974), pp. 14-24.

P.112   "instinctively avoiding the coarseness. . . .": Otto Jespersen, *Language: Its Nature, Development and Origin* (1922), pp. 237-254.

P.112   "The new circumstances . . ." wrote Thomas Jefferson. . . .": As quoted in *Our Own Words* by Mary Helen Dohan (1975), p. 3.

P.113   correctly mirrors: ibid.

P.113   "The use of language . . . bottom nonsense. . . .": Edwin Newman, *A Civil Tongue* (1976).

P.113   *Bitch* when used as a verb has no sex. It is a common word in the vernacular of women in the Women's Movement. Buttons and T-shirts carrying the message "Bitch, Sister, Bitch" were popular in 1973. This is an example of taking a negative word and turning it around, as it were, and making it positive. The case of *Black, dyke, old,* and *menopause* have the same linguistic histories.

P.113   delineates strategies and laws: Constantina Safilios-Rothschild, *Women and Social Policy* (1974), p. 126.

P.114   "The implications of all this. . . .": Haig A. Bosmajian, *Language of Oppression* (1974), p. 133.

P.115   "I am the living mind . . .": Adrienne Rich, "The Stranger" *Diving into the Wreck: Poems 1971-72* (1973).

11. Masturbation

P.116   "We are all apt to expect too much. . . .": Jane Austen, "Mansfield Park," *The Complete Novels of Jane Austen* vol. 1 (1950), p. 601.

P.117   35 million women . . . over age 45. *Statistical Abstract of the U.S. for 1974,* US Government Printing Office (1975).

P.117   82 percent said they had masturbated: Shere Hite, *The Hite Report* (1976), p. 3.

P.117 "children have absorbed. . . .": William H. Masters, Virginia E. Johnson, and Robert J. Levin, *The Pleasure Bond* (1975), pp. 230-231.

P.118 "Masturbation is not childish. . . .": David Stonecypher, *Getting Older and Staying Young* (1974), p. 244.

P.118 "to rest is to rust": ibid., p. 74.

P.119 "the use of an artificial penis. . . .": Havelock Ellis, *Psychology of Sex* vol. 1, p. 169.

P.119 Nineteenth-century America . . . women's sexual "voraciousness". . . .: G. J. Barker-Benfield, *Male Attitudes Toward Women and Sexuality in Nineteenth-Century America* (1976).

P.119 "Masturbation was seen . . . character defect. . . .": Barbara Ehrenreich and Deirdre English, *Complaints and Disorders* (1973), p. 30.

P.119 "masturbation . . . development of frigidity. . . .": Frank Caprio, *Sexually Adequate Female* (1975), p. 124-125.

P.120 "Surprisingly, most researchers have not shown interest. . . .": Hite, p. 3-4.

P.120 "Masturbation is not something. . . .": Boston Women's Health Book Collective, *Our Bodies, Ourselves* (1973), p. 31.

P.120 "can be a useful part. . . .": Marjorie W. Hackmann, *Practical Sex Information,* p. 16-17.

P.120 "to explore, define and celebrate. . . .": National Organization for Women, New York, *Proceedings of the Women's Sexuality Conference* (1974).

P.120 Individual women spoke. . . .: Lindsay Miller, "Women Confer on Sex," *New York Post* (June 11, 1973).

P.120 "portraits of women": Betty Dodson, *Liberating Masturbation: A Meditation on Self Love* (1975), p. 28.

P.121 "the social approval to be aggressive. . . ." ibid., p. 13.

P.121 "I didn't look funny or awful": ibid., p. 8.

P.121 "There is a vast range. . . .": ibid., p. 5.

P.121 "It is not a dirty thing. . . .": Jane Wallace, *Masturbation: A Woman's Handbook* (1975), p. 5.

P.121 "It's a woman's right. . . .": ibid., p. 16.

P.123 "Remember to take it easy. . . .": ibid., p. 40.

P.124 "While it is true that vibrators. . . .": Barbara Seaman, *Free and Female* (1973), p. 74.

P.124 *"Touch is an end in itself. . . .":* Masters, Johnson, and Levin, p. 238.

P.127 "The more orgasms a woman has. . . ." Mary Jane Sherfey, *The Nature and Evolution of Female Sexuality* (1972), p 12.

P.128 "even when sexual love exists before the mar age. . . .": Simone de Beauvoir, *Second Sex* (1961), p. 420.

P.128 "Coition is a far more complex. . . .": Simone de Beauvoir, *The Coming of Age* (1973), p. 479.

P.129 "Many modern women exhibit. . . .": Gail Sheehy, *Passages* (1976), p. 357.

12. Sex Is Better When You're Older

P.130 "Sexual activities have a plurality of ends. . . .": Simone de Beauvoir, *The Coming of Age* (1973), p. 472-473.

P.130 women over 40 in "The Aging Female": William H. Masters and Virginia E. Johnson, *Human Sexual Response* (1966), pp. 223-247.

P.130 Freud's biological mistake: Freud spells it out when he says "With the change to femininity, the clitoris must give up to the vagina its sensitivity, and, with it, its importance. . . ." Sigmund Freud, *New Introductory Lectures on Psycho-Analysis* (1946) pp. 151-152.

P.130 "The clitoris is a woman's sexually most sensitive organ. . . .": Jane E. Brody, "Personal Health," *New York Times* (January 12, 1977).

P.130 clitoris contains the same number of nerves: Ruth Herschberger, *Adam's Rib* (1948), p. 31.

P.130 It is not pictured on anatomical charts: Alix Shulman, "Organs and Orgasms," *Women in Sexist Society,* edited by Vivian Gornick and Barbara K. Moran (1972), p. 295.

P.130 vaginal orgasm was . . . a misunderstanding: Ruth and Edward Brecher, *An Analysis of Human Sexual Response* (1966), p. 84.

P.131 The case for the clitoris: Ann Koedt, *The Myth of the Vaginal Orgasm* (1970).

P.131 "I disagree with the claim that sex is better. . . .": Sherwin A. Kaufman, *The Ageless Woman* (1967), p. 116.

P.134 "The terror of felt sexuality. . . .": Vivian Gornick, "Women as Outsiders," in *Woman in Sexist Society,* edited by Vivian Gornick and Barbara K. Moran (1972), p. 137.

P.136 "The popular idea that a woman. . . ." and "The nearly universal sentiment. . . .": Mary Jane Sherfey, *The Nature and Evolution of Female Sexuality* (1972), p. 112.

P.136 Kinsey was . . . biased: Masters and Johnson, p. 214.

P.137 Edith Wharton: Her erotic writing can be found in the appendix to *Edith Wharton: A Biography* by R. W. B. Lewis (1975).

P.138 Moll Flanders . . . an embarrassment: Virginia Woolf, *The Common Reader* (1953), p. 90.

P.138 Doris Lessing and June Arnold: See Doris Lessing, *The Golden Notebook* (New York: Simon & Schuster, 1962) for a view of middle-aged male and female, and June Arnold, *Sister Gin* (Plainfield, VT: Daughters, Inc., 1975) for one of middle-aged female and female.

P.138 "Woman must put herself into the text. . . ." and "For what they have said so far. . . .": Helene Cixous, "The Laugh of the Medusa," *Signs: Journal of Women in Culture and Society* vol. 1, no. 4 (Summer 1976), pp. 875-893.

P.141 "Estrogen replacement therapy has come seductively. . . .": Jane Ocle, "Sex Begins at Forty," *Harper's Bazaar* (August 1973), p. 87.

P.142 "To all intents and purposes. . . .": Sherfey, p. 134-135.

P.142 "can be brought to orgasm again. . . .": Helen Singer Kaplan, *The New Sex Therapy* (1974), p. 31.

P.143 Shere Hite reports that the women in her study: Shere Hite, *The Hite Report* (1976), p. 85.

P.143 "There is good evidence that androgens. . . .": Estelle R. Ramey, "Sex Hormones and Executive Ability," in *Women & Success,* edited by Ruth B. Kundsin (1974), p. 253.

P.144 "progesterone is the one. . . .": Kaufman, p. 120.

P.144 A very fine book on the subject: Lonnie Garfield Barbach, *For Yourself* (1976), available in paperback.

P.144 "Orgasm, for women as for men. . . .": Brody, "Personal Health."

P.144 "a mere collection of reflexes. . . .": Simone de Beauvoir, *The Coming of Age* (1973), p. 472.

P.145 "Generally speaking it is an adventure. . . .": ibid., p. 473.

P.145 "People confuse sex with friction": Edward Field, personal interview, February 6, 1977.

P.145 "sexual activity helps to get rid of. . . .": Abraham I. Friedman, *Fat Can Be Beautiful* (1974), p. 189.

P.145 "advantage as far as exercise. . . .": ibid., p. 194.

P.145 complain of burning on urination: Masters and Johnson, p. 223-247.

P.147 "While these uterine contractions occur. . . .": ibid., 241.

P.147 "endocrine starvation" and "steroid starvation": ibid., p. 242.

13. Our Hormones

P.158   "What comes out is what I feel. . . .": Billie Holiday, as quoted in *Billie Holiday: The Golden Years,* by Ralph J. Gleason (1962), p. 7.

P.158   "There is not a day in a woman's life. . . .": Katharina Dalton, *The Menstrual Cycle* (1969), p. 12.

P.159   disquieting side effects: Rosetta Reitz, "What Doctor's Won't Tell You About Menopause," *Majority Report* (October 3, 1974), p. 1.

P.160   "it is important to remember the limitations. . . .": *The Merck Manual of Diagnosis and Therapy,* 11th ed. (1966), p. 435.

P.160   Estrogens . . . broken down. . . . job of the liver: M. S. Biskind, "Nutritional Therapy of Endocrine Disturbances," in *Vitamins and Hormones* vol. 4, edited by Robert S. Harris and Kenneth V. Thimann (1946), pp. 147-180.

P.160   the ovaries also produced progesterone: Edmund R. Novak, Georgeanna Seegar Jones, and Howard W. Jones, Jr., *Novak's Textbook of Gynecology* 7th ed. (1965).

P.160   adrenalin . . . defense mechanisms of flight, fight, and fear: Hans Selye, *The Stress of Life* (1956).

P.161   Hormones are a crucial factor. . . .: Thomas H. Green, *Gynecology: Essentials of Clinical Practice* (1971).

P.161   "It seems . . . true that an increase . . . of one hormone. . . .": John Yudkin, *Sweet and Dangerous* (1973), p. 163-164.

P.161   Sugar is all around us . . . : William Dufty, *Sugar Blues* (1975), p. 143.

P.161   "A high sugar diet. . . .": ibid., p. 150.

P.161   "the disturbance of the equilibrium. . . .": J. R. Willson, C. T. Beecham, and E. R. Carrington, *Obstetrics and Gynecology* (1971).

P.161   "rather, to some unknown factors. . . .": ibid.

P.163   "Numerous studies in postmenopausal. . . .": Pentti K. Siiteri and Paul C. Mac-Donald, "The Role of Extraglandular Estrogen in Human Endocrinology," in *Handbook of Physiology,* edited by R. O. Greep and E. B. Astwood (1973), sec. 7, vol. 2, pt. 1, p. 619.

P.163   "The major source of estrogen in the postmenopausal. . . .": ibid., p. 620.

P.164   "The exact tissue site(s) . . . is presently unknown.": Jay M. Grodin, Pentii K. Siiteri, and Paul C. MacDonald, "Source of Estrogen Production in the Postmenopausal Woman," *Journal of Clinical Endocrinology and Metabolism* vol. 36 (February 1973), pp. 207-214.

P.164   "In normal premenopausal women, the extraglandular. . . .": Siiteri and Mac-Donald, p. 627.

P.164   "I believe that the female hormone. . . .": As quoted in Siiteri and MacDonald, p. 615.

P.164   "The increased incidence of human female breast and endometrial cancer. . . .": Kenneth J. Ryan, "Cancer Risk and Estrogen Use in the Menopause," *New England Journal of Medicine* vol. 293 (1975), p. 1199.

P.165   "where estrogen may be elevated. . . .": Saul B. Gusberg, et al., "Carcinogenesis and Estrogen," in *Menopause and Aging* (1971), p. 5.

P.165   "This peripheral estrogen production increases. . . .": Ryan, p. 1199.

P.165   "The postmenopause cannot be considered . . . quiescence. . . .": Siiteri and MacDonald, p. 627.

P.166   "the potential women leaders . . . have cycles. . . .": Estelle Ramey, "Men's Cycles," *Ms. Magazine* (Spring 1972), p. 14.

14. Hormones and Cancer

P.167   "The modern era of steroid metabolic. . . .": Saul B. Gusberg, "The Individual at

High Risk for Endometrial Carcinoma," *American Journal of Obstetrics and Gynecology* vol. 126 (November 1976), p. 537.

P.167   33,000 women died. . . .: Jane E. Brody, "Estrogen After Menopause Held No Bar to Cancer," *New York Times* (August 17, 1976).

P.167   Cancer of the breast is a malignant tumor: George Crile, Jr., *What Women Should Know About the Breast Cancer Controversy* (1974), p. 15.

P.167   The study of 1,891 women in Louisville. . . .: Robert Hoover, et al., "Menopausal Estrogens and Breast Cancer," *New England Journal of Medicine* vol. 295 (1976), pp. 401-405.

P.168   "The female hormones have no significant role. . . .": Alan E. Nourse, "Hormones and Cancer, Is There a Connection?" *Woman's Day* (February 1976), p. 38.

P.169   "men treated with estrogens for prostatic carcinoma. . . .": Saul B. Gusberg, et al., "Carcinogenesis and Estrogens," in *Menopause and Aging* (1971), p. 6.

P.169   Breast Cancer Profile: Adapted from the report of Dr. H. P. Leis, Jr., New York Medical College, to the International College of Surgeons, San Diego Meeting (1974).

P.169   "meaningless because they had been used. . . .": Hoover, et al.

P.170   As much as 15 or 20 years may elapse. . . .: Testimony of Roy Hertz and U. Saffrotti, US Congress, House of Representatives, Government Operations Committee, *Regulation of Diethylstilbestrol: Its Use as a Drug in Humans and in Animal Feeds.* 92nd Cong., 1st sess. (November 11, 1971), pt. 1, pp. 37-73.

P.170   ERT is associated with an increase of 5 to 14 times. . . .: Kenneth J. Ryan, editorial, "Cancer Risk and Estrogen Use in the Menopause," *New England Journal of Medicine* vol. 293 (1975), p. 1200.

P.170   "there had been no carefully conducted studies. . . .": Noel S. Weiss, editorial, "Risks and Benefits of Estrogen Use," *New England Journal of Medicine* vol. 293 (1975), p. 1200.

P.170   Endometrial cancer . . . struck 27,000 . . . killing 3,000: Barbara Yuncker, "Link Hormone Pills to a Cancer of the Uterus," *New York Post* (December 4, 1975), p. 12.

P.170   One of the studies, conducted in Los Angeles. . . .: Harry K. Ziel and William D. Finkle, "Increased Risk of Endometrial Carcinoma among Users of Conjugated Estrogens," *New England Journal of Medicine* vol. 293 (1975), pp. 1167-1170.

P.170   "that the incidence rate . . . increased. . . .": ibid., p. 1169.

P.170   By 1968, the rate of hysterectomy . . . was 31 percent: J. P. Bunker and B. W. Brown, Jr., "The Physician-Patient as an Informed Consumer of Surgical Services," *New England Journal of Medicine* vol. 290 (1974), pp. 1051-1055.

P.171   "studies have indicated this operation. . . .": Jane E. Brody, "Incompetent Surgery Is Found Not Isolated," *New York Times* (January 27, 1976), p. 1.

P.171   "the risk of endometrial cancer was 4.5 times greater. . . .": Donald C. Smith, et al., "Association of Exogenous Estrogen and Endometrial Carcinoma," *New England Journal of Medicine* vol. 293 (1975), p. 1164.

P.171   Dr. Donald Austin . . . California Tumor Registry . . . 50 percent increase: Mat Clark, "Warning on Estrogen," *Newsweek* (December 8, 1975), pp. 92A-92B.

P.171   27.2 cases per 100,000 population to 41.4: Jane E. Brody, "Coast Study Finds Sharp Rise in Uterine Cancer," *New York Times* (November 1, 1975).

P.172   "Racial and environmental factors. . . .": Ryan, pp. 1199-1200.

P.172   "patients with cervical cancer. . . .": Smith, p. 1165.

P.172   The disease is related to the habits of the affluent: Saul B. Gusberg, "A Strategy for the Control of Endometrial Cancer," *Proceedings of the Royal Society of Medicine* vol. 68 (March 1975), p. 163.

P.172   trend toward more animal fats: Brody, "Coast Study Finds Sharp Rise in Uterine Cancer."

P.172 "as the Japanese have adopted a Western-type. . . .": Saul B. Gusberg, "The Individual at High Risk for Endometrial Carcinoma," pp. 535-542.

P.172 ranges reported . . . hypertension (30-50 percent). . . . : Smith, p. 1164.

P.172 "Dr. Saul B. Gusberg has suspected. . . .": Statement by Dr. Sheldon Cherry, "The
Estrogen Controversy," *The Pat Collins Show,* WCBS-TV, New York (December
11, 1975).

P.173 "Further consideration leads one to the speculation. . . .": Gusberg, "A Strategy for
the Control of Endometrial Cancer," p. 164.

P.173 "copious intake of vitamin B complex. . . .": Carlton Fredericks, "The Estrogen
Tragedy," *Prevention* (May 1976), p. 167.

P.173 "Our group has reported . . . aspiration curettage. . . .": Gusberg, "A Strategy for
the Control of Endometrial Cancer," p. 166-167.

P.174 "cancer's catch-22": "Cancer's Catch-22," *Newsweek* (August 2, 1976), p. 49.

P.174 "one of the worst iatrogenic disasters. . . .": As quoted in "Doctors Failed to Warn
Women about Mammography Risk," by Anna Mayo, *The Village Voice* (August
23, 1976), p. 15.

P.174 "I warn women to have mammograms. . . .": ibid.

P.176 "massive promotion and advertising": As quoted in "F.D.A. Chief Suspicious of
Estrogens," by Frances Cerra, *New York Times* (January 22, 1976).

P.176 "We are not convinced. . . .": ibid.

P.176 "charged with acting to please. . . .": Lesley Stahl, *Face the Nation,* CBS-TV and
Radio, Washington, D.C. (December 28, 1975).

P.176 "an informed consent law. . . .": Morton Mintz, *Face the Nation,* CBS-TV and
Radio, Washington, D.C. (December 28, 1975).

P.177 At the Chicago Lying-In Hospital, a new study. . . . : Nadine Brozan, "Repercussions of a Drug," *New York Times* (June 17, 1976).

P.177 "By 1953 . . . DES didn't work. . . .": Barbara Seaman, "The Dangers of Sex
Hormones," *Playgirl* (July 1976), p. 72.

P.177 "about 40 million women . . . given . . . DES . . .": Kay Weiss, "Cancer and
Estrogens—A Review," *Women & Health* vol. 1, no. 2 (March/April 1976), p. 3.

P.177 growth inhibitor for tall girls: Nadine Brozan, "The Use of Estrogen as a Growth
Inhibitor," *New York Times* (February 11, 1976), p. 55.

P.178 withdrawal of sequential oral contraceptives: "Sequential Pills Being Withdrawn,"
New York Times (February 26, 1976).

15. Estrogen Replacement Therapy

P.179 "Eight million prescriptions. . . .": Kay Weiss, "Cancer and Estrogens—A Review,"
Women & Health vol. 1, no. 2. (March/April 1976), p. 3.

P.180 $80 million in 1975: "Estrogen Therapy: The Dangerous Road to Shangri-La,"
Consumer Reports (November 1976), p. 642.

P.180 "The consensus of informed opinion. . . .": As quoted in "Estrogen Therapy: The
Dangerous Road to Shangri-La," p. 643.

P.181 their need has never been proven: W. D. Holsten, "Protecting Patients from Drugs,"
New England Journal of Medicine vol. 285 (1971), p. 1202.

P.181 An estimated 25 million prescriptions a year: Jane E. Brody, "Estrogen after
Menopause Held No Bar to Cancer," *New York Times* (August 17, 1976).

P.181 "Of these one quarter . . . negative side effects.": Louise Silverstein, et al., *Survey on
Menopause* (unpublished paper, May 1975), p. 13.

P.183 *It's A Matter of Time:* The 17-page booklet that came from the Ayerst front, the
Information Center on the Mature Woman. No name or publishing information
given except 97-0030/RI-200- June 1972.

P.183 *Your Menopause* by Ruth Carson: Public Affairs Pamphlet No. 447 (June 1973). I
called them up to ask them if they were aware of how destructive and outdated

their pamphlet was. They said they revised it and sent me another (December 1976). It was revised and an improvement, but nothing I would recommend.

P.183 subject of . . . a regularly featured column: Mary Reinholz, "The Liberated Woman," *New York Sunday News* (March 16, 1975).

P.184 The language used by Dr. Wilson: Detailed notes are in Chapter 1. If you pick up the book you will find these quotes or ones just like them on every page.

P.184 "Only hot flashes . . . and genital atrophy. . . .": Kenneth J. Ryan and Don C. Gibson, ed., *Menopause and Aging* (1971), p. 10.

P.185 The Wilson Research Foundation: It received in 1964 $17,000 from the Searle Foundation, $8,700 from Ayerst Laboratories, and $5,600 from the Upjohn Company as reported by James Ridgeway and Nancy Sommers in *New Republic* (March 19, 1966) and cited in Morton Mintz, *The Pill* (1969), p. 30.

P.185 Dr. Wilson . . . pushing the contraceptive pill: Mintz, p. 30.

P.185 100 percent greater risk of heart attack: Jerry L. Weaver, "Government Response to Contraceptive and Cosmetic Health Risks," *Women & Health* vol. 1, no. 2 (March/April 1976), p. 6.

P.185 "It is only the faculty of childbearing. . . .": Katharina Dalton, *The Menstrual Cycle* (1969), p. 87.

P.185 "Dr. Roland and other gynecologists. . . .": "Should Hormone Therapy Be Used in Menopause?" *Good Housekeeping* (May 1973), p. 201.

P.186 "I'm not such a great believer in minimal dosage. . . .": Robert Greenblatt and Edmund Novak, "Treating Menopausal Women and Climacteric Men," *Medical World News* (June 28, 1974).

P.186 "It is more likely that an emotional reaction. . . .": Saul Gusberg, as quoted in "Should Hormone Therapy Be Used in Menopause?" p. 201.

P.186 "the total number of women . . . positive experience (68%). . . .": Silverstein, et al., p. 15.

P.186 "criticized it as a fad. . . .": Matt Clark, "Warning on Estrogen," *Newsweek* (December 8, 1975), p. 92B.

P.187 For over 50 years, controversy. . . .: Pentti K. Siiteri and Paul C. MacDonald, "The Role of Extraglandular Estrogen in Human Endocrinology," in *Handbook of Physiology*, edited by R. O. Greep and E. B. Eastwood (1973), sec. 7, vol. 2, pt. 1, p. 623.

P.187 "profound widespread metabolic effects": Chull S. Song and Paul Beck, "Metabolic Effects of Steroid Hormones," in *Menopause and Aging* (1971), p. 10.

P.187 "evidence is strong that estrogens can contribute. . . .": ibid., p. 11.

P.187 "The acceleration of coronary artery disease. . . .": Robert H. Furman, "Coronary Heart Disease and the Menopause," in *Menopause and Aging* (1971), p. 52.

P.188 "If by 'success' we mean. . . .": Robert P. Heaney, "Menopausal Effects on Calcium Homeostasis and Skeletal Metabolism," in *Menopause and Aging* (1971), p. 66.

P.188 "she may be subjected to additional hazards. . . .": William H. Inman, "The Relationship Between Estrogens and Progestogens and Thromboembolic Disease," in *Menopause and Aging* (1971), p. 99.

P.188 "scientific studies to date have not established. . . .": *Menopause: The Experts Speak* (1975), p. 7.

P.188 "This is not an innocuous drug. . . .": As quoted in "Use of Estrogen Linked to Cancer," *New York Times* (December 4, 1975), p. 1 and p. 55.

P.189 prescription recommended: Pauline B. Bart and Marlyn Grossman, "Menopause," in *The Woman as Patient,* edited by Malka T. Notman and Carol Nadelson, forthcoming.

P.190 Betty Lee Morales: Ms. Morales is a nutritionist activist who is constantly fighting for better health legislation.

P.190 "The rationalization for using these two supplements. . . .": James Leathem, "Sex and Nutrition," *Life and Health* (July 1973), p. 63.

16. The Menopausal Woman as Hero

P.192 "there is a general consensus. . . .": Jessie L. Weston, *From Ritual to Romance* (1957), p. 20.

P.193 $80-million worth of estrogen: "Estrogen Therapy: The Dangerous Road to Shangri-La," *Consumer Reports* (November 1976), p. 642.

P.195 "I have your questions in front of me. . . .": I mailed three questions to Dr. Gusberg with my request for an interview. We spoke on the telephone on January 13, 1977, and he graciously answered more questions.

17. Nutrition and Middle Age

P.203 "maybe we should all be vegetarians.": Enid Nemy, "Nutritional Problems of Women Discussed by Medical Experts," *New York Times* (November 22, 1975).

P.204 "Persons on seemingly adequate diets. . . .": Adelle Davis, *Let's Eat Right to Keep Fit* (1954), p. 39.

P.207 "increases oxygen efficiency. . . .": G. Edward Griffin, *World Without Cancer* (1974), p. 140.

P.208 "Irregular or excessive menses. . . .": Harold Rosenberg and A. N. Feldzamen, *The Book of Vitamin Therapy* (1975), p. 155.

P.209 recommends 1,000 to 2,000 mg per day: Linus Pauling, *Vitamin C and the Common Cold* (1970), p. 84.

P.210 "hot flashes, night sweats. . . .": Davis, p. 153.

P.210 "They are the basic spark-plugs. . . .": Henry A. Schroeder, *Trace Elements and Man* (1973), p. vii.

P.212 "sugar irritates the lining. . . .": John Yudkin, *Sweet and Dangerous* (1973), p. 130.

P.212 "sugar . . . alterations . . . hormones": ibid., p. 156. See also William Dufty, *Sugar Blues* (1975), and E. M. Abrahamson and A. W. Pezet, *Body, Mind and Sugar* (1974), for other convincing evidence that sugar is poison.

P.212 "the appetite of tumors for sugar.": Dr. Otto Meyerhoff, as quoted in Linda Clark, *Get Well Naturally* (1972), p. 221.

P.212 Our B vitamins . . . are ravaged by alcohol: Roger J. Williams, *Alcoholism: The Nutritional Approach* (1973).

P.213 No one denies coffee has an invigorating. . . .: Richard F. Demfewolff, "The Truth About Coffee and Your Health," *Science Digest* (June 1975), pp. 31-35.

P.213 studies by Dr. Philip Cole . . . bladder cancer: Sonny Kleinfield, "Coffee Is," *New Times* (October 3, 1975), p. 47.

P.213 "[cocoa] . . . 2,214 cal. per pound.": *Encyclopedia Brittanica* (1972), vol. 6, p. 4.

P.217 "Rolled oats . . . lower cholesterol.": Clark, p. 315.

P.220 still prescribing estrogen . . . can raise the risk of uterine cancer: Harry K. Ziel and William D. Finkle, "Increased Risk of Endometrial Carcinoma Among Users of Conjugated Estrogens," *New England Journal of Medicine* vol. 293 (1975), pp. 1167-1170.

P.221 "sets the foundations. . . .": Carlson Wade, as quoted in P. E. Norris, *Everything You Want to Know About Yogurt* (1974), p. vii.

P.221 The Jewish Memorial Hospital . . . studies: Barry Cunningham, "The Yogurt Explosion," *New York Post* (October 2, 1976), p. 25.

P.221 "their serum cholesterol was reduced. . . .": Judith Hennessee, "Yogurt: Getting into the Culture," *New Times* (July 23, 1976), p. 49.

P.222 Assimilation of calcium . . . the enzymes in yogurt: Carlson Wade, *Helping Your Health with Enzymes* (1966), p. 193.

P.222 "who had found that administration . . . to animals. . . .": As quoted in Carlton Fredericks, *Look Younger, Feel Healthier* (1972), p. 217.

P.222 Ilya Metchnikoff: *Yogurt and You,* booklet from Dannon Milk Products (1976), p. 2.

P.222 Doctors commonly prescribe yogurt. . . .: Alan H. Nittler, *A New Breed of Doctor* (1975), p. 45.

P.223 "the normal acidity of the vagina. . . .": ibid., p. 50.

P.225 hypophyseal hormone . . . from protein.: "Sex and Nutrition," *Life and Health* (July 1973), p. 64.

18. Male Menopause

P.226 "My brain I'll prove. . . .": William Shakespeare, *Richard II,* act 5, scene 5, line 6.

P.226 "the organism of male supposes that. . . .": As quoted in Simone de Beauvoir, *Second Sex* (1961), p. 150.

P.227 "Even without a comparable. . . .": Theodore Isaac Rubin, "Dr. Rubin," *Ladies' Home Journal* (November 1971), p. 52.

P.227 "A well-integrated man adjusts. . . .": Helen Kaplan, as quoted in Martha Weinman Lear, "Is There a Male Menopause?" *New York Times Magazine* (January 28, 1973), p. 19.

P.227 "male menopause is . . . faintly silly": Peter Chew, *The Inner World of the Middle-Aged Man* (1976), p. 117. An excellent book which I recommend.

P.228 "At 50 . . . 'No more bullshit.'": Gail Sheehy, *Passages* (1976), p. 403.

P.228 "nervousness, decrease or loss. . . .": Lear, p. 7.

P.228 Do men have monthly cycles? . . .: Judith Randal, "The Monthly Cycle: Not for Women Only," *Sunday News* (September 5, 1976), p. 98.

P.228 "Men *do* have monthly cycles. . . .": Estelle Ramey, "Men's Cycles," *Ms. Magazine* (Spring 1972), pp. 8-14.

P.229 "cyclic change is so unexpected. . . .": Gay Gaer Luce, *Body Time* (1971).

P.229 "The hormone-production levels are dropping. . . .": Lear, p. 21.

P.229 there are those who are for . . . and others . . . against it.: Robert Greenblatt and Edmund Novak, "Treating Menopausal Women—and Climacteric Men, *Medical World News* (June 28, 1974), p. 53.

P.229 "the true climacteric is a physiological cessation. . . .": Herbert S. Kupperman, as quoted in Greenblatt and Novak, p. 53.

P.230 Kupperman . . . prescribes testosterone. . . . He claims that . . . the use of placebos.: Greenblatt and Novak, p. 53.

P.230 "that raising his testosterone level. . . .": Lear, p. 7.

P.230 "they create a dependency. . . .": Ivan Popov, *Stay Young* (1975), p. 83.

P.231 What is impotence?: Philip Nobile, "What Is Impotence, and Who's Got It?" *Esquire* (October 1974), p. 95-98.

P.232 Well over half of the American male: Chew, p. 107.

P.232 "cancer originating in this gland. . . .": Gilbert Cant, "Male Trouble," *New York Times Magazine* (February 16, 1975), p. 15.

P.232 As many as 60,000 men. . . .: ibid.

P.233 "The most common. . . .": Cant, p. 65.

P.233 "is like pouring gasoline. . . .": Statement by Jay Rosenblum on "Impotence," *Pat Collins Show,* WCBS-TV (June 9, 1976).

P.233 some slight discomfort with erection: Cant, p. 65.

P.233 "when the hormonal loss is gradual. . . .": Lear, p. 20.

P.233 Hunzas of the Himalayas: Read *Hunza Health Secrets* by Renee Taylor (1965) and find out about reverence of age.

P.234 Dan Levinson . . . study: Cited in Chew, pp. 40-41.

P.234 "the individual has stopped growing up. . . .": Elliot Jaques, "Death and the Mid-Life Crisis," *International Journal of Psychoanalysis* vol. 46 (1965), p. 506.

P.234 "because they're looking for that fountain of youth. . . .": statement by John Revson on "Male Menopause: The Pause that Perplexes," *National Public Affairs Center for Television* (NPACT) (June 24, 1974).

P.235   "The idea of death, the fear of it. . . .": Ernest Becker, *The Denial of Death* (1973), p. ix.

P.235   Medical research . . . heavy stress as a prime cause: David C. Glass, "Stress, Competition and Heart Attacks," *Psychology Today* (December 1976), pp. 54-57.

P.236   We are born with a specific amount. . . .: Hans Selye, "Remaking Your Idea," *Vogue* (January 1957).

P.236   "a great deal more research. . . .": Ramey, "Men's Cycles," pp. 8-14.

Bibliography

Abrahamson, E.M. and Pezet, A.W. *Body, Mind and Sugar.* New York: Pyramid Books, 1974.

Asimov, Isaac. *Human Body.* New York: New American Library, 1964.

Austen, Jane. "Mansfield Park." In *The Complete Novels of Jane Austen,* vol. 1. New York: Random House, 1950.

Barbach, Lonnie Garfield. *For Yourself: The Fulfillment of Female Sexuality.* New York: Doubleday Anchor Press, 1976.

Barker-Benfield, G.J. *Male Attitudes Toward Women and Sexuality in Nineteenth-Century America.* New York: Harper & Row, 1976.

Bart, Pauline B. "Depression in Middle-Aged Women." In *Women in Sexist Society.* Edited by Vivian Gornick and Barbara K. Moran. New York: New American Library, 1972.

Bart, Pauline B., and Grossman, Marlyn. "Menopause." In *The Woman as Patient.* Edited by Malka T. Notman and Carol Nadelson. New York: Plenum Press, forthcoming.

Beauvoir, Simone de. *The Coming of Age.* New York: Warner Paperback Library, 1973.
_____. *Second Sex.* New York: Bantam Books, 1961.

Becker, Ernest. *The Denial of Death.* New York: Free Press, 1973.

Beckett, Samuel. *Endgame.* New York: Grove Press, 1958.

Bell, I.P. "The Double Standard." *Trans-Action* vol. 8, no. 1–2 (1970), pp. 69-74.

Benedek, Therese. "Climacterium, a Developmental Phase." *Psychoanalytic Quarterly* vol. 19 (1950), pp. 1-27.

Bernard, Jessie. *The Sex Game.* New York: Atheneum, 1972.

Bishop, Helen Gary. *Orgasm: The Ultimate Female Experience.* New York: Pinnacle Books, 1976.

Biskind, M.S. "Nutritional Therapy of Endocrine Disturbances." *Vitamins and Hormones.* Vol. 4. Edited by Robert S. Harris and Kenneth V. Thimann. New York: Academic Press, 1946, pp. 147-80.

Bosmajian, Haig A. *Language of Oppression.* Washington, D.C.: Public Affairs Press, 1974.
_____. "The Language of Sexism," *ETC.* vol. 29 (1972), pp. 305-313.

Boston Women's Health Book Collective. *Our Bodies, Ourselves: A Book By and For Women.* New York: Simon and Schuster, 1973. [rev. ed., 1976.]

Brecher, Ruth, and Brecher, Edward. *An Analysis of Human Sexual Response.* New York: New American Library, 1966.

Brody, Jane E. "Coast Study Finds Sharp Rise in Uterine Cancer." *New York Times,* November 1, 1975.

———. "Estrogen After Menopause Held No Bar to Cancer." *New York Times,* August 17, 1976.

———. "Incompetent Surgery Is Found Not Isolated." *New York Times,* January 27, 1976.

———. "Personal Health." *New York Times,* January 12, 1977.

Brownmiller, Susan. *Against Our Will: Men, Women and Rape.* New York: Simon and Schuster, 1975.

Brozan, Nadine. "Repercussions of a Drug." *New York Times,* June 17, 1976.

———. "The Use of Estrogen as a Growth Inhibitor." *New York Times,* February 11, 1976.

Bunker, J.B., Brown, W.W., Jr., "The Physician-Patient as an Informed Consumer of Surgical Services." *New England Journal of Medicine* vol. 290 (1974), pp. 1051-1055.

Burke, Kenneth. *Permanence and Change, An Anatomy of Purpose.* New York: Bobbs-Merrill, 1965.

"Cancer's Catch-22." *Newsweek,* August 2, 1976, p. 49.

Cant, Gilbert. "Male Trouble." *New York Times Magazine,* February 16, 1975.

Caprio, Frank. *Sexually Adequate Female.* North Hollywood, Calif.: Wilshire, 1975.

Carson, Ruth. *Your Menopause.* New York: Public Affairs Pamphlet No. 447, 1973. [Revised 1976.]

Castelton-Thomas, Virginia. *My Secrets of Natural Beauty.* New Canaan, Conn.: Keats Publishing, 1972.

Cerra, Frances. "F.D.A. Chief Suspicious of Estrogens." *New York Times,* January 22, 1976.

Cheraskin, E.; Ringsdorf, W.M.; and Brecher, Arline. *Psychodietetics.* Briarcliff Manor, N.Y.: Stein and Day, 1974.

Chernosky, Marvin. "Dry Skin and Its Consequences." *Journal of the American Medical Women's Association* vol. 27, no. 4 (March 1972), pp. 133-145.

Cherry, Sheldon H. *The Menopause Myth.* New York: Ballantine, 1976.

Chesler, Phyllis. *Women and Madness.* New York: Avon Books, 1972.

Chew, Peter. *The Inner World of the Middle-Aged Man.* New York: Macmillan, 1976.

Cixous, Helene. "The Laugh of the Medusa." Translated by Paula Cohen and Keith Cohen. In *Signs: Journal of Women in Culture and Society* vol. 1, no. 4 (Summer 1976), pp. 875-893.

Clark, Linda. *Get Well Naturally.* New York: Arc Books, 1972.

Clark, Matt. "Warning on Estrogen." *Newsweek,* December 8, 1975, p. 92A.

Comfort, Alex. *A Good Age.* New York: Crown, 1976.

———. *Joy Of Sex.* New York: Simon and Schuster, 1972.

———. *More Joy Of Sex.* New York: Simon and Schuster, 1974.

Cooper, David. *The Grammar of Living.* New York: Pantheon, 1974.

Cowan, Belita. "Estrogen Therapy Linked to Endometrial Cancer in Postmenopausal Women." *her-self,* December/January 1976, p. 10.

Crile, George, Jr. *What Women Should Know About the Breast Cancer Controversy.* New York: Pocket Books, 1974.

Cunningham, Barry. "The Yogurt Explosion." *New York Post,* October 2, 1976.

Dalton, Katharina. *The Menstrual Cycle: An Essential Guide for Women and Men.* New York: Pantheon, 1969.

———. *The Premenstrual Syndrome.* Springfield, Ill.: Charles Thomas, 1964.

Daly, Mary. *Beyond God the Father: Toward a Philosophy of Woman's Liberation.* Boston: Beacon Press, 1973.

Dannon Milk Products. *Yogurt and You.* Long Island City, N.Y.: Dannon Milk Products, 1976.

Davis, Adelle. *Let's Eat Right to Keep Fit.* New York: Harcourt, Brace, 1954.

Day, Harvey. *About Middle Age and After.* London: Thorsons Publishers, 1966.

Demfewolff, Richard F. "The Truth About Coffee and Your Health." *Science Digest,* June 1975, p. 31-35.

Dickinson, Emily. *Final Harvest: Emily Dickinson's Poems.* Edited by Thomas H. Johnson. Boston: Little, Brown, 1961.

Deutsch, Helene. *The Psychology of Women* vols. 1 and 2. New York: Grune and Stratton, 1945.

Dodson, Betty. *Liberating Masturbation: A Meditation on Self Love.* New York: Bodysex Designs, 1975.

"Does Low Calcium Intake Cause Osteoporosis?" *Journal of American Medical Association* vol. 218, no. 2 (October 11, 1971), p. 263.

Dohan, Mary Helen. *Our Own Words.* Baltimore: Penguin Books, 1975.

Dorland's Illustrated Medical Dictionary, 24th ed. Philadelphia: W.B. Saunders, 1965.

Dufty, William. *Sugar Blues.* Radnor, Pa.: Chilton, 1975.

Ehrenreich, Barbara, and English, Deirdre. *Complaints and Disorders.* Old Westbury, N.Y.: The Feminist Press, 1973.

Eliot, George. *Middlemarch.* New York: New American Library, 1964.

Eliot, T.S. *Collected Poems and Plays, 1909-1950.* New York: Harcourt, Brace, 1952.

Ellis, Havelock. *Psychology Of Sex.* Buchanan, N.Y.: Emerson Books [no date].

Ellis, John M. *The Doctor Who Looked at Hands.* New York: Arc Books, 1971.

Embey, Philip. *Woman's Change of Life.* London: Thorsons Publishers, 1955.

Empson, William. *Seven Types of Ambiguity.* New York: New Directions, 1947.

"Estrogen Therapy: The Dangerous Road to Shangri-La." *Consumer Reports,* November 1976, pp. 642-645.

Farb, Peter. *Word Play: What Happens When People Talk.* New York: Knopf, 1973.

"F.D.A. Warnings on Hexachlorophene." *New York Times,* December 12, 1971, pt. 4.

Felstein, Ivor. *Sex in Later Life.* Baltimore, Md.: Penguin Books, 1970.

Firestone, Shulamith. *The Dialectic of Sex.* New York: Bantam Books, 1971.

Flint, Marcha. "The Menopause: Reward or Punishment?" *Psychosomatics* vol. 16 (4th quarter 1975), p. 163.

Frankfort, Ellen. *Vaginal Politics.* New York: Bantam Books, 1973.

Fredericks, Carlton. "The Estrogen Tragedy." *Prevention,* May 1976, p. 167.

_____. *Look Younger, Feel Healthier.* New York: Grosset & Dunlap, 1975.

Freud, Sigmund. *New Introductory Lectures on Psycho-analysis.* London: Hogarth Press, 1946.

Friday, Nancy. *Forbidden Flowers.* New York: Pocket Books, 1975.

_____. *My Secret Garden.* New York: Pocket Books, 1974.

Fried, Barbara. *The Middle-Age Crisis.* New York: Harper & Row, 1967.

Friedan, Betty. *The Feminine Mystique.* New York: Dell Publishing, 1963.

Friedman, Abraham I. *Fat Can Be Beautiful.* New York: Berkley Publishing, 1974.

Friedman, Arnold P., Frazier, Shervert H., Jr., and Shultz, Dodi. *The Headache Book.* New York: Dodd, Mead, 1973.

Furman, Robert H. "Coronary Heart Disease and the Menopause." In *Menopause and Aging.* US Dept. of Health, Education, and Welfare Publ. No. (NIH)73-319 (1971).

Glass, David C. "Stress, Competition and Heart Attacks." *Psychology Today,* December 1976.

Glass, Robert H., and Kase, Nathan G. *Woman's Choice.* New York: Basic Books, 1970.

Gleason, Ralph J. *Billie Holiday: The Golden Years.* Columbia Records, 1962 [booklet].

Goleman, Daniel. "Why Your Temples Pound." *Psychology Today,* August 1976.

Gornick, Vivian. "Women as Outsiders." In *Women in Sexist Society.* Edited by Vivian Gornick and Barbara K. Moran. New York: New American Library, 1972.

Gray, Madeline, *Changing Years: The Menopause Without Fear.* Garden City, N.Y.: Doubleday, 1958.

Green, Thomas H., Jr. *Gynecology: Essentials of Clinical Practice.* 2nd ed. Boston: Little, Brown, 1971.

Greenblatt, Robert, and Novak, Edmund. "Treating Menopausal Women—and Climacteric Men." *Medical World News,* June 28, 1974.

Griffin, G. Edward. *World Without Cancer: The Story of Vitamin B₁₇.* Thousand Oaks, Calif.: American Media, 1974.

Grodin, Jay M.; Siiteri, Pentti K., and MacDonald, Paul C. "Source of Estrogen Production in the Postmenopausal Woman." *Journal of Clinical Endocrinology and Metabolism* vol. 36 (February 1973), pp. 207-214.

Gusberg, Saul B. "The Individual at High Risk for Endometrial Carcinoma." *American Journal of Obstetrics and Gynecology* vol. 126 (November 1976), pp. 535-542.

_____. "A Strategy for the Control of Endometrial Cancer." *Proceedings of the Royal Society of Medicine* vol. 68 (March 1975), pp. 163-168.

Gusberg, Saul B., et al. "Carcinogenesis and Estrogens." In *Menopause and Aging.* US Dept. of Health, Education, and Welfare Publ. No. (NIH)73-319 (1971).

Hackmann, Marjorie W. *Practical Sex Information.* Corvallis, Ore.: Waking Woman Press [no date].

Hanks, Laura; Demers, Joanne; and Alic, Margaret. "Vaginal Ecology." *Portland Scribe,* 4 parts, August 5, 1976 to September 2, 1976.

Harding, Esther M. *Woman's Mysteries.* New York: Bantam Books, 1973.

Hart, C.W.M., and Pilling, Arnold R. *The Tiwi of North Australia.* New York: Holt, Rinehart and Winston, 1969.

Heaney, Robert P. "Menopausal Effects on Calcium Homeostasis and Skeletal Metabolism." In *Menopause and Aging.* US Dept. of Health, Education, and Welfare Publ. No. (NIH)73-319 (1971).

Heaney, Robert P.; Eisenberg, Eugene; and Johnston, C. Conrad, Jr. "Postmenopausal Osteoporosis." In *Menopause and Aging.* US Dept. of Health, Education, and Welfare Publ. No. (NIH)73-319 (1971).

Heilbrun, Carolyn G. *Toward a Recognition of Androgyny.* New York: Harper & Row, 1974.

Hennessee, Judith. "Yogurt: Getting into the Culture." *New Times,* July 23, 1976.

Herschberger, Ruth. *Adam's Rib.* New York: Pellegrine & Cudahy, 1948.

Hertz, Roy and Saffrotti, U. Testimony, US Congress, House of Representatives, Government Operations Committee. *Regulation of Diethylstilbestrol: Its Use as a Drug in Humans and in Animal Feeds.* 92nd Cong., 1st sess. November 11, 1971, pt. 1. Washington, D.C.: US Government Printing Office, pp. 37-73.

Hitchcock, John T. *The Magars of Banyan Hill.* New York: Holt, Rinehart and Winston, 1969.

Hite, Shere. *The Hite Report: A Nationwide Study of Female Sexuality.* New York: Macmillan, 1976.

Holsten, W.D. "Protecting Patients from Drugs." *New England Journal of Medicine* vol. 285 (1971), p. 1202.

Hoover, Robert, et al. "Menopausal Estrogens and Breast Cancer." *New England Journal of Medicine* vol. 295 (1976), pp. 401-405.

Horney, Karen. "The Dread of Women." *International Journal of Psychoanalysis* vol. 3 (1932), p. 359.

_____. "The Flight from Womanhood: The Masculinity Complex in Women, As Viewed by Men and by Women." *International Journal of Psychoanalysis* vol. 7 (1926), p. 338.

"How Strong Is the Skin?" *Medical World News,* October 2, 1970.

Hrachovec, Josef P. *Keeping Young & Living Longer: How to Stay Active & Healthy Past 100.* Los Angeles: Sherbourne Press, 1972.

Huber, Joan, ed. *Changing Women in a Changing Society.* Chicago: University of Chicago Press, 1973.

Hunt, Bernice, and Hunt, Morton. *Prime Time.* New York: Stein and Day, 1975.

Hutton, Isabel. *Woman's Prime of Life.* New York: Emerson Books, 1937.

Huxley, Aldous. *Words and Their Meaning.* Los Angeles: Ward Ritchie, 1940.

Inman, William H. "The Relationship Between Estrogens and Progestogens and Thromboembolic Disease." In *Menopause and Aging.* US Dept. of Health, Education and Welfare Publ. No. (NIH)73-319 (1971).

Jackson, Mildred, and Teague, Terri. *The Handbook of Alternatives to Chemical Medicine.* Oakland, Calif.: Laugton-Teague Publications, 1975.

James, Henry. *The Sacred Fount.* New York: Grove Press, 1953.

Jaques, Elliott. "Death and the Mid-Life Crisis." *International Journal of Psychoanalysis* vol. 46 (1965), p. 506.

Jespersen, Otto. *Language: Its Nature, Development and Origin.* London: Allen & Unwin, 1922.

Kaplan, Helen Singer. *The New Sex Therapy.* New York: Brunner/Mazel, 1974.

Kase, Nathan. "Estrogens and the Menopause." *Journal of American Medical Association* vol. 227, no. 3 (January 21, 1974), pp. 318-319.

Kaufman, Sherwin A. *The Ageless Woman: Menopause, Hormones and the Quest For Youth.* Englewood Cliffs, N.J.: Prentice-Hall, 1967.

Keim-Loughran, Joan T. "Condition Your Condition." *Well-Being: A Healing Magazine* no. 1 (February 7, 1977), p. 11. [Published in San Diego.]

Key, Mary Ritchie. "Linguistic Behavior of Male and Female." *Linguistics* vol. 88 (August 15, 1972), pp. 15-31.

Kinsey, A.C., Pomeroy, W.B. and Martin, C.E. *Sexual Behavior in the Human Male.* Philadelphia: W.B. Saunders, 1948.

———. et al. *Sexual Behavior in the Human Female.* New York: Pocket Books, 1970.

Kirsch, Jonathan. "Can Your Mind Cure Cancer?" *New West,* January 3, 1977, p. 40-45.

Kittler, Glenn D. *Control for Cancer.* New York: Warner Paperback Library, 1963.

Kleinfeld, Sonny. "Coffee Is." *New Times,* October 3, 1975, p. 47.

Koedt, Ann. *The Myth of the Vaginal Orgasm.* Boston: New England Free Press, 1970.

Korzybski, Alfred. *Science and Sanity.* 4th ed. Lakeville, Conn.: International Non-Aristotelian Library, 1958. [1st ed. 1933].

Kramer, Cheris. "Women's Speech: Separate But Unequal?" *Quarterly Journal of Speech* vol. 60, (February 1974), pp. 14-24.

Krassner, Zonia P. "Review of the Symposium on Nutritional Disorders of American Women." *Women & Health* vol. 1, no. 2. (March/April 1976), published at SUNY College at Old Westbury, New York, p. 27.

Kraus, Hans. *Backache, Stress and Tension: Their Cause, Prevention and Treatment.* New York: Pocket Books, 1972.

Kroger, W.S., and Freed, S.C., *Psychosomatic Gynecology.* Glencoe, Ill.: Free Press, 1956.

Laing, R.D. *The Politics of Experience.* New York: Ballantine, 1967.

Lakoff, Robin. "Language and Women's Place." *Language in Society* vol. 2 (1973), pp. 45-79.

Lamb, Lawrence E. *Stay Youthful and Fit, A Doctor's Guide.* New York: Harper-Row, 1974.

Larned, Deborah. "Do You Take Valium?" *Ms. Magazine,* November 1975, pp. 26-30.

———. "The Selling of Valium." *Ms. Magazine,* November 1975, p. 32.

Lear, Martha Weinman. "Is There a Male Menopause?" *New York Times Magazine,* January 28, 1973.

Leathem, James. "Sex and Nutrition." *Life and Health,* July 1973, p. 63.

Leavitt, Ruby. "The Older Woman: Her Status & Role." In *On Older Women By Older Women.* Printed for OWL (Older Women's Liberation) Conference, Spring 1972.

Leonard, George. "The Search for Health: From the Fountain of Youth to Today's Holistic Frontier." *New West,* January 3, 1977, pp. 14-15.

LeShan, Eda. *The Wonderful Crisis of Middle Age.* New York: Warner Paperback Library, 1974.

Levine, Lena, and Doherty, Beka. *The Menopause.* New York: Random House, 1952.

Lewis, R.W.B. *Edith Wharton: A Biography.* New York: Harper & Row, 1975.

Lincoln, Miriam. *You'll Live Through It.* New York: Harper and Brothers, 1950.

Lolly, James J. *The Over Fifty Health Manual.* Englewood Cliffs, N.J.: Prentice-Hall, 1963.

Luce, Gay Gaer. *Body Time: Physiological Rhythms and Social Stress.* New York: Pantheon, 1971.

Mahoney, Kathryn, and Mahoney, Michael J. "Fight Fat with Behavior Control." *Psychology Today,* May 1976, p. 39.

Masters, William H., and Johnson, Virginia E. *Human Sexual Response.* Boston: Little, Brown, 1966.

———. *Human Sexual Inadequacy.* Boston: Little, Brown, 1970.

Masters, William H.; Johnson, Virginia E.; and Levin, Robert J. *The Pleasure Bond: A New Look at Sexuality and Commitment.* Boston: Little, Brown, 1974.

Mayo, Ann. "Doctor's Failed to Warn Women About Mammography Risk." *Village Voice,* August 23, 1976.

Mems, Gordon. "The Menopause and Breast Cancer." *The Lancet,* March 2, 1974.

Menopause and Aging. Edited by Kenneth J. Ryan and Don C. Gibson. US Dept. of Health, Education, and Welfare Publ. No. (NIH) 73-319 (1971).

Menopause: The Experts Speak. US Dept. of Health, Education, and Welfare Publ. No. (NIH) 75-756 (1975).

Merck Manual of Diagnosis and Therapy. 10th ed. Edited by Charles E. Lyght, et al. Rahway, N.J.: Merck & Co., 1961.

Merck Manual of Diagnosis and Therapy, 11th ed. Edited by Charles E. Lyght, et al. Rahway, N.J.: Merck & Co., 1966.

Merck Manual of Diagnosis and Therapy, 12th ed. Edited by David N. Holvey, et al. Rahway, N.J.: Merck & Co., 1972.

Merriam, Eve. *Sex and Semantics: Some Notes on BOMFOG.* Pittsburgh, Pa. KNOW, Inc.

Miller, Casey, and Swift, Kate. "One Small Step for Genkind." *New York Times Magazine,* April 16, 1972.

Miller, Lindsay. "Women Confer on Sex." *New York Post,* June 11, 1973.

Mintz, Morton. *The Pill.* Boston: Beacon Press, 1969.

Mitchell, Juliet. *Psychoanalysis and Feminism.* New York: Pantheon, 1974.

Monthly Extract, An Irregular Periodical vol. 3, no. 1 (March/April 1974).

Morrison, Margaret. "The Great Feminine Spray Explosion." *F.D.A. Consumer,* October 1973.

Moss, Z. "It Hurts to Be Alive and Obsolete: The Aging Woman." In *Sisterhood Is Powerful.* Edited by Robin Morgan. New York: Vintage, 1970.

Murray, Jessica. "Male Perspective in Language." *Women: A Journal of Liberation* vol. 3, no. 2 [no date], p. 50.

National Organization for Women, New York. *Proceedings of the Women's Sexuality Conference.* New York: NOW, NY, 1974.

Nemy, Enid. "Nutritional Problems of Women Discussed by Medical Experts." *New York Times,* November 22, 1975.

Neugarten, Bernice L., ed. *Middle Age and Aging.* Chicago: University of Chicago Press, 1968.

Neugarten, Bernice L., and Dowty, Nancy. "The Middle Years." In *American Handbook of Psychiatry.* 2nd ed. Vol. 1. Edited by S. Arieti. New York: Basic Books, 1974.

Neugarten, Bernice L., and Kraines, Ruth J. "Menopausal Symptoms in Women of Various Ages." *Psychosomatic Medicine* vol. 27 (1965), pp. 266-73.

"New Medicine & Holistic Healing." *New West,* May 10, 1976.

Newman, Edwin. *A Civil Tongue.* New York: Bobbs-Merrill, 1976.

Newman, J. Hynes. *Our Own Harms.* Newport Beach, Calif.: Quail Street Publishing Co., 1976.

Nilsen, Alleen Pace. "Sexism in English: A Feminist View." In *Female Studies 6.* Edited by Nancy Hoffman, Cynthia Secor, and Adrian Tinsley. Old Westbury, N.Y.: Feminist Press, 1972.

Nittler, Alan H. *A New Breed of Doctor.* New York: Pyramid Books, 1975.

Nobile, Philip. "What Is the New Impotence, and Who's Got It?" *Esquire,* October 1974.

Norris, P.E. *Everything You Want to Know About Yogurt.* New York: Pyramid Books, 1974.

Nourse, Alan E. "Hormones and Cancer: Is There a Connection?" *Women's Day,* February 1976, p. 38.

Novak, Edmund R.; Jones, Georgeanne Seegar; and Jones, Howard W., Jr. *Novak's Textbook of Gynecology.* 7th ed. Baltimore: Williams and Wilkins, 1965.

Ocle, Jane. "Sex Begins at Forty." *Harper's Bazaar,* August 1973.

One, Varda. *Manglish,* Pittsburgh, Pa.: KNOW, Inc.

Orwell, George. "Politics and the English Language." In *The Borzoi Reader.* Edited by C. Muscatine and M. Griffith. New York: Knopf, 1971.

Page, Louise, and Fincher, Lillian J. *Food and Your Weight.* Home and Garden Bulletin #74. US Department of Agriculture, 1960.

Pauling, Linus. *Vitamin C and the Common Cold.* San Francisco: W.H. Freeman, 1970.

Pitkin, Walter B. *Life Begins at Forty.* 1932.

Popov, Ivan. *Stay Young.* New York: Grosset & Dunlap, 1975.

Prensky, Joyce, ed. *Healing Yourself.* 6th rev. ed. Seattle, Wash.: Healing Yourself Collective, 1976.

Ramey, Estelle. "Men's Cycles." *Ms. Magazine,* Spring 1972, pp. 8-14.

_____. "Sex Hormones and Executive Ability." In *Women and Success.* Edited by Ruth B. Kundsin. New York: William Morrow, 1974.

Randal, Judith. "The Monthly Cycle: Not for Women Only." *Sunday News,* September 5, 1976.

Reinholz, Mary. "The Liberated Woman." *New York Sunday News,* March 16, 1975.

Reitz, Rosetta. "Is Nixon In His Menopause?" *Village Voice,* July 11, 1974, p. 81.

_____. (pseudonym: Rachael Goldman). "The Liberation of the Yiddisha Mama." *Village Voice,* February 11, 1971, p. 26.

_____. "Love My Menopause? You Must Be Crazy!" *Prime Time* vol. 4, no. 3 (April 1976), p. 17.

_____. "What Doctor's Won't Tell You About Menopause." *Majority Report,* October 3, 1974, p. 1.

Reuben, David. *Everything You Always Wanted to Know About Sex.* New York: David McKay, 1970.

Rich, Adrienne. *Diving Into The Wreck: Poems 1971-72.* New York: W.W. Norton, 1973.

_____. *Poems: Selected and New 1950-1974.* New York: W.W. Norton, 1975.

Richards, Ivor A., and Ogden, Charles K. *The Meaning of Meaning.* New York: Harcourt, Brace, 1959.

Rodale, J.I. *The Prevention System for Better Health.* Emmaus, Pa.: Rodale Press, 1974.

Rosenberg, Harold, and Feldzamen, A.N. *The Book of Vitamin Therapy.* New York: Berkley Publishing, 1975.

Root, Leon. *Oh, My Aching Back: A Doctor's Guide to Your Back Pain and How to Control It.* New York: David McKay, 1973.

Roth, Philip. *Portnoy's Complaint.* New York: Bantam Books, 1970.

Rubin, Theodore Isaac. "Dr. Rubin." *Ladies' Home Journal,* November 1971.

Ruebsaat, Helmut, and Hull, Raymond. *The Male Climacteric.* New York: Hawthorn Books, 1975.

Rush, Florence. "Woman in the Middle." In Notes from the Third Year. Edited by Anne Koedt. P.O. Box 8A, Old Chelsea Station, N.Y., 10011, 1971.

_____. "A Woman Of That Age," *Prime Time* vol. 4, no. 3 (April 1976), p. 3.

Ryan, Kenneth J. "Cancer Risk and Estrogen Use in the Menopause." *New England Journal Of Medicine* vol. 293 (1975), p. 1199.

Safilios-Rothschild, Constantina. *Women and Social Policy.* Englewood Cliffs, N.J.: Prentice-Hall, 1974.

Schaefer, Leah Cahan. *Women and Sex.* New York: Pantheon, 1973.

Schroeder, Henry A. *Trace Elements and Man.* Old Greenwich, Conn.: Devin-Adair Co., 1973.

Schuckman, Terry. *Aging Is Not for Sissies,* Philadelphia: Westminster Press, 1975.

Seaman, Barbara. "The Dangers of Sex Hormones." *Playgirl,* July 1976.

_____. *Free and Female.* Greenwich, Conn.: Fawcett World Library, 1973.

Seldin-Schwartz, Ethel. "Diary of a Middle-Aged Divorce." *Ms. Magazine,* April 1976, p. 86.

Selye, Hans. "Remaking Your Idea." *Vogue,* January 1975.

_____. *The Stress of Life.* New York: McGraw Hill, 1956.

"Sequential Pills Being Withdrawn." *New York Times,* February 26, 1976.

Sheehy, Gail. *Passages.* New York: Dutton, 1976.

Shelmire, Bedford Jr. *The Art of Looking Younger.* New York: Dell, 1975.

Sherfey, Mary Jane. *The Nature and Evolution of Female Sexuality.* New York: Random House, 1972.

"Should Hormone Therapy Be Used in Menopause?" *Good Housekeeping,* May 1973.

Shulman, Alix. "Organs and Orgasms." In *Women in Sexist Society: Studies in Power and Powerlessness.* Edited by Vivian Gornick and Barbara K. Moran. New York: New American Library, 1972.

Siiteri, Pentti, and MacDonald, Paul C. "Role of Extraglandular Estrogen in Human Endocrinology." In *Handbook of Physiology,* vol. 2. Edited by R.O. Greep and E.B. Eastwood. Washington, D.C.: American Physiological Society, 1973.

Silverstein, Louise, et al. *Survey on Menopause.* New York University: unpublished paper, May 19, 1975.

Smith, Bessie. "Wasted Life Blues." © 1957 by Frank Music Corp., New York, NY. In *Bessie Smith: Empress of the Blues.* A Schirmer Songbook. Edited by Clifford Richter. New York, 1957.

Smith, Donald C., et al. "Association of Exogenous Estrogen and Endometrial Carcinoma." *New England Journal of Medicine* vol. 293 (1975), p. 1164.

Smith, S.L. and Sauder, C. "Food Cravings, Depression, and Premenstrual Problems." *Psychosomatic Medicine* vol. 31 (1969), pp. 281-287.

Smith-Rosenberg, Carroll. "Puberty to Menopause: The Cycle of Femininity in Nineteenth Century America." *Feminist Studies* vol. 1, no. 1 (1973), pp. 3-4.

Snider, Arthur J. "The Magnetism of Middle-Aged Men." *New York Post,* May 7, 1976.

Snively, William D., Jr., and Thuerback, Jan. *The Sea of Life.* New York: David McKay, 1969.

Snyder, Solomon H. *Madness and the Brain.* New York: McGraw Hill, 1974.

Soddy, Kenneth with Kidson, Mary C. *Men in Middle Life.* Philadelphia: J.B. Lippincott, 1967.

Solomon, Joan. "Menopause: A Rite Of Passage." *Ms. Magazine,* December 1972, pp. 16-18.

Sommers, Tish, and Guracar, Genny. *The Not-So-Helpless Female.* New York: David McKay, 1973.

Song, Chull S., and Beck, Paul. "Metabolic Effects of Steroid Hormones." In *Menopause and Aging.* Publ. No. (NIH) 73-319 (1971).

Statistical Abstract of the U.S. for 1974. Washington, D.C., US Government Printing Office, 1975.

Stedman's Medical Dictionary, 22nd ed. Baltimore, Md.: Williams and Wilkins, 1972.

Stein, Gertrude. *The Making of Americans*. New York: Something Else Press, 1966.

Stonecypher, David D., Jr. *Getting Older and Staying Young: A Doctor's Prescription for Continuing Vitality in Later Life*. New York: W.W. Norton, 1974.

Strainchamps, Ethel. "Our Sexist Language. "In *Women in Sexist Society, Studies in Power and Powerlessness*. Edited by Vivian Gornick and Barbara K. Moran. New York: New American Library, 1972.

Taylor, Renee. *Hunza Health Secret for Long Life and Happiness*. Englewood Cliffs, N.J.: Prentice-Hall, 1965.

Thompson, Clara. "Middle Age." In *Women: Body and Culture*. Edited by Signe Hammer. New York: Harper & Row, 1975.

"Use of Estrogen Linked to Cancer." *New York Times,* December 4, 1975, p. 1.

Wade, Carlson. *Helping Your Health with Enzymes*. New York: Arc Books, 1966.

Wallace, Jane. *Masturbation: A Woman's Handbook*. Brooklyn: Side Hill Press, 1975.

Weaver, Jerry L. "Government Response to Contraceptive and Cosmetic Health Risks." *Women & Health* vol. 1, no. 2 (March/April 1976), pp. 5-11. Published at SUNY/College at Old Westbury, N.Y.

Weideger, Paula. *Menstruation & Menopause*. New York: Knopf, 1976. Rev. ed.: Dell, 1977.

Weiss, Kay. "Cancer and Estrogens—A Review." *Women & Health* vol. 1, no. 2 (March/April 1976), p. 3. Published at SUNY/College at Old Westbury, N.Y.

Weiss, Noel S. "Risks and Benefits of Estrogen Use." Editorial. *New England Journal of Medicine* vol. 293 (1975), p. 1200.

Weston, Jessie L. *From Ritual to Romance*. Garden City, N.Y.: Doubleday Anchor Books, 1957.

Wharton, Edith. *A Backward Glance*. New York: Appleton-Century, 1934.

White, Paul Dudley. "The Role of Exercise in the Aging." In *Health Aspects of Aging*, American Medical Association booklet, 1965.

Whorf, Benjamin Lee. *Language, Thought and Reality: Selected Writings of Benjamin Lee Whorf*. Edited by John B. Carroll. Cambridge, Mass.: MIT Press, 1956.

Williams, Roger J. *Alcoholism: The Nutritional Approach*. Austin, Texas: University of Texas Press, 1973.

Willson, J.R.: Beecham, C.T.: and Carrington, E.R. *Obstetrics and Gynecology*. St. Louis, Mo.: C.V. Mosby, 1971.

Wilson, Robert A. *Feminine Forever*. New York: M. Evans, 1966.

Winter, Ruth. *Ageless Aging*. New York: Crown, 1973.

Woolf, Virginia. *The Common Reader*. New York: Harcourt, Brace & World, 1953.

_____. *A Room of One's Own*. New York: Harcourt, Brace, 1944.

Yudkin, John. *Sweet and Dangerous*. New York: Bantam Books, 1973.

Yuncker, Barbara. "Link Hormone Pills to a Cancer of the Uterus." *New York Post,* December 4, 1975.

Ziel, Harry K., and Finkle, William D. "Increased Risk Of Endometrial Carcinoma Among Users of Conjugated Estrogens." *New England Journal of Medicine* vol. 293 (1975), pp. 1167-70.

Zinberg, Norman E. "The War Over Marijuana." *Psychology Today,* December 1976.

Zohman, Lenore R. *Beyond Diet*. Coventry, Conn.: Best Foods Exercise Booklet.

Index

workshops, 7–9, 80, 98, 112, 133
Menopause and Aging (HEW publication), 184
Menstrual Cycle, The (Dalton), 13–14
Menstrual record, 21ff.
Menstruation
  artificial, 159
  cessation of, 19–24
  flooding in, 20
  frequent, 20
  heavy, 20
  irregularity in, 22
  staining, 20
Merck Manual, The, 11, 12, 22, 107, 160
Metchnikoff, Ilya, 222
Metzger, Joseph, 220
Meyerhoff, Dr. Oscar, 212
Middle-age
  for men, 109, 139, 140, 234–236
  for women, 1, 17, 64, 71, 83, 140, 193–194
Migraine. *See* Headache
Minerals, 205, 206–207, 210
Mini-menopause, 68
Mintz, Morton, 176, 185
Molasses, blackstrap, 216
Moll Flanders (Defoe), 138
Molmar, Dr. Joseph, G., 212
Monilia fungi, in vagina, 223
Monthly cycles, in men, 228, 229
Monthly Extract, The, 72, 100
Morales, Betty Lee, 190
"Morning-after" pill, 177
Morrow, Dr. Paul, 186
Mouth, sore and dry, 22
Ms. Magazine, 79, 111
Munter, Carol, 37
My Secret Garden (Friday), 124
Myth of the Vaginal Orgasm, The (Koedt), 131

Naps, 61
National Cancer Institute, 172
National Organization for Women. *See* NOW
Natural cosmetics, 44–50
Natural foods, 190, 219. *See also specific foods*
Nature and Evolution of Female Sexuality (Sherfey), 127, 129

Nausea, 22, 75
"Nervous disorders," 65
New England Journal of Medicine, 164, 167, 170, 172, 176, 195, 220
Newman, Edwin, 113
New Medicine, 61, 62
New Sex Therapy (Kaplan), 142
Niacin, 102, 207
Niehmans, Dr. Paul, 230
Night sweats, 21, 31
  and calcium, 210
Nipples, 146
Nourse, Dr. Alan E., 168
NOW (National Organization for Women), 97, 120
Nowack, Carol, 64
Numbness, 22
Nurturing, 32, 47, 77, 112
Nutrition
  and menopause, 14, 33–35, 77–78, 200–225
  related to cancer, 197
Nuts, 216, 217
"Nymphomania," 142

Oatmeal, 46, 48, 217
Obesity. *See* Overweight; Weight gain
Obstetrics and Gynecology (Willson, et al.), 161
Oh, My Aching Back (Root), 57
Oil. *See* Fat(s)
Oiling of skin, 44, 47, 121–122
"Old lady," 139–140
"Old maid," 66, 111
Onanism, 117–118
Oophorectomy. *See* Ovaries
Oral contraceptives. *See* Birth-control pills
Orgasm, 117, 127, 130, 136–137, 142–144
  multiple, 127, 136, 142–143
Osteoporosis, 22, 56ff., 186, 188, 210
Our Bodies, Ourselves (Boston Book Collective), 120
Ova. *See* Eggs (human)
"Ovarian dysfunction," 11ff.
Ovaries, 12, 15–16, 65, 159, 163, 171, 181
"Oversexed," 142, 144
Overweight, 34, 37, 38, 201. *See also* Weight gain